VASOPRESSIN: DISTURBED SECRETION AND ITS EFFECTS

DEVELOPMENTS IN NEPHROLOGY

Volume 25

For a list of titles in this series see last page of this volume

Vasopressin:
Disturbed Secretion and Its Effects

by
L. KOVÁCS

Comenius University Medical School
Department of Pediatrics
Bratislava, Czechoslovakia

and
B. LICHARDUS

Institute of Experimental Endocrinology
Center of Physiological Sciences of the Slovak Academy of Sciences
Bratislava, Czechoslovakia

Springer Science+Business Media, B.V.

Library of Congress Cataloging in Publication Data

Kovács, L.
    Vasopressin : disturbed secretion and its effects / by L. Kovács
and B. Lichardus.
        p.   cm. -- (Developments in nephrology)
    Bibliography: p.
    Includes index.
    ISBN 0-7923-0249-4 (U.S.)
    1. Vasopressin--Pathophysiology.   2. Vasopressin--Physiological
effect.   3. Body fluid disorders.   I. Lichardus, Branislav.
II. Title.   III. Series.
    [DNLM: 1. Vasopressins.   W1 DE998EB / WK 520 K88v]
RC630.K68   1989
616.4'7--dc20
DNLM/DLC
for Library of Congress   89-15335

ISBN 978-94-010-6686-0   ISBN 978-94-009-0449-1 (eBook)
DOI 10.1007/978-94-009-0449-1

Kluwer Academic Publishers incorporates the publishing programmes of Dr W. Junk
Publishers, MTP Press, Martinus Nijhoff Publishers, and D. Reidel Publishing Company.

Distributors
---

for the United States and Canada: Kluwer Academic Publishers, 101 Philip Drive,
Norwell, MA 02061, USA
*for Albania, Bulgaria, China, Cuba, Czechoslovakia, German Democratic Republic,
Hungary, Democratic People's Republic of Korea, Mongolia, Poland, Rumania, U.S.S.R.,
Democratic People's Republic of Vietnam, and Yugoslavia:* Avicenum, Czechoslovak
Medical Press, Prague, Czechoslovakia
for all other countries: Kluwer Academic Publishers Group, P.O. Box 322, 3300 AH
Dordrecht, The Netherlands

Joint edition published by
Kluwer Academic Publishers, Dordrecht, The Netherlands and Avicenum, Czechoslovak Medical Press, Prague, Czechoslovakia

Copyright

© 1989 by Avicenum, Czechoslovak Medical Press, Prague

Softcover reprint of the hardcover 1st edition 1989

Translated by Milan Erban, M.D.

CONTENTS

PREFACE

The mechanisms by which animals regulate the volume and composition of their body fluids has long had a particular fascination for students of biology. As a consequence, the subject can lay claim to an impressive record of ground-breaking scientific achievements as well as a provocative body of philosophical speculation concerning the role of the system in the origin and evolution of life. Indeed, the entire concept of homeostasis on which so much of our current biologic thinking is based, derives from Claude Bernard's pioneering exploration of the forces that determine the composition of this 'internal sea'. Other seminal achievements credited to this area of inquiry include the first description of a genetically transmitted human disease (familial neurogenic diabetes insipidus); the first isolation sequencing and synthesis of a peptide hormone (vasopressin and oxytocin); the first demonstration of peptide hormone synthesis by way of a larger protein precursor; the first description of resistance to the biologic actions of a hormone (nephrogenic diabetes insipidus); and the conceptual realization of the unique counter-current mechanism that permits concentration of the urine. This record of far reaching and fundamental advances has been distinguished by many fruitful inter-actions between clinical and basic science. Indeed, the basic studies that led to discovery of an antidiuretic hormone in the posterior pituitary were based upon prior clinical observations that the syndrome of diabetes insipidus was often associated with pathology localized to the base of the brain and could be treated by administering aqueous extracts of the gland!

In the last twenty years, research in water metabolism has taken a different direction but is again positioned on the cutting edge of significant scientific advance. The diversity and elegance of these recent accomplishments reflect the growth of biomedical science as a whole. Thus, the last two decades witnessed the development and application of sensitive and specific immuno-assays for vasopressin, the creation of new techniques to describe normal and abnormal regulation of hormone secretion, the discovery of several new influences on secretion, preliminary description of the location and functional properties of the control systems, the synthesis of vasopressin analogues with highly selective agonist or antagonist properties, the demonstration of different classes of receptors and post receptor mechanisms by which the hormone exerts its various effects, the discovery of vasopressin in extra hypophyseal neurons and even some peripheral tissues, the discovery of an experimental animal with an inherited form of vasopressin deficiency, and last but not least, the determination of the chromosomal location, structure, transcription and translation products of the genes that code for the precursor proteins of both vasopressin and oxytocin. As before, many of these accomplishments have been fostered by a mutually beneficial interaction between the basic and clinical sciences.

This book on vasopressin by László Kovács and Branislav Lichardus fulfills a major need by providing an up-to-date and comprehensive overview of current knowledge, unsolved mysteries and continuing controversies in the area of water metabolism.

It lives up fully to the exemplary traditions of its subject matter by ranging easily from clinical to basic science with a most skilful effort made to synthesize the two. At the same time, it is organized in such a way that it is easy to locate information on very specific topics. Its pedagogical value is further enhanced by a generous use of illustrations and tables. But the book is also much more than a handy up-to-date text or reference source because it is spiced here and there with the kinds of personal thoughts and philosophical speculations that have distinguished the literature in this field for nearly a century. Hence, it is as likely to be of interest to the general scientific reader as well as to beginning students or experts in the field.

Because recent studies of vasopressin function have begun to carry far beyond the traditional bounds of fluid homeostasis and into the realm of baroregulation, hemostasis, hypothalamic releasing hormones, genetics and neurochemical transmission or modulation, this book should also be of interest to clinical and basic scientists working in areas as diverse as cardiovascular function, hematology, neuroendocrinology, neurology, developmental biology and clinical and molecular genetics. Even the recent growth in interest of the important physiologic role played by the thirst mechanism that is so well presented in this book should be of value to disciplines ranging from behavioral biology to psychiatry to internal medicine and pediatrics. This kind of continuing broad appeal to biologists from many disciplines is amply illustrated in this book. It provides comforting reassurance that this area of inquiry will remain in the forefront of biomedical progress for many years to come.

July 28, 1989

Gary L. Robertson, M. D.
Department of Medicine,
University of Chicago,
Chicago, Illinois, U.S.A.

INTRODUCTION

Altogether it is not exaggerated to claim that the original designing of the world-famous synthetic vasopressin analog dDAVP in 1967 in Prague at the Institute of Organic Chemistry and Biochemistry, Czechoslovak Academy of Sciences, opened up a qualitatively new era in both basic and clinical research of vasopressin function. It was this outstanding invention that prompted from the very outset the interest in the experimental and clinical aspects of vasopressin secretion and its effects at the Institute of Experimental Endocrinology, Centre of Physiological Sciences, Slovak Academy of Sciences, Bratislava (Czechoslovakia).

For more than a decade, the key-player in the clinical part of our research activity was Vilma Némethová, M. D., a highly initiative, industrious, devoted, friendly and unselfish personality, who pioneered pediatric endocrinology in Slovakia. This book should be a modest tribute in her honor.

Later on, the clinical basis of our working team widened to involve other colleagues from Departments of Pediatrics I and II, Comenius University Medical School, Bratislava, as well as from other institutions from this country and from Hungary. The experience obtained during the activity of this working team have laid the basis of the present book. We highly appreciate the valuable contribution of all team members, as well as that of Professors Heinz Valtin, M. D. (Hanover, New Hampshire) and Vratislav Schreiber, M. D., D. Sc., Corresponding Member of the Academy (Prague) for having served as reviewers of the annotation and the final manuscript respectively.

Our thanks are due in particular to staff members of the Institute of Experimental Endocrinology, Ing. Nikolaj Michajlovskij, C. Sc., RNDr. Jozef Ponec, C. Sc. and Mrs. Mária Tordová and Anna Zemánková, for their excellent and skilful laboratory assistance sine qua non.

We are also deeply obliged to all those authors of publications on vasopressin which served us as a rich source of ideas and illustrations; we have absorbed and internalized them, to avoid their distortion by major modifications. At the same time we would like to apologize to all those whose works have not been referred to in the present book, either due to the limited space or to our unintentional failure.

We feel especially honored by the fact that Professor Gary L. Robertson,

M. D. (Chicago, Illinois), whose decisive contribution to the pathophysiology and clinics of vasopressin is generally highly appreciated, was ready to kindly write the Preface to this book.

Last but not least, we would like to express our appreciation of the helpful attitude of Avicenum, Medical Publishing House (Prague, Czechoslovakia) and Kluwer Academic Publishers (Dordrecht, The Netherlands), and of the understanding and reliable background for our work offered by our families.

We will be grateful for any critical comments on the present work; they will stimulate and promote our future research.

Branislav Lichardus, M. D., D. Sc.

Corresponding Member of the Academy

László Kovács, M. D., D. Sc.

1 BASAL MECHANISMS OF WATER AND SALT HOMEOSTASIS

More than 100 years ago Claude Bernard pointed out that it is body fluids washing all the cells in an organism rather than the atmosphere surrounding the body that represents the environment all mammals (including man) live in. He therefore termed the extracellular fluid "the internal milieu" which is perfectly isolated from, and protected against, erratic oscillations of the external inanimate world thanks to a number of homeostatic mechanisms. The maintenance of a steady relationship of water and solutes (principally sodium chloride) is just one example of such homeostatic mechanisms.

At the single cell level, life most probably started developing in primeval oceans during the Precambrian era. Decisive for a favorable fate of life was that both the chemical composition and the physical characteristics of the oceanic environment surrounding the early living cells were more or less constant. Continuous movement of the sea waters warranted perpetual renewal of the external environment and removed metabolic products of the cells from their environment.

To a great extent biological evolution was determined by changes in the inanimate nature. The electrolyte concentrations of the sea waters gradually increased, in particular due to erosion of mainland. Two principal possibilities of adaptation to new conditions opened up before the organisms living in the changing primeval oceans. One of them was to increase the density of the intracellular fluid in parallel with the changing composition of the external environment. This however required restructuration of a whole system of deep rooted regulatory mechanisms that proved effective during the foregoing development. Alternatively the cells could take a portion of the external environment for their own internal milieu and establish at the same time organs and systems to ensure maintenance of both the composition and the volume of this internal environment. Both the above possibilities have found their way in evolution (Yancey et al. 1982). Nevertheless, the highest level of evolution could reach that branch of multicellular organisms which instead of taking the way of cellular adjustment, figuratively speaking, enclosed a portion of Precambrial ocean into themselves in form of their own extracellular fluid representing some kind of an "internal sea" in which the cells live (Smith 1951).

1.1 BODY WATER DISTRIBUTION AND OSMOTIC CONCENTRATION

Water is the basis of all life. We purposefully repeat this as all biochemical processes in the organism occur in water solution which represents the major single component of living matter, and no other one is so indispensable as water for its survival. The water content of the human organism is strongly age-dependent: it decreases from 96% of total body weight in a two-week embryo to 55—60% body weight in older age (Friis-Hansen 1983).

Ingenious as he was, Claude Bernard considered the body a two-compartment system composed of an intracellular and an extracellular compartment separated from each other by the cell membrane which is freely permeable to water, but to a lesser or greater extent remains "impermeable" to most water soluble substances. (The term "impermeability" is a simplification of the underlying process: in reality, solutes are kept in the intracellular or extracellular compartment due to their dimensions and/or their electric charge, and mainly due to transmembrane transport mechanisms.)

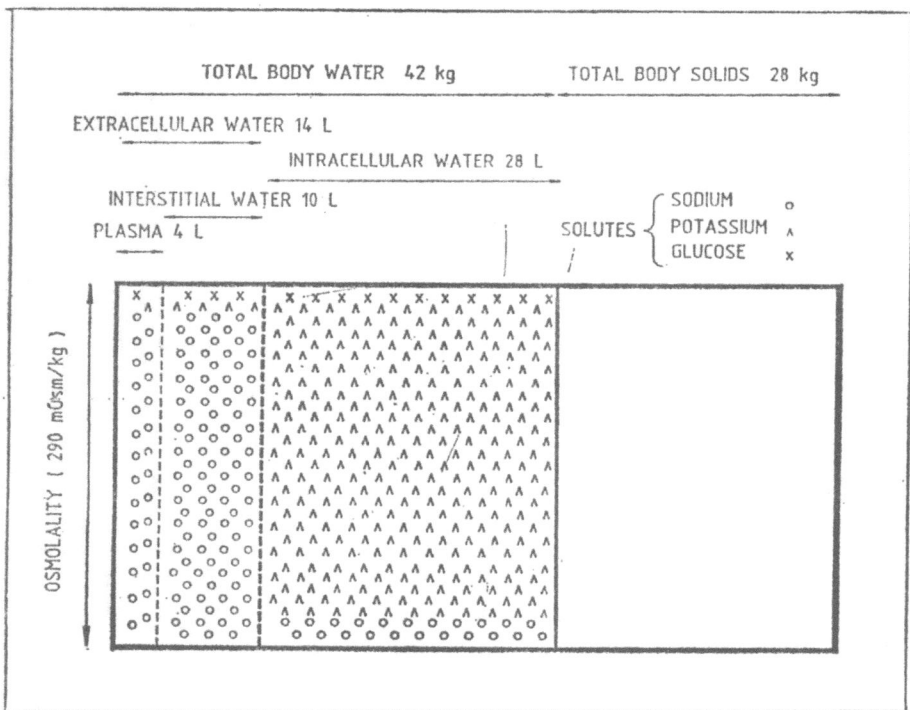

Fig. 1.1. Scheme of the distribution and composition of body water in healthy adult. Volume is shown on the horizontal axis and solute concentration (or osmolality) is indicated by the vertical dimension (by Robertson 1983 with kind permission).

2

Osmotic concentrations — the number of impermeable solute particles in a unit of body fluids — are important in determining the distribution of water between the compartments. Since mammalian cell membranes are freely permeable to water, body fluids are in osmotic equilibrium and body water is distributed between the body fluid compartments according to the osmotic concentration gradient, i.e. according to the relative amounts of "impermeable" substances in the individual compartments. Normally, intracellular fluid (ICF) contains about two thirds of total body osmotic solute, while the remaining one third is in extracellular fluid (ECF). Consequently, ICF normally contains two thirds and ECF one third of total body water, while one fourth of the ECF compartment is intravascular (Fig. 1.1).

Each compartment contains a single major solute. The predominant solutes inside the cell are potassium and its anions. By contrast, more than 90 per cent of the osmolality of plasma and other extracellular fluid is due to sodium and its anions. Thus the plasma osmolality can be appreciated as:

$$P_{osm}(mOsm/kg) = 2 \times P_{Na} + P_{urea} + P_{glucose} \qquad \text{(equation 1.1)}$$

where 2 reflects the osmotic contribution of anions accompanying sodium ions, and plasma concentrations (P) of all solutes are expressed in mmol/l. Although urea contributes to the absolute values of P_{osm}, measured by the freezing point depression, it does not act to hold water in the extracellular space because of its membrane permeability. Therefore urea is an ineffective osmole and does not contribute to the effective P_{osm}. Hence, the effective osmolality (tonicity) in body fluid is virtually synonymous with the plasma concentration of sodium and its anions:

$$P_{osm} \text{ eff } (mOsm/kg) \approx 2 \times P_{Na} \text{ (mmol/l)} \qquad \text{(equation 1.2)}$$

(the above estimation is invalid if other impermeant solutes, e.g. glucose or mannitol, are present in excess in extracellular compartment).

1.2 BALANCE STATE

Despite wide variations in dietary intake, the volume and composition of body fluids are maintained in an extremely narrow physiological range as excretion is adjusted to match intake. Thus the amount of a substance added to the body each day by dietary ingestion or endogenous production normally is equal to the amount eliminated from the body by excretion or endogenous utilization (Table 1.1). This is referred to as balance state or **steady state**. The balance is achieved thanks to several very complex homeostatic mechanisms adjusting intake and excretion of solutes and water.

In this regard it is important to understand the differences between **volume regulation** and **osmoregulation**. Volume regulation is achieved mainly by

Table 1.1. Typical daily water balance in a healthy human

Water intake (ml/day)		Water output (ml/day)	
drinking water	1,500	renal	1,500
water content of food	800	gastrointestinal	200
water of oxydation	300	insensible (skin, respiratory)	900
Total	2,600	Total	2,600

adjusting renal sodium excretion, while osmolality is maintained by regulating both water intake via thirst and water excretion via vasopressin. Because of the relative independence of the regulatory mechanisms from each other, both volume and osmolality are subjects of alterations independently of the other variable. These alterations may be manifested in several clinical forms (Fig. 1.2). Absolute or relative water deficit (in relation to body solutes) means **dehydration**, while absolute or relative water excess is marked as **hyperhydration**. Deficit of body sodium content means ECF volume contaction, while increased total body sodium content is associated with ECF **volume expansion**. Note that of the nine possible combinations eight are abnormal and six are associated with abnormal plasma osmolality (sodium concentration).

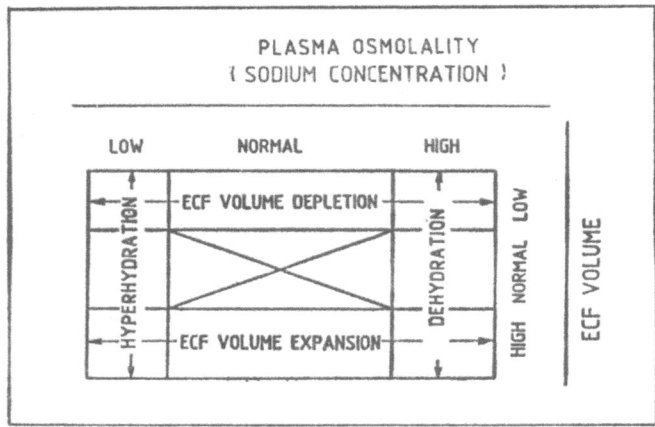

Fig. 1.2. Disturbances in extracellular fluid (ECF) volume and osmolality. Osmolality changes, represented as serum sodium concentration, are shown on the horizontal axis while volume changes are indicated by the vertical dimension.

1.3 REGULATION OF EXTRACELLULAR FLUID VOLUME (THE CONTROL OF SODIUM BALANCE)

Adequate tissue perfusion is essential for normal cell metabolism providing nutrients and removing waste products. It is not surprising therefore that multiple sensors and multiple effectors are involved in the maintenance of effective circulating blood volume, i.e. of that part of the extracellular fluid (ECF) volume which is in the vascular space effectively perfusing the tissues. It is important to realize that the effective circulating volume is not a measurable entity, but refers to the rate of perfusion of the capillary circulation. It varies with the extracellular fluid volume in healthy subjects; both of these parameters are dependent on total body Na^+ stores since sodium salts are the primary extracellular solutes which act to hold the appropriate volume of water within the extracellular space. As a result, the regulation of sodium balance by modifying urinary sodium excretion and the maintenance of the effective circulating volume are closely related functions.

1.3.1 REFLEX ARC

Thus changes in effective circulating volume constitute the signal that allows urinary sodium excretion to vary approximately with fluctuations in sodium intake. These changes are sensed by **low pressure** receptors located in the cardiopulmonary circulation, and by the **high pressure** receptors in the carotid sinus, in the aortic arch and the afferent glomerular arteriole (JGA, the juxtaglomerular apparatus). Although it is volume that is being regulated, these receptors are in nature pressure-(stretch-) receptors that record the fullness of the vascular bed by intravascular pressure and/or by stretch acting on vascular walls. This allows an effective volume control, since pressure and/or vascular distension and volume are directly related to each other. It may well be that the net volume status is normally determined in the brain where the individual afferent signals from the different peripheral receptors are integrated and transformed in an efferent signal regulating systemic and, in particular, renal hemodynamics (by changing the activity of the sympathetic nervous system), renal sodium and water excretion and also thirst and (in animals rather than in humans) sodium appetite (Lichardus 1978).

1.3.2 VOLUME DEPLETION

The immediate first line response to reduction in effective circulating volume involves enhancement of the sympathetic neural tone and secretion of catecholamines (norepinephrine and epinephrine) (Fig. 1.3). The resulting

5

venous constriction decreases the venous blood pool, which normally contains approx. 70% of the total intravascular volume, and this augments the blood delivery to the heart. This enhanced venous return in combination with increased myocardial contractility and heart rate raises the cardiac output. In addition there is arterial vasoconstriction, increasing systemic vascular resistance which raises the blood pressure toward normal. Renin secretion is enhanced by hypotension, partly by increasing the sympathetic tone and partly by changes of the renal perfusion pressure. This results in the generation

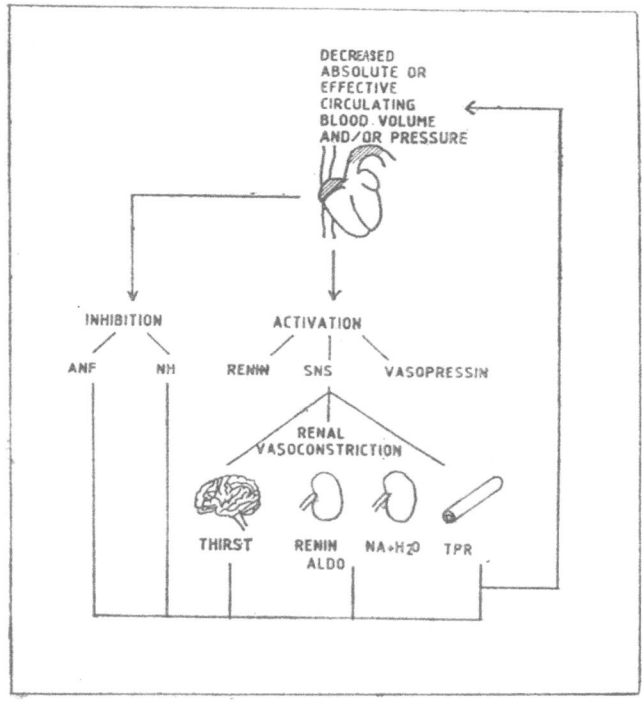

Fig. 1.3. Schematic representation of hormonal mechanisms activated in response to extracellular fluid volume depletion. (SNS-sympathetic nervous system, TPR-total peripheral resistance, ALDO- aldosterone, ANF- atrial natriuretic factor, NH-natriuretic hormone, circulating sodium transport inhibitor.) (Johnston 1985 with permission.)

of the vasoconstrictor angiotensin II. Furthermore, the enhanced adrenergic effects of neural function contribute to the increase in renal tubular reabsorption. These cardiovascular changes are reversed by volume expansion as sympathetic activity is reduced. It should be noted that these alterations in sympathetic tone with changes in effective circulating volume are mostly compensatory and that appropriate changes in renal sodium excretion are required to restore normal volume balance (Rose 1984).

1.3.3 VOLUME EXPANSION

Renal sodium excretion varies directly with the effective circulating blood volume (ECBV). When ECBV is expanded the urine Na concentration can exceed 100 mmol/l; in contrast, urine can be rendered virtually sodium-free (U_{Na} as low as 1 mmol/l) in the presence of volume depletion and normal renal function. These homeostatic changes in sodium excretion can result from alterations both in the filtered load (i.e. the glomerular filtration rate, GFR), and in tubular reabsorption which is affected by multiple factors, including the mineralocorticoid hormone aldosterone which promotes sodium retention. Although GFR varies with volume status (it tends to increase with volume expansion and decreases with volume contraction, both of which can contribute to the associated changes in sodium excretion) alterations in GFR are not required to maintain sodium balance. The prevailing importance of tubular reabsorption is illustrated by the phenomenon of **glomerulo-tubular balance** in which a primary alteration in GFR without changes in volume does not lead to a substantial change in urinary Na^+ excretion since tubular reabsorption varies in the same direction. Thus it appears that variations in tubular reabsorption constitute the main adaptive response to fluctuations in ECBV (DeWardener et al. 1961).

1.3.3.1 Natriuretic hormone(s)

Expansion of ECF volume with a sodium load results in an appropriate increase in renal sodium excretion. For some years it has been recognized that this natriuretic response cannot be attributed entirely to the increase in GFR (first factor) and/or the decrease in aldosterone secretion (second factor). Thus the hypothetical factor responsible, at least partly, for enhanced tubular sodium rejection has been termed "third factor". It is now clear that the "third factor" itself is composed of several factors including intrarenal hemodynamics and humoral natriuretic substances.

A humoral compound capable of promoting natriuresis, probably by inhibiting the activity of the transporting enzyme Na^+, K^+-ATPase, has been considered important in sodium, volume and pressure homeostasis for the last three decades. Evidence in support of the existence of a **natriuretic hormone**, an endogenous inhibitor of Na^+, K^+-ATPase (a digitalis-like substance), probably released from the hypothalamus in response to volume expansion has been documented in all mammals studied including humans (e.g. newborns, preterm infants, low-renin arterial hypertension) (Graves and Williams 1987, Kovács et al. 1988). However, so far efforts to isolate and identify the postulated hormone have been ineffective (deWardener et al. 1961, Lichardus and Pearce 1966, Lichardus et al. 1965, 1968, Lichardus and Ponec 1971, deWardener and McGregor 1983, Schreiber 1985, Kramer and Lichardus 1987, Kramer et al. 1989).

The search for the natriuretic hormone led nevertheless to an important but rather unexpected finding: de Bold et al. (1981) reported that the cardiac myocytes produce and release a natriuretic and vasodilator (blood pressure decreasing) substance which was later identified as a polypeptide and named atrial natriuretic peptide (ANP, alpha human ANP is composed of 28 amino-acid (AA) residues, m.w. 3,500). The natriuretic mechanism of ANP is not known in detail (Table 1.2). It probably promotes renal sodium excretion, at least partly, by increasing the medullary blood flow and thereby washing out the cortico-medullary osmotic gradient. Plasma levels of ANP (approx. 50 pg/ml under resting conditions) have to vary in direct proportion to changes in atrial pressure, independently of the atrial innervation or any other humoral signal (Kramer and Lichardus 1986, Cody et al. 1987).

Table 1.2. Characteristics of the atrial natriuretic peptide (ANP) and the digoxin-like natriuretic hormone (circulating sodium transport inhibitor)

	Atrial natriuretic peptide	Circulating sodium transport inhibitor
Molecular weight	high	low (cca 500 daltons)
Structure	polypeptide	steroid(?); polypeptide (?)
Vascular effect	vasodilation	vasoconstriction
Renal effect	increased renal blood flow and GFR	inhibitor of Na^+, K^+ - ATPase
Digoxin-like immunoreactivity	— —	+ + +

The synthesis and release of ANP was also identified in the brain. Moreover, a specific **brain natriuretic peptide** (BNP) was discovered later which is composed of 26 AA. It differs by its immunoreactivity from ANP, with the natriuretic and vasodilator activities being identical in both factors (Matsuo 1988). Brain ANP and BNP, similarly as vasopressin and angiotensin II in the brain, are believed to play a role also in the central regulation of sodium, water and circulatory homeostasis (Goetz 1988, Kramer et al. 1989).

1.4 REGULATION OF EXTRACELLULAR FLUID OSMOLALITY (THE CONTROL OF WATER BALANCE)

Osmoregulation means a complex of processes in the organism occurring on relative or absolute deficit or excess of body water, with the final aim to maintain isotonicity of body fluids (280—300 mOsm/kg). Ideally operating osmoregulation is thus based on a rigorous qualitative parallelism of body water and salt contents:

$$P_{osm} \text{ eff.} = \frac{\text{total body sodium content}}{\text{total body water content}} \qquad \text{(equation 1.3)}$$

This concept finds its clinical application in patients with hyponatremia ($P_{Na} < 135$ mmol/l) or hypernatremia ($P_{Na} > 150$ mmol/l). **Hyponatremia** usually represents hypoosmolality, i.e. absolutely or relatively more total body water content in relation to the total body sodium content. Conversely, **hyper-natremia** represents hyperosmolality, i.e. a relative or absolute deficit of total body water in relation to osmotically active solutes (see Fig. 1.2).

1.4.1 IMMEDIATE, "FIRST LINE" RESPONSE TO ALTERATIONS IN ECF OSMOLALITY

Thanks to their chemical composition, body fluids are able to respond to changes in ECF osmolality mainly by reducing the load through "buffer" mechanisms. Alterations of osmotic concentration of fluid at one side of the semipermeable cell membrane are rapidly abolished through water redistribution between the body spaces. Upon an increase in extracellular concentrations of osmotically active agents (e.g. due to water loss or to increased content of solutes), a portion of water is rapidly shifted from cells into the extracellular space until osmotic equilibrium is attained, although at a higher level than previously. If on the other hand, osmotic concentration of ECF decreases, water rapidly permeates into the cells until new equilibrium is reached. Thanks to these characteristics of the cell membrane rapid shifts of the ECF osmotic concentration are immediately transferred into total volume of body water, thereby considerably reducing the extent of the osmotic load of the individual cells.

This first line "buffer" defence associated with volume control of cells themselves has its significant limitations. Rapid and excessive osmotic loads can cause irreversible damage to the cells. Thus, excessive water intake and the resulting cell swelling secondary to extracellular hypoosmolality can result in cell bursting and death, whereas dehydrated (due to extracellular hyperosmolality) and shrunken cells can no longer fully meet their original function owing to increased viscosity and increased electrolyte concentration of the cytoplasm. To prevent these undesirable changes, complex and slow-acting osmoregulatory systems have to be simultaneously activated both at cellular level and at the level of the organism as a whole.

1.4.2 OSMOREGULATION AT THE CELLULAR LEVEL

Cellular adaptation mechanisms to changes in extracellular osmotic concentration developed as early as in primitive single cell organisms (Frömter 1987). Osmotic shifts of water are reduced through modifications of the intracellular amounts of osmotically active substances, thus producing a more favorable osmotic gradient. This results in normalization of cell volume, though at the expense of cell osmolality.

In face of osmotic stress there are essentially two ways of how the regulatory changes in intracellular solute content can proceed. The first of them, shifts of ions across the cell membrane, are involved in the acute response of a cell to water challenge (Kregenow 1981, Cserr et al. 1987). The other mechanism, generation or dissipation of intracellular organic osmoles by modifying intracellular metabolic pathways, is much slower to respond. Nonelectrolyte solutes with a relatively complex structure and higher molecular weights are known to make up some proportion of intracellular osmolality even under physiological conditions. Sustained increase in extracellular osmolality induces enzymatic cleavage of the larger molecules (polymers) into numerous smaller molecules which the larger molecules are composed of (e.g. amino acids, sucrose, mannitol, polyhydric alcohols, glycerol, etc.). This results in an enrichment of the cytoplasm in soluble particles, thus producing additional " idiogenic" osmoles and eventually leading to increased intracellular osmolality. On the other hand, adaptational reduction of intracellular osmolality upon sustained hypoosmolality of ECF very probably results from inverse processes. Smaller nonelectrolyte particles undergo condensation giving rise to larger molecules, and the associated decrease in "idiogenic" osmoles results in decrease of intracellular osmolality (Thurston et al. 1987).

An important point is that the above cellular adaptational processes to both increased or decreased ECF tonicity as well as the readaptation after the withdrawal of the osmotic challenge are time consuming, taking several hours before they can manifest themselves in their fully developed forms (Pollock and Arieff 1980). This fact becomes of clinical importance if the therapeutical returning of ECF osmolality to the original, "normal" state occurs so rapidly that readaptation cannot take place (chapters 18.1 and 20.2).

1.4.3 OSMOREGULATION AT THE LEVEL OF THE ORGANISM

The ability to regulate cell volume through a special system of extracellular osmolality control is one generally accepted capacity of animals living on dry land. Excessive shifts in plasma concentrations of sodium and/or other osmotically active substances are neutralized by increasing or decreasing the body water content (on hyperosmolality or hypoosmolality respectively). In other words, the stability of body fluid composition is mainly determined by the balance between intake and metabolically produced water on one hand, and that removed or lost through the kidneys and the intestines, lung and skin on the other hand (the Verney's mechanism) (Fig. 1.4).

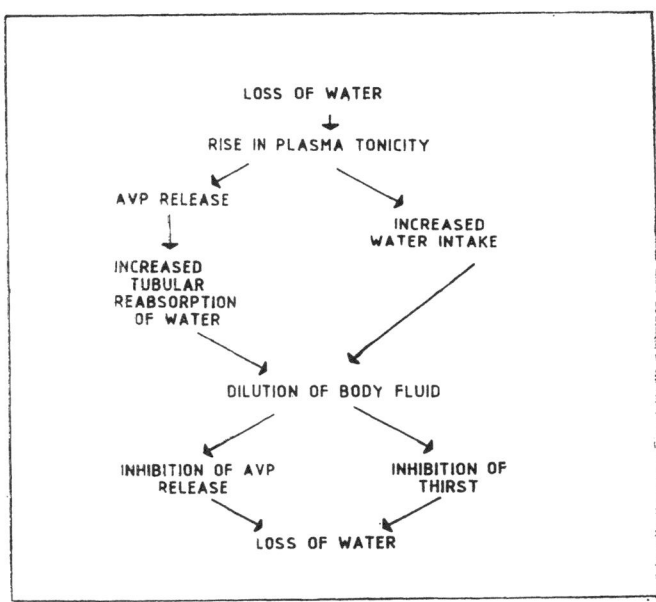

Fig. 1.4. Summary of the role of the vasopressin — thirst complex in regulation of body fluid composition (Verney's mechanism).

1.4.3.1 Water intake (thirst)

No organism can live without supplementing renal and extrarenal losses of fluids by the intake of adequate amounts of water. Under basal conditions, water intake is "prophylactic" as it mainly serves to anticipate a future need for water. The amounts of water ingested vary considerably from one individual to another and are determined largely by custom and diet. However, when water intake ceases water losses result in the sensation of thirst which, as dehydration progresses, becomes more and more severe, until it dominates all feelings and thoughts of the individual (Fitzsimmons 1985).

The control of water intake and that of renal water excretion are two mutually dependent aspects of the body's osmoregulatory system (see Fig. 1.4). The osmoregulatory importance of thirst can be easily demonstrated by recalling the well known experience that in patients with complete central diabetes insipidus the plasma osmolality as a rule remains normal or only slightly decreased despite huge renal water losses. This indicates that effective renal water conservation is not indispensable for an effective osmoregulation, provided the thirst mechanism is working properly and water is readily available.

1.4.3.2 Renal water conservation (vasopressin secretion)

With regard to body water conservation there is no doubt that the major homeostatic regulation is affected by the action of the antidiuretic hormone (vasopressin) on the kidney. In contrast to some other hormones (such as insulin or mineralocorticoids) vasopressin is not directly indispensable for the organism to survive. The main contribution of the vasopressin-mediated renal regulation of water excretion is mainly that the hormone reduces the dependence of the individual on the feeling of thirst, thus enabling him to be "independent" of water source, at least for a certain interval of time. The importance of vasopressin increases upon challenging conditions associated with extensive extrarenal water loss and transient inaccessibility of water. To appreciate the significance of vasopressin for osmoregulation it is sufficient to just once see the suffering of a patient with complete central diabetes insipidus formally "hanging" on the tap day and night due to exhaustive imperative of drinking 8 to 12 or more liters of water, and then to observe a conspicuous reduction of diuresis following vasopressin substitution leading to a dramatic improvement in his condition.

As a matter of fact, the most common knowledge on vasopressin barely exceeds the fact that the hormone is produced by the hypothalamic neuro-secretory cells and is stored in the posterior pituitary and that lesion of this brain area or of the pituitary is clinically manifested by nonglycosuric solute-free polyuria (central diabetes insipidus). Nevertheless, did our knowledge about this hormone be no more than it is operative in the primary control of renal water excretion, we should be aware of its extraordinary homeostatic importance. Today, however, much more is known about vasopressin. A review of this newly accumulated knowledge will be the main topic of the following chapters.

2 HYPOTHALAMO-NEUROHYPOPHYSEAL HORMONES AND NEUROPHYSINS

We know with certainty that ancient Greeks had known the neurohypophysis and that they assumed this brain structure to play a role of a certain filter serving to pass the mucous substance produced by the brain ("pituita") to the nose. This idea seems to have been generally accepted until the turn of our century when vasopressoric, antidiuretic, uterotonic, and milk ejecting effects of neurohypophyseal extracts were all disclosed within a short interval. These findings prompted characterization, isolation and synthesis of biologically active and phylogenically close neurohypophyseal peptides and their protein carriers, neurophysins.

From the viewpoint of comparative endocrinology, the neurohypophyseal peptides are perhaps the most thoroughly characterized hormonal systems in vertebrates. They belong to the most ancient type of internal secretion; in effect, they replaced the primitive neurohormones occurring in lower animals (e.g. in insects). However, neurohypophyseal peptides are already coordinators of a higher nature. They interfere with broader areas of control of important functions such as brain activity, reproduction, circulation, stress response, and water and electrolyte equilibrium.

So far, neurohypophyseal peptides have been thoroughly characterized in more than 40 different mammalian and nonmammalian (lung fishes, amphibians, reptiles, birds) species. In general, these peptides operate on the following principles: 1. the neurohypophysis of any species produces two kinds of hormones; 2. the hormones are nonapeptides with disulfide bridges between the cysteine residues in positions 1 and 6 with glycine-amide attached to the carboxy-end of the molecule; 3. any zoological class (mammals, birds, etc.) possesses hormones typical of that class; 4. the amino acids in positions 1, 5, 6, 7, and 9 have remained unchanged throughout the evolution, whereas changes (mutations) concerning amino acids in positions 3, 4, and 8 resulted in the development of various neurohypophyseal peptides with typical biological activities; 5. the zoological classes differ from each other in one or mostly two positions of the hormone molecule.

Although none of the naturally occurring neurohypophyseal hormones has absolutely selective biological activity, each one is characterized by some prevailing action: either oxytocic or vasopressin-like. Considerations about the available data on comparative biochemistry from the viewpoint of paleontological data led Acher (1980) to postulate the existence of two developmental lines of the naturally occurring neurohypophyseal hormones (Fig. 2.1). Their origin could have been in duplication of the original gene encoding a common ancestral molecule. The **oxytocin line** involves three developmental steps (isotocin, mesotocin, and oxytocin), while the **vasopressin line** has two independent peptides (arginine-vasotocin and vasopressin).

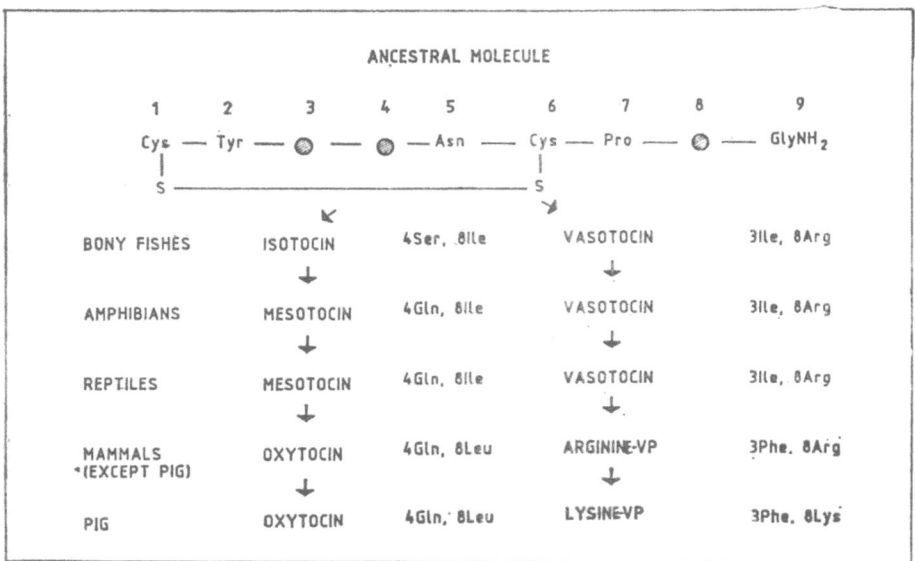

Fig. 2.1. Hypothetical scheme of the evolution of neurohypophyseal hormones compiled by Acher (1980). One gene duplication and a series of subsequent single substitutions in position 3, 4 and 8 produce two distinct molecular lines. The substituted amino-acids and their positions in the hormone are listed to the right of each hormone.

2.1 ARGININE-VASOPRESSIN (AVP) AND LYSINE-VASOPRESSIN (LVP)

In most mammals and also in humans this hormone occurs in form of arginine-vasopressin (AVP). In the pig and hippopotamus (and possibly in other members of the order Suina) these effects are mediated by lysine-vasopressin (LVP); in marsupials this role plays phenypressin (Acher 1980, Chauvet et al. 1980) (see Fig. 2.1).

Investigations of this hormone in the past often helped unravel several fundamental aspects of physiology. Vasopressin has become an archetype of all agents of humoral nature synthesized and produced by nerve cells, i.e. neurotransmitters and neurohormones (Bargmann 1949, Scharrer and Scharrer 1954). Also it was the first peptide hormone which has been shown to be synthesized in form of a larger precursor molecule together with its protein carrier (neurophysin), i.e. prohormone (Sachs and Tabatake 1964). Moreover, vasopressin and oxytocin were the first biologically active peptides to be synthesized in vitro (DuVigneaud et al. 1954a, 1954b). Also, vasopressin was one of the first humorally active substances which could be shown to develop their activity on the periphery mediated by an intracellular second messenger — cyclic adenosine monophosphate, cAMP (Orloff and Handler 1962). Several new aspects of vasopressin regarding its anatomy, biosynthesis and effects apparently fall into the line of this beautiful tradition.

In endocrinology there is an increasing number of examples of hormones that were originally identified and named on the basis of some particular effects and then subsequently found to exert other effects as well, some of which turn out to be of greater physiological importance than the original ones. Vasopressin is a classic example of a similar development of knowledge. Vasopressin, as its name implies, was originally extracted as a pressor substance from the posterior pituitary (Oliver and Schaffer 1895); since the time its antidiuretic property was documented by Farini (1913) and Van den Velden (1913) and definitively confirmed by Starling and Verney in 1924, the function of this hormone in the regulation of water homeostasis has begun dominating the scientific scene. Accordingly, it was baptized a second time and given the second name of "antidiuretic hormone", ADH, which has been used indiscriminately with its previous name. Besides these major actions of vasopressin, which still serve as endpoints for the bioassay of AVP and evaluation of agonistic and antagonistic properties of its numerous synthetic analogs, recently a variety of other, clinically important effects of the hormone (hemostatic, ACTH-releasing and metabolic actions, involvement in brain processes etc.) could be discovered.

2.2 OXYTOCIN (OT)

The structure of oxytocin (OT) differs from that of vasopressin only in positions 3 and 8 with isoleucine and leucine replacing phenylalanine and arginine respectively (see Fig. 2.1). It is generally accepted that the hormone acts on the specific oxytocin receptors in the myoepithelial cells to affect milk ejection, and in the myometrium to elicit uterine contraction. Physiologic concentrations of oxytocin do not stimulate uterine muscle; towards the end of gestation however uterine oxytocin receptors increase and the myometrium becomes more excitable (Fuchs et al. 1983). In contrast, vasopressin that acts on distinct AVP receptors in the myometrium is more active on nonpregnant than on pregnant uterus; owing to this AVP has been suggested to play an important role in dysmenorrhea (Akerlund et al. 1979, Guillon et al. 1987).

Although the role of oxytocin in reproductive function has been known for decades, there has been little progress in identifying any clearly defined physiological role for oxytocin in nonpregnant state. The observation that known stimuli of vasopressin secretion (infusion of hypertonic saline, hemorrhage, vomitus, surgical stress and also endotoxin) simultaneously stimulate oxytocin release (Weitzman et al. 1978b, Kasting 1986, Nussey et al. 1988a, 1988b) indirectly suggests that this hormone may have additional, so far little understood, biological activities. Some of these effects are known to be synergistic with the action of vasopressin, while others act in opposite direction. Because of their similar structures, both oxytocin and vasopressin can react with the renal vasopressin receptors. Oxytocin possesses relatively weak antidiuretic properties, which, however may reach the level of clinical importance in certain circumstances (chapter 20.3.1.10). Recently oxytocin could be shown to affect brain processes involved in memory in a way opposite to that of vasopressin. In fact oxytocin impairs memory acting as an "amnestic" peptide, whereas vasopressin acts antiamnestically (chapter 12.2.2). As various kinds of stress induce oxytocin release in both male and cyclic or ovariectomized female rats, a proposal has been made to classify oxytocin as a "stress hormone" (Lang et al. 1983). Also a role of oxytocin as a potential hypophyseotropic factor has been suggested recently. Oxytocin appears as a full agonist on the anterior pituitary receptors of the rat, but it is about 10 times less effective than vasopressin. Thus it is likely that oxytocin plays a role in ACTH secretion only when vasopressin is not available (Antoni et al. 1983).

2.3 OTHER NATURALLY OCCURRING NONAPEPTIDES IN MAMMALS

In addition to vasopressin and oxytocin, at least two other neurohypophyseal peptides, arginine vasotocin (AVT) and a novel oxytocin-vasotocin-like material (OT-VT) have been recently detected in mammals and humans. The true physiological significance of these putative peptides is unclear, and any assertion as to this topic at present would be highly speculative.

2.3.1 ARGININE VASOTOCIN (AVT)

Interestingly enough, this hybrid peptide containing the cyclic moiety of oxytocin together with the side chain of vasopressin in the same molecule (see Fig. 2.1) was first synthesized and only subsequently found in its natural form in nonmammalian tetrapods in which it has been found to have oxytocic, vasopressoric and water saving effects. In amphibians, the latter effect is manifested by an increased permeability of the apical (outer serosal) membranes of the urinary bladder cells to water. Nevertheless, it cannot be ruled out that the original, primitive peripheral function of AVT may have been associated with circulation control, and possibly (secondarily) also with the regulation of the renal excretory function via alteration of renal perfusion pressure and glomerular filtration (Chan 1977).

Recent reports have demonstrated the presence of immunoreactive AVT, which was primarily considered a purely neurohypophyseal principle of nonmammalian tetrapods, in the neurohypophysis, the plasma, the cerebrospinal fluid and the urine of fetuses and the pineal gland of mammals, and its presence in the human fetal pituitary has now been confirmed radioimmunologically and chromatographically (Skowsky and Fisher 1977, Pavel 1980, Ervin et al. 1985). These are provoking and so far unique data concerning the hypothesized role of the phylogenetically older nonapeptide in the ontogeny of species at a higher level of evolution.

2.3.2 NOVEL OXYTOCIN-VASOTOCIN-LIKE MATERIAL (OT-VT-LIKE MATERIAL)

Amico et al. (1986) reported that the plasma of human adults contains an oxytocin-vasotocin-like material, with an elution profile on high performance liquid chromatography that is different from those of AVP, AVT or oxytocin. This novel OT-VT-like material appears to be estrogen responsive in both males and females; its levels are elevated during pregnancy. Newborn plasma also contains a compound, that is immunologically and chromatographically identical with the novel OT-VT material observed in estrogen primed adults (Ervin et al. 1988). In vitro metabolism studies employing cystine aminopeptidase of human pregnancy plasma, trypsin or chymotrypsin indicate that OT-VT is not a metabolic product of AVP or oxytocin. Owing to the estrogen sensitivity of this material it is tempting to hypothesize that it may be involved in the biology of human reproduction.

2.4 NEUROHYPOPHYSEAL PEPTIDES WITHOUT ESTABLISHED HORMONAL ACTIVITY

Two other peptides, the hormone-associated neurophysin and the glycopeptide, are consistently present in the neurohypophysis. They are synthesized, packed into neurosecretory granules, to undergo axonal transport, and to be released into the circulation together with vasopressin and oxytocin (chapter 4).

2.4.1 HORMONE-ASSOCIATED NEUROPHYSINS (NP)

Each of the mammalian species investigated so far has two independent neurophysins, one for vasopressin and another for oxytocin. The neurophysins so far found in each species consist of roughly 95 amino acids, of which the central 60 or so are highly conserved in all the known neurophysin sequences. The differences between the individual neurophysins concern differences in amino acid sequences in the N-terminal (posititons 1—9 of the residue) and C-terminal (positions 75—96 of the residue) molecule moieties. In humans the secretion of **vasopressin**-linked neurophysin (the nicotine-stimulated neurophysin) increases under the action of the same secretory stimuli that also stimulate AVP secretion. The secretion of the other, oxytocin-linked (i.e. estrogen-stimulated) neurophysin increases in women in the period of lactation (Robinson 1984).

The functional significance of neurophysins remains an unresolved issue. This is even more surprising in the light of the extremely conserved primary sequence of both the above principles. One possible role of neurophysin is that of carrier protein for the nonapeptide hormones within the neurosecretory granules, although such a carrier system seems not necessary for other peptide hormones traveling from the hypothalamus to the hypophysis. Alternatively the biological role of neurophysin might be related to protection of the hormones against intracellular proteolytic degradation. Although neurophysin has been reported to possess natriuretic and even proteoanabolic activities, these most likely are of minor, if any, importance (Ponec and Lichardus 1977). The clinical significance of neurophysins, for the present at least, lies in their more pronounced immunogenicity as compared to that of the active hormones (i.e. AVP or OT), allowing to estimate, by determining their plasma levels, the actual state of neurohypophyseal function (Verbalis and Robinson 1985).

2.4.2 VASOPRESSIN-ASSOCIATED GLYCOPEPTIDE

Not until the amino acid sequence of the vasopressin precursor could be identified became the origin of the neurohypophyseal glycopeptide clear. Probably, it is a phylogenetically new peptide product; its enzymatic cleavage from the C terminal part of the neurophysin in the course of the intracellular processing of the precursor molecule is likely to occur only in species that synthesize vasopressin (see Fig. 2.1) (Acher et al. 1988). This fact along with the evidence that glycopeptide is released from the posterior pituitary together with vasopressin into the systemic circulation indicate a specific, albeit still unknown biological function for this neuronal product (Nagy et al. 1988).

3   NEUROSECRETION

Since the initial discovery by Bargmann (1949) and Scharrer and Scharrer (1954) that the neurohypophyseal peptides vasopressin and oxytocin are initially synthesized in the hypothalamic neurosecretory neurons with subsequent transport to and secretion from axon terminals in the posterior pituitary, this neuroendocrine system has been the essential model for studying neurosecretion of peptides. Today, the concept of the neurosecretory cell extends far beyond the original ideas, i.e. that neurons secrete hormones directly into the bloodstream. With the emergence of the "peptidergic neuron" as major cellular component in the nervous system, the question arises whether there is such a cell type as the "conventional neuron". As the neurons share so many morphological, biochemical and electrophysiological properties with other cell types, it appears that the only really unique feature of the neuron is its axon, i.e. the long process devoid of ribosomes which is specialized in axonal transport and rapid conduction of action potentials.

During the past decade it has become clear that neurons throughout the CNS produce a large number of different peptides which upon release are thought to affect the activity of other neurons. Many of these peptides were initially identified on the basis of peripheral effects, but are now known to have central as well as peripheral functions, often in unrelated systems under separate control mechanisms. Thus the vasopressinergic and oxytocinergic neurosecretory cell is no longer a unique phenomenon. It simply represents one of the diverse forms in which peptidergic neurons occur. It is in this context that the classic neurosecretory system, the hypothalamo-neurohypophyseal system, has become more than a subject of historical interests. Because of the background that has accumulated about this system and its peptides it remains an especially valuable model for the study of various aspects of peptidergic neuron function (Zimmerman et al. 1987).

3.1   NEURAL ORGANIZATION OF THE VASOPRESSINERGIC SYSTEM

The relative ease with which neurons of the hypothalamo-neurohypophyseal vasopressinergic system can be stained has resulted in numerous neuroanatomical studies. Initial studies with the Gomori staining technique (based on the

19

identification of S-S groups of cysteine and originally employed for the determination of insulin content in pancreatic Langerhans islets) have been followed by immunohistochemical techniques using specific antisera to the neurophysins and later to arginine vasopressin and oxytocin. This approach has provided extensive new information concerning the organization of the system.

The most striking new information concerning this system has centered around four main areas: 1. the complex cytoarchitecture of vasopressinergic and oxytocinergic nuclei in and outside the hypothalamus, involving numerous other neuropeptides within the nuclei, and in some cases, colocalization of more than one peptide in neurosecretory neurons; 2. the projection of vasopressinergic and oxytocinergic neurons to areas of the central nervous system other than the posterior pituitary, specifically to the median eminence and extrahypothalamic structures; 3. the multiple diverse afferent inputs to the vasopressinergic neurons, in particular brainstem projections to the PVN; and finally 4. the peripheral vasopressin producing cells (Sofroniew 1983, Swanson and Sawchenko 1983, Zimmermann et al. 1987).

3.1.1 NEURONS PRODUCING VASOPRESSIN AND OXYTOCIN

Immunohistological studies have confirmed the existence of two clearly distinguishable types of vasopressin and oxytocin producing neurons: greater, magnocellular neurons (15—35 μm in diameter) as opposed to smaller, parvocelular perikarya (10—15 μm in diameter). These neurons differ not only histologically, but also functionally. The term magnocellular refers mainly to posterior pituitary perikarya in origin, while parvocellular neurons project to numerous hypothalamic and extrahypothalamic areas other than the neurohypophysis (Sofroniew 1983).

3.1.1.1 Magnocellular perikarya of the supraoptic (SON) and paraventricular (PVN) nuclei

The magnocellular neurons of the hypothalamic supraoptic and paraventricular nuclei have long been recognized as major sources of the vasopressin and oxytocin released from the neurohypophysis. It has also become clear that each neuron synthesizes and secretes only one neurohypophyseal hormone, vasopressin or oxytocin, and its associated neurophysin. This could be demonstrated in Brattleboro rats (chapter 4.4) showing no vasopressin or vasopressin-neurophysin immunoreactivity, but normal oxytocin and oxytocin-neurophysin immunoreactivity. SON contains only magnocellular perikarya. The cytoarchitectonic structure of PVN is more complex and composed of several nuclear groups: three of them being magnocellular (anterior, posterior and medial), and five parvocellular (anterior, medial, lateral, dorsal and paraventricular). Probably every magnocellular neuron contains either vasopressin or oxytocin and projects to the neural lobe (Swanson and Kuypers 1980, Silverman and Zimmermann 1983). Vasopressingergic and oxytocinergic neurons are present in both the SON and the PVN, but sited at fairly discrete areas within each nucleus and with some variation in the exact distribution between SON and PVN in different species. (Fliers et al. 1985).

With the detection of rapidly increasing numbers of newly discovered peptides in the central and peripheral nervous system several additional neuroactive peptides have been found to be localized within the magnocellular hypothalamic nuclei, in particular in the paraventricular nucleus (angiotensin II, glucagon, gastrin/cholecystokinin etc.). So far, the coexistence of dynorphin with vasopressin and of oxytocin with cholecystokinin has been demonstrated in the same magnocellular perikarya and their fibres and terminals in the neural lobe (Watson et al. 1982; Kiss et al. 1984).

3.1.1.2 Accessory magnocellular perikarya

Additional magnocellular vasopressin and oxytocin neurons have been identified in a number of so-called accessory nuclei scattered through various regions of the hypothalamus (rostral periventricular nucleus, anterior and posterior fornicate nuclei, nucleus circularis, etc.) (Fisher et al. 1979, Silverman and Zimmerman 1983). Similarly as SON and PVN, these accessory nuclei contain intermingled populations of magnocellular vasopressin and oxytocin neurons which for most part project to the posterior pituitary. It appears that these accessory neurons resemble the magnocellular neurons of the SON and PVN not only by their microstructure, but also by both their electrophysiological and functional characteristics.

3.1.1.3 Parvocellular vasopressinergic perikarya

Several groups of parvocellular vasopressin and oxytocin neurons have now been identified both inside and outside the hypothalamus; these neurons do not appear to project to the posterior pituitary. In the hypothalamus parvocellular perikarya were found in 5 subdivisions of the PVN (Swanson and Kuypers 1980). In the human material approximately 16 per cent of cells in the suprachiasmatic nucleus can be stained with anti-vasopressin (Swaab et al. 1985). Outside the hypothalamus a large number of clearly parvocellular vasopressin/neurophysin-containing neurons were discovered in the bed of the nucleus stria terminalis, the septal region and the medial amygdala, and smaller numbers in the region of locus ceruleus (Sofroniew 1983). These new findings suggest that the vasopressin system in the brain does not originate solely in the hypothalamus and its environs.

In the paraventricular nucleus and, to a lesser degree, in the suprachiasmatic nucleus subpopulations of perikarya containing other neuropeptides along with AVP (corticotropin-releasing factor, neurotensin, opioid peptides, angiotensin II, etc.) were identified (Sawchenko 1987).

3.1.2 FIBER PROJECTIONS OF VASOPRESSINERGIC NEURONS

It is now recognized that neurons containing vasopressin and its neurophysin project to various vascular and neural target areas in the brain (Fig. 3.1) : 1. The best known projection is the classic hypothalamo-neurohypophyseal system, from which vasopressin is released into the bloodstream to exert its hormonal effects in the periphery (Silverman and Zimmermann 1983). 2. Separate parvocellular neurons release vasopressin into the hypophyseal-portal vessels of the median eminence, where AVP is thought to affect the anterior pituitary function (Sawchenko 1987). 3. It has become clear that

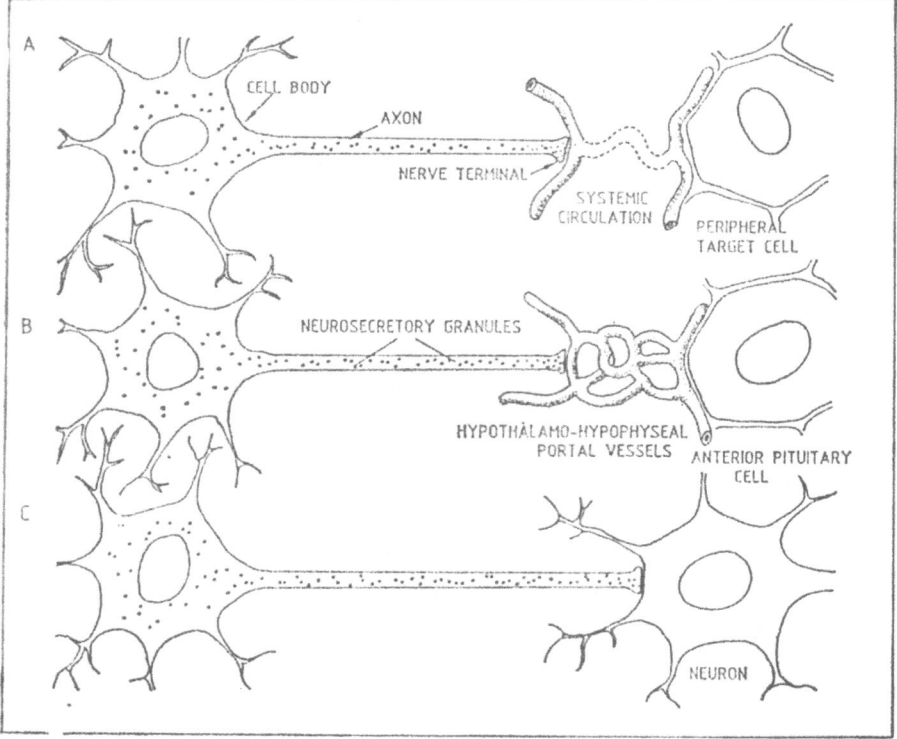

Fig. 3.1. Schematic representation of vasopressinergic neurons and their different target sites.

vasopressin immunoreactive parvocelular cell bodies send projections to numerous areas within the brain; in these locations vasopressin may act either as neurotransmitter or neuromodulator (Riphagen and Pittman 1986).

3.1.2.1 The classic hypothalamo-neurohypophyseal neurosecretory system

The neurohypophysis is the most generally known vascular target area of vasopressinergic (and oxytocinergic) neurosecretory cells; this area contains the largest concentrations of readily releasable peptides within the central nervous system. Since SON contains only magnocellular neurons, and since the main, if not the sole, projection of the SON is to the neurohypophysis, this nucleus is the major contributor of vasopressin and oxytocin to the systemic circulation. PVN projects fewer fibres to this region; they originate from the magnocellular subdivisions of the nucleus. The importance of the contribution of the accessory magnocellular projections to the posterior pituitary in the rat has been pointed out by Fisher et al. (1979). These authors observed that accessory magnocellular elements, at least in the animal species they studied, were as important in number as those concentrated in PVN and SON in terms of projections to the

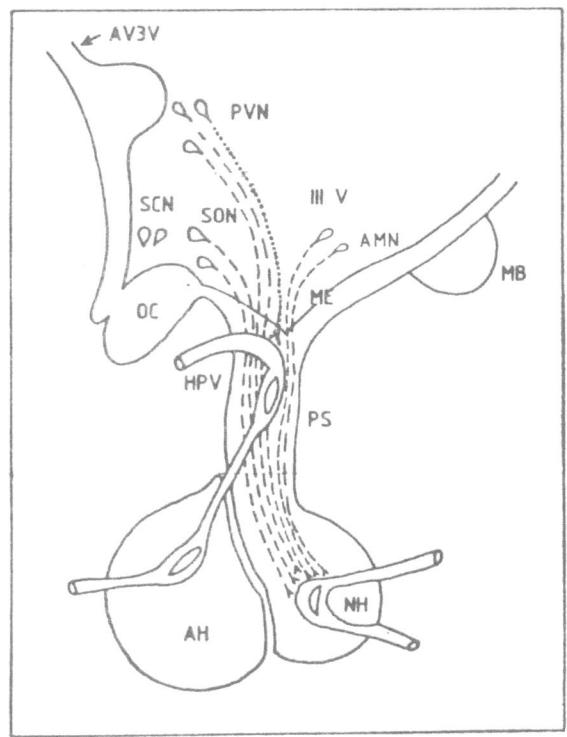

Fig. 3.2. Diagram of the hypothalamo-neurohypophyseal system.
(PVN: paraventricular nucleus, SON: supraoptic nucleus, SCN: suprachiasmatic nucleus, AMN: accessory magnocellular nuclei, IIIV: third cerebral ventricle, MB: mammalian body, OC: optic chiasm, ME: median eminence, PS: pituitary stem, AH: adenohypophysis, NH: neurohypophysis, HPV: adenohypophyseal portal vessel, AV3V: anteroventral third ventricle region). (From Legros 1979, modified.)

posterior pituitary gland. Large-diameter, mostly nonmyelinized axons o magnocellular vasopressinergic neurons converge in the region of the internal zone of the rostral median eminence and reach within the pituitary stalk the neurohypophysis. In this organ axons bilaterally form specific nerve endings, the neurohemal organs, on fenestrated protein-permeable walls of systemic capillaries (Fig. 3.2).

This extensive distribution of magnocellular vasopressinergic neurons provides sufficient redundancy in the neurohypophyseal system to make simple neurogenic diabetes insipidus unlikely to result from an isolated hypothalamic lesion, since preservation of only 10 to 20 per cent of the magnocellular neurons will provide sufficient vasopressin to prevent the development of clinical diabetes insipidus. Therefore vascular infiltrative or neoplastic lesions in the hypothalamus must produce near-total bilateral destruction of SON, PVN and accessory magnocellular elements, or their output tracts, to cause sufficient vasopressin deficiency to result in pituitary diabetes insipidus. Consequently, lesions of the posterior pituitary, pituitary stalk and infundibulum are much more likely to produce clinical diabetes insipidus than isolated hypothalamic disease (Verbalis et al. 1985).

3.1.2.2 Parvocellular projections to the median eminence

The first clear demonstration of nonpituitary projections of vasopressinergic neurons was the discovery of hormone-associated neurophysin terminals around portal capillaries in the zona interna of the median eminence (Parry and Livett 1973) (see Figs. 3.1 and 3.2). The hormone-containing granules in terminals on or near the portal capillaries are smaller than those in the posterior pituitary gland, and they originate mainly from cells of the median parvocellular division of PVN. Measurements of neurophysin and vasopressin levels in the portal blood of monkeys confirmed markedly elevated concentrations, thousandfold higher than those measured in the peripheral circulation (Zimmerman et al. 1973), indicating that the hormone is released directly into the portal blood.

A function for vasopressin in portal blood has been suggested by long standing observations of the ability of exogenous vasopressin to stimulate, both in vivo and in vitro, adrenocorticotropin (ACTH) release (for review see Hedge and Huffmann 1987) (chapter 11). Interestingly, the PVN is also the site of the perikarya of corticotropin-releasing factor (CRF) producing neurons that project to the median eminence with evidence for co-localization of vasopressin and CRF within the same neurons in a particular (the median parvocellular) subdivision of the PVN (Whitnall and Gainer 1988). Thus vasopressin and CRF in these subsets of parvocellular neurosecretory neurons appear to share a functional association as stimulators of corticotropin secretion, seemingly being regulated by circulating adrenal steroids (Sawchenko 1987). In the light of their well established physiologic roles as initiators of the stress response

(Makara 1985) it seems that this population of parvocellular neurosecretory neurons will provide a useful model for the understanding of the overall organization economy of the hypothalamus and for providing at least one framework in which the significance of the apparently widespread phenomenon of peptide co-localization may be approached in a meaningful functional context.

3.1.2.3 Parvocellular extrahypothalamic projections

A major new development in the study of neurohypophyseal peptides in the last few years has been that vasopressin and oxytocin containing fibers project to a large number of brain areas where they terminate by means of synapses that cannot be morphologically distinguished from other peptidergic terminals (Buijs and Swaab 1979) (see Fig. 3.1). The areas containing vasopressin and oxytocin fibres are quite diverse, ranging from autonomic centers in the brainstem and spinal cord to forebrain limbic centers, and even to the neocortex. However, the density of fibres of terminals within the different areas vary considerably from single isolated fibres as seen in the neocortex to very dense innervation as found in the structures of the dorsomedial medulla (the area postrema, the nucleus tractus solitarius, and the dorsal motor nucleus of the vagus) (Weindl and Sofroniew 1985).

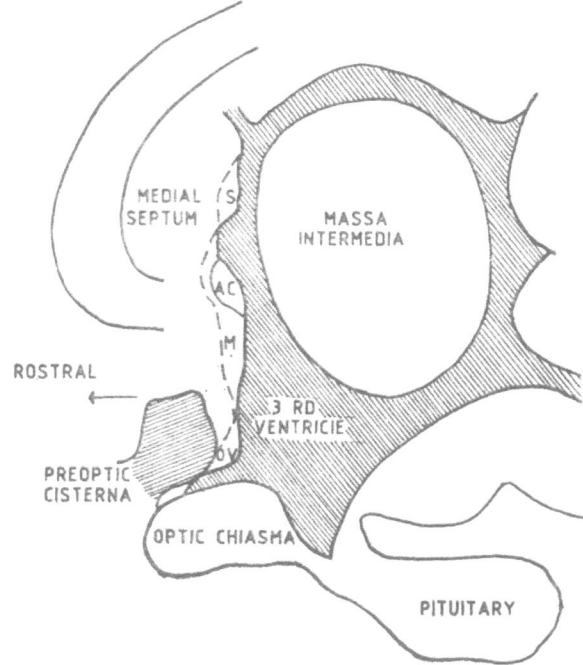

Fig. 3.3. Diagram of the midsagittal section through the mammalian brain, indicating position of structures in anterior wall of the 3rd ventricle. The 3rd ventricle is shaded; boundaries of the subfornical organ (S), median preoptic nucleus (M) and organum vasculosum of lamina terminalis (OV) are shown by the interrupted line. AC: anterior commissure. (From McKinley 1987 with kind permission.)

25

At present, the parvocellular subdivisions of PVN, the suprachiasmatic nucleus (SCN) and the bed nucleus of the stria terminalis (BST) appear to be the source of the majority of extrahypothalamic AVP (Fig. 3.3). Observations that AVP is released into the brain, that specific binding sites (receptors) occur in brain areas congruent with known vasopressinergic terminals, and the physiological and behavioral effects induced by central administration of this peptide (van Leeuven 1987) indicate that AVP has become a strong candidate for a neurotransmitter within the CNS (chapter 12). Furthermore, it is apparent that certain acute stimuli that alter circulating levels of AVP may also be effective in altering its CNS levels (Riphagen and Pittmann 1986). AVP may therefore be released simultaneously in the brain and in the periphery to provide a coordinated neural and endocrine response to homeostatic perturbations.

3.1.3 AFFERENT INPUTS TO THE SUPRAOPTIC AND PARAVENTRICULAR NUCLEI

Both SON and PVN are densely innervated by neural projections originating from various brain sites. Perhaps the richest afferentation to both the supraoptic and the paraventricular nucleus is projected from other hypothalamic nuclei, including SON-PVN interconnections.Among others patways have been established that project to SON and PVN from the anteroventral third ventricle (AV3V) region and from the brainstem autonomic centers (Figs. 3.3 and 3.4).

3.1.3.1 Neural inputs from the anteroventral third ventricle (AV3V) region

Significant evidence has accumulated suggesting that the SON and PVN neurons themselves are not the principal osmoreceptors; rather, the role of osmoreceptors is played by anatomically separated neurons located on the blood side of the blood-brain barrier and synaptically communicating with vasopressinergic neurosecretory neurons. Two circumventricular organs — the subfornical organ (SFO) and organum vasculosum laminae terminalis (OVLT) — located in the AV3V area, outside the blood-brain barrier (see Fig. 3.3) are the likely sites of the type of systemic central interaction necessary for the brain to be "informed" on the concentration of blood-borne stimuli (McKinley et al. 1985).

Electrolytic ablation of the OVLT interrupts neural inputs that stimulate magnocellular system to release vasopressin in response to normal humoral stimuli and thus produces a profound disruption in the system controlling body fluid homeostasis (Gruber et al. 1976, Thrasher and Keil 1987). However, such lesions do not entirely suppress either drinking or vasopressin secretion to nonphysiologic increases of plasma osmolality indicating that OVLT is the principal, though not the only, site of the osmosensitive elements in the CNS. Whether there is a single discrete set of osmoreceptor neurons or a heterogenous group of central osmoreceptive neurons with varying sensitivities in different nuclei which should provide some degree of expected redundancy to this regulatory system awaits better characterization of the afferent inputs to SON and PVN.

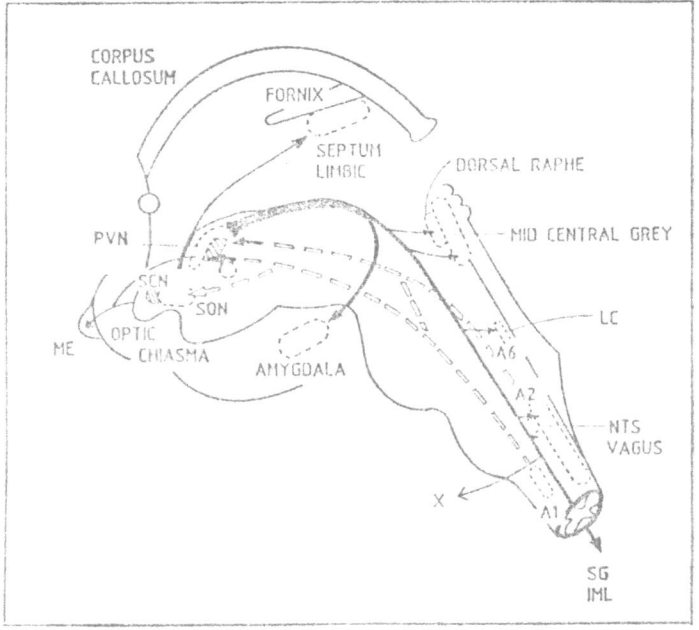

Fig. 3.4. Descending vasopressinergic projections (dotted arrows) from the paraventricular nucleus (PVN) to forebrain structures and midbrain autonomic and cardiovascular centres, including the locus ceruleus (LC), the nucleus tractus solitarius (NTS) and the dorsal nucleus of the vagus (X) as well as to the substania gelatinosa (SG) and intermediolateral bundle (IML) of the spinal cord. Ascending catecholaminergic pathways (interrupted arrows) from the A1 area of the ventromedullary region of the midbrain and the A2 and A6 regions to the supraoptic (SON) and paraventricular (PVN) nucleus in the hypothalamus (from Johnston 1985 with kind permission).

The second circumventricular nucleus, the subfornical organ (SFO), is believed to play a contributory role in central sensing of volume depletion via circulating angiotensin II levels. This pathway provides a potential mechanism whereby volume depletion can trigger vasopressin secretion (and thirst) via humoral (angiotensin) stimuli independent of classic baroreceptor pathways. At the same time, this would provide a measure of redundancy for vasopressin secretion in response to volume stimuli. Thus it is likely that, as with osmoreception, multiple pathways are involved in transmitting information about blood pressure and volume to the hypothalamo-neurohypophyseal system (McKinley 1987).

3.1.3.2 Neural inputs from extrahypothalamic brain areas

In fact each extrahypothalamic region which is innervated by vasopressinergic parvocellular neurons projects back to the hypothalamus, mostly to the paraventricular nucleus (PVN). Perhaps the most thoroughly studied reciprocal link of this kind is that between PVN and catecholaminergic centers in the brainstem (see Fig. 3.4). Efferents from predominantly parvocellular subunits of PVN terminate on catecholamine containing neurons in 1. the ventro-lateral medulla, the A1 group; 2. the dorsal vagal complex, the A2 group; and 3. the locus ceruleus, the A6 group. In turn, ascending fibres from these catecholamine groups terminate on neurons in PVN and SON. Visceral afferent stimuli from volume and baroreceptors and probably also nausea stimuli acting both peripherally via the vagus nerve or centrally in the area postprema may affect vasopressin release by these pathways. However, the organisation of these ascending pathways is notably complex. For example, catecholamine neurons of the A1 group appear to project substantially to the magnocellular neurons of both PVN and SON. In contrast, catecholamine neurons of the A2 group of the dorsal vagal complex and of the A6 group of the locus ceruleus appear to terminate mostly on parvocellular subdivisions of PVN (Swanson and Sawchenko 1983). Therefore, separate links between the brainstem and the vasopressinergic nuclei may exist for the regulation of plasma vasopressin (via magnocellular neurons), and for the regulation of autonomic functions such as circulation (via parvocellular neurons).

Another important afferentation to vasopressinergic nuclei, in particular PVN, originates in the limbic system, including the hippocampus, the septum and the amygdala. Reciprocal links of vasopressin containing neurons with these regions are of special interest since these areas are thought to be involved in memory and other behavioral processes.

The above summary of the major new neuroanatomical data suggests that SON and PVN should no longer be regarded simply as two identical vasopressinergic nuclei in different parts of the hypothalamus but rather as nuclei with different roles in coordinating body functions. The fact that PVN receives significant synaptic input from a number of extrahypothalamic regions in addition to those from the hypothalamus and that it projects to the median eminence, the brainstem and the spinal cord (in contrast to SON which primarily projects to the neurohypophysis) led Swanson and Sawchenko (1983) to hypothesize the role of this nucleus as being an integrator and modulator of a wide range of visceral responses: the neurohypophyseal and the adeno-hypophyseal secretion (specifically ACTH release via vasopressin/CRF projections to the median eminence) as well as the autonomic reflexes via descending brainstem and spinal cord projections ("autonomic visceral effector nucleus of the central nervous system").

3.1.4 IMMUNOREACTIVE VASOPRESSIN IN PERIPHERAL TISSUES

Until recently the hypothalamus was considered the only site of vasopressin synthesis. This view had to be revised in the light of studies demonstrating vasopressin biosynthesis not only in brain regions outside the hypothalamus but also in the light of evidence that vasopressin and parts of its precursor (i.e. neurophysin and glycopeptide) could be identified in a number of nonneural, mostly steroidogenic peripheral tissues, including testis, ovary, uterus, fetal and adult adrenal, sympathetic ganglia and thymus (Clements and Funder 1986). By many physico-chemical and bioactivity criteria this peripheral AVP behaved as authentic AVP. Moreover, the demonstration of AVP/neurophysin messenger RNA in these "nontraditional tissues" (Ivell et al. 1986) gives evidence for peripheral synthesis of AVP. In addition, some peripheral tissues known to contain AVP possess specific binding sites for the hormone, which are similar (but not necessarily identical) to the subtype of vasopressin receptors present in vascular smooth muscle cells (Maggi et al. 1987).

The function of tissue AVP remains unknown. The levels of the vasopressin peptide in the peripheral tissues are in general 2—3 orders of magnitude lower than those in the hypothalamus suggesting that the nonapeptide at these sites can only have a local modulatory (paracrine) function but does not substantially contribute to circulating AVP. The ability of the hormone to stimulate testicular progesterone synthesis and inhibit androgen biosynthesis (Kasson et al. 1986) is consistent with its proposed paracrine role in the gonads. A role in the regulation of catecholamine synthesis in the adrenal gland has been also suggested (Nussey et al. 1987). Similarly, thymic AVP may play a role in the modulation of the immune response, as it was reported that AVP can replace the interleukin II requirement for the production of gamma interferon in murine spleen cultures (Markwick et al. 1986).

4 BIOSYNTHESIS, TRANSPORT AND RELEASE OF VASOPRESSIN

The idea that vasopressin and oxytocin, although composed of only a few amino-acids, are synthesized on ribosomes as common precursors together with their respective neurophysins derives from the work of Sachs and Tabatake (1964). Their original concept concerning the synthesis of biologically active peptides in form of precursor molecules was postulated long before the discovery of proinsulin, and has become a milestone in the development of neurosciences. The exact details of this biosynthetic pathway came with the isolation of cDNA clones from a hypothalamic cDNA library. It contained the entire sequence corresponding to the vasopressin messenger RNA (mRNA) and hence the polypeptide it encoded. Later DNA probes derived from these hypothalamic cDNA clones were used to isolate and sequence the vasopressin gene itself (Schmale et al. 1987). The data obtained proved unambiguously that the vasopressin precursor is composed of several distinct peptides: the hormone, its carrier protein neurophysin, and a glycopeptide. The precursor can be considered a typical representative of a class of proteins termed cellular polyproteins in analogy with viral polyproteins composed of several viral entities. Another example of cellular polyproteins in eukaryotic cells is the prohormone proopiomelanocortin which becomes proteolytically cleft to produce ACTH and a number of other biologically active agents (Hebert 1981).

The question may arise whether it is not a "squander of the strength of nature" to produce large molecules if the biologically active fragment represents but a small fraction (approximately one tenth for vasopressin) of the original molecule (Schreiber 1979). One should however bear in mind that the contemporaneous peptide hormones had their origin in gene products originally serving other purposes for the cell (enzymes, cell membrane constituents, etc.). Proteolytic cleavage of the original molecules produced fragments possessing significant biological activities; the preservation of these fragments was biologically advantageous. This gave rise to hormones with marked activities throughout the organism and/or at sites (target organs) distant from the sites of production. In turn one may wonder why the production of the "useless" part of the molecule (e.g. neurophysin or glycopeptide) has not been eliminated during evolution. This may be explained — at least partially — by the fact that a relatively long chain of the peptide molecule must be formed on ribosomes located on the surface of the granular endoplasmic reticulum, to overcome the dimensions of the ribosome itself and most likely also the distance between the ribosome and the cisternae of the endoplasmic reticulum by which the hormone is then taken up. Thus to be synthesized at all, the peptide molecule must have a certain minimal length; this minimal length for linear molecules is assumed to be about 70 amino acids.

In addition, the existence of cellular polyproteins provides the possibility of posttranslational regulation via different proteolytic cleavage to yield different biologically active end-products in various cells of the organism as it is the case for example with the proopiomelanocortin-prohormone (Herbert 1981). There is some evidence that also neurohypophyseal prohormones may be further processed to different final products in different areas of the brain: within the CNS a fragment of vasopressin has been identified which has enhanced vasopressin-like memory consolidation effects (chapter 12.2.3).

4.1 STRUCTURAL ORGANIZATION OF THE VASOPRESSIN GENE

The structurally identical human genes for vasopressin and oxytocin prohormones are separated by only 12 kilobases on chromosome 20, but coded by inversely arranged DNA strands (Sausville et al. 1985). The vasopressin precursor gene is approximately 2 kilobases long and includes three exons (making up approximately 30 per cent of the total gene length and encoding the amino acid sequence of the precursor) and two mediating segments (introns) (Fig 4.1). The introns thus divide the gene into three independent functional domains encoding vasopressin, neurophysin and glycopeptide. The first exon is composed of nucleotide bases which encode the signal peptide (a hydrophobic sequence of 19 amino acids, a typical component of all the secreted peptides), the vasopressin molecule itself, and a phylogenically relatively poorly preserved N-terminal portion of neurophysin. The central, phylogenically highly preserved moiety of the neurophysin molecule (aminoacids in positions 10—76 of the peptide) is encoded by the second exon, whereas the remaining C-terminal portion of neurophysin and the glycopeptide are encoded by the third exon.

The second neurohypophyseal nonapeptide, oxytocin, whose synthesis was once thought to be linked with that of vasopressin in the form of the Van Dyke protein, has been shown to be the product of another, quite discrete gene. Nevertheless genes which encode vasopressin and oxytocin precursor are essentially identical in organization; they probably evolved by point mutation and duplication of a common ancestral gene (see Fig. 2.1), and they are expressed via quite comparable but distinct biosynthetic pathways. The only apparent structural distinction of the oxytocin prohormone from the vasopressin precursor is its lack of the glycopeptide sequence. This might indicate that the DNA sequence corresponding to this C-terminal peptide, once part of the oxytocin precursor, has been "lost" during evolution.

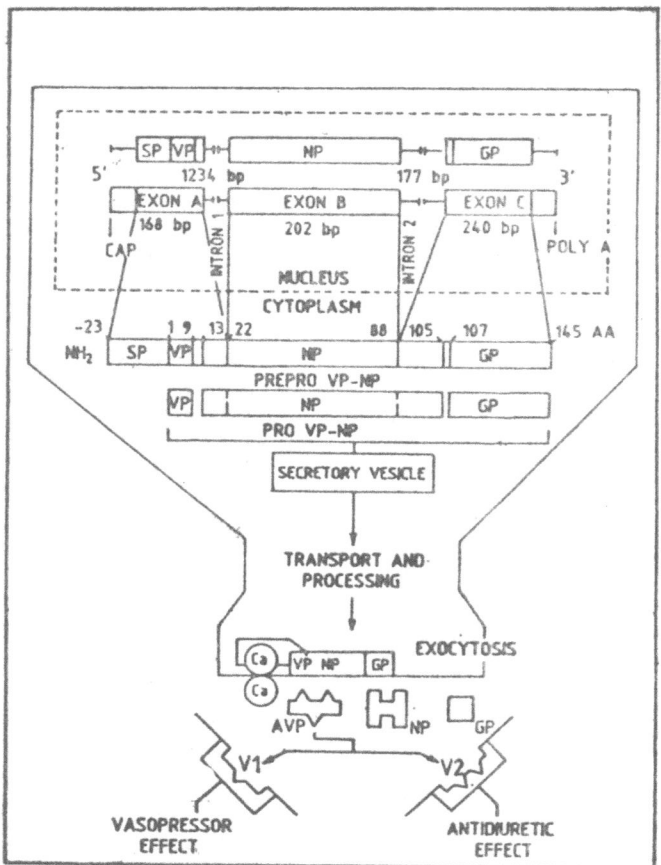

Fig. 4.1. Synthesis, transport and release of vasopressin in a hypothetical neurosecretory neuron (data withdrawn from Brownstein et al. 1980, Richter 1985, Sausville et al. 1985; adapted from Cacabelos 1986) (VP—vasopressin, NP—neurophysin, GP—glyco-peptide, SP—signal peptide, bp—base pairs, AA—amino-acids).

4.2 POSTTRANSLATIONAL PROCESSING OF THE VASOPRESSIN PRECURSOR

The process of vasopressin biosynthesis involves a number of intricate intra-cellular mechanisms (see Fig. 4.1). The expression of the genetic information aimed at the production of a biologically active polypeptide starts in the cell nucleus by the activation of the process of transcription. This is followed by a cascade of events including processing of the initial RNA transcripts, excision of the mediating RNA segments (introns), relinkage of specific RNA segments (exons), and modification of the 3′-terminal region by polyadenylation, and of the 5′-terminal region by the addition of 7-methyl guanosine caps. The mature, fully equipped preproVPNpmRNA is then transported to the cytoplasm and serves, on the surface of the rough endoplasmic reticulum, as a pattern model for the translation of the genetic information from polynucleotides into a 166 aminoacid precursor, prepropressorphysin (preproVPNp). However, to become the final biologially active proteins, the precursor must undergo a series of modifications in its primary structure. The precursor passes via the Golgi to be packed into neurosecretory granules and axonally transported in a colchicine sensitive fashion to nerve terminals. During this transport, lasting 12—24 h in average, the primary structure of the precursor becomes the subject of a series of enzymatic modifications resulting in the conversion of the precursor into vasopressin, neurophysin and glycopeptide.

Multiple enzymatic activities have been identified in neurosecretory granules (trypsin-like converting enzymes, carboxypeptidase-like enzymes, and amidation-like enzymes) which may be responsible for the "packing" of the prohormone into secretory granules and for its intragranular processing. Owing to the complexity of this process it is quite obvious that any disturbance of any individual enzymatic step may be the cause of failure of the neurosecretory cells to produce and release vasopressin into the circulation. It may be therefore expected that certain forms of congenital neurogenic diabetes insipidus will be identified in future in which the cause underlying the deficient production of vasopressin will be secondary not to the lack of the proper genetic message for the prohormone, but rather to deficiency of enzymes necessary for intragranular processing of the precursor molecule.

Moreover, incomplete processing of the molecule might be manifested by the release into the blood of certain imperfect fragments of prohormone cleavage in addition to vasopressin, neurophysin and glycoprotein. The latter possibility should not be considered unusual as similar observations have been reported in relation to other endocrine systems. For example, as many as 5 per cent of the hormonal content of pancreatic beta- cells are made up by incompletely processed proinsulin fragments which are subsequently released into the circulation and can be detected by radioimmunological methods. It may seem surprising at first sight that, according to recent reports, peptides with higher molecular weight, probably suggesting their incomplete enzymic cleavage, account for as many as 10—15 per cent of the total neurophysin immunoreactivity in the human posterior pituitary (Verbalis and Robinson 1983). The detection of circulating prohormone might in future provide further information of the pathways of intragranular processing of neurohypophyseal peptides in physiological and pathophysiological conditions in humans. Such a test might eventually be of great interest for the detection and monitoring of ectopic production of vasopressin and neurophysin in patients with oat cell carcinoma of the lung associated with the syndrome of inappropriate vasopressin secretion. The observation of a large proportion of high-molecular vasopressin in the circulation of patients with oat cell carcinoma of the lung (Yamaji et al. 1981, Smitz et al. 1985), a finding consistent with the general opinion about disordered protein processing in many neoplastic tissues, might also be in support of this view. The determination of incompletely processed precursor forms of vasopressin and neurophysin may therefore perspectively become a diagnostic marker enabling early detection of ectopic AVP secretion, in analogy to the widely used determination of proinsulin in the diagnosis of insulinomas (Rubinstein and Steiner 1971, Verbalis and Robinson 1985).

4.3 REGULATION OF THE VASOPRESSIN GENE EXPRESSION

More recent methods of investigation enable to evaluate relative intensities of simultaneous processes of production, transport and secretion of AVP at least at three different levels. Radioimmunnoassay of plasma or urine AVP provides information about the intensity of AVP secretion; the immunohistochemical technique following colchicine administration (resulting in accumulation of the peptide in the perikaryon due to the inhibition of axonal transport) provides insight into the synthetic activities of the nonapeptide and its precursors; finally, using the in situ hybridization technique for the determination of vasopressin mRNA levels it is now possible to study the gene regulation at the transcriptional level.

The available data concerning expression of the vasopressin gene fully agree with the current concepts of the function of the individual groups of vasopressinergic neurons (chapter 3.1.2). Plasma hyperosmolality in experimental animals induces a 2—5-fold elevation of vasopressin mRNA levels in all SON neurons and in a part of PVN neurons, while leaving mRNA levels in vasopressinergic cells of the suprachiasmatic nucleus unchanged (Burbach et al. 1984a). On the other hand, adrenalectomy is associated with elevated mRNA levels in the medial parvocellular subdivision of PVN neurons but not in other hypothalamic vasopressinergic cells, implying that the release from glucocorticoid feedback is ultimately a transregulatory factor for the expression of the AVP gene in this particular subpopulation of neurons (Wolfson et al. 1985). Vasopressin mRNA levels in the suprachiasmatic nucleus display an intrinsic circadian rhythm present since the early fetal life suggesting the involvement of the hormone in the circadian timekeeping system (Reppert and Uhl 1987). In addition, for most peripheral tissues in which immunoreactive AVP has been reported (chapter 3.1.4) demonstration of specific mRNA has confirmed the local gene expression. Interestingly, in all peripheral tissues studied, the vasopressin encoding mRNA appears consistently shorter than its hypothalamic counterpart; the smaller size is apparently due to tissue specific differences in the length of the poly (A) tails (see Fig. 4.1) (Ivell et al. 1986).

4.4   THE BRATTLEBORO RAT — AN ANIMAL MODEL OF HEREDITARY NEUROGENIC (CENTRAL) DIABETES INSIPIDUS

Hereditary central diabetes insipidus in man is caused by the absence of vasopressin from the posterior pituitary. An ideal model system for studying this disorder and other functions of AVP seemed to be available when the rat strain "Brattleboro" was discovered (Valtin 1967, Sokol and Valtin 1982). This mutant rat derived from the normal Long-Evans strain carries an autosomal recessive defect to synthesize properly vasopressin, its corresponding neurophysin and glycopeptide, but has an unaffected ability to produce and release oxytocin and its associated neurophysin.

The genetic defect has been attributed to a single base deletion in exon B (see Fig. 4.1), the neurophysin encoding domain of the Brattleboro vasopressin gene (Schmale and Richter 1984). This deletion sequence would predict an mRNA which would be translated incorrectly due to the frameshift. In addition, loss of the stop codon could prevent normal runoff the ribosomes, blocking them on the mRNA. However recent data reported by Majzoub et al. (1987) suggest that in the hypothalamus of the Brattleboro rat vasopressin mRNA is expressed at a low level that fails to increase appropriately with osmotic stress and that vasopressin and its associated precursor products are synthesized in subnormal, but detectable amounts. The regulatory defect demonstrated by these authors could be due to decreased transcription of the vasopressin gene and/or increased degradation of vasopressin mRNA. Moreover, there is now evidence that a small but distinct population of magnocellular neurons in homozygous Brattleboro rats (s.c. di/di rats) are vasopressin positive (Richards et al. 1985). Furthermore, in contrast to earlier reports, normal quantities of what appears by biochemical and immunological criteria to be vasopressin have been found in the appropriate cells of Brattleboro ovaries and adrenals (Lima et al. 1984, Nussey et al. 1984). Thus, the vasopressin deficiency in the Brattleboro rat can no longer be regarded a simple model of a genetic deficiency disease, for the etiology of this defect may be multifaceted and its expression tissue specific.

4.5   VASOPRESSIN RELEASE FROM THE NEUROHYPOPHYSIS

The relatively slow processes of the synthesis and axonal transport of the neurohypophyseal nonapeptides are insufficient to explain rapid changes in the peptide levels occurring following secretory stimuli. Axons of the magnocellular neurosecretory cells fulfil a double function: they transport neuro-secretory granules into the neurohypophysis, and they transmit secretomotoric stimuli triggering the release of the neurosecrete from its pituitary stores. Thus one fundamental process in the functioning of the magnocellular neurons is the mechanism of **stimulus-secretion coupling**, i.e. the translation of action potentials which are generated at the perikaryon in response to synaptic release of neuroactive agents from nerve terminals ending on the cell bodies in the hypothalamus, into the release of the neurosecretory product from the posterior pituitary.

As outlined in chapter 3.1.3, multiple neuropathways have been descri-bed to project to the magnocellular neurons. In each of these path-ways different neurotransmitters may be operative in the stimulation and/or inhibition of the release of the hormone. In addition, vasopressin release may be regulated also by neuroactive agents released from nerve terminals in the posterior pituitary. Countless substances have been reported to influence the release of vasopressin (catecholamines, acetylcholine, angio-tensin II, atrial natriuretic factor, gamma-aminobutyric acid — GABA, histamine, substance P, etc.), but our understanding of the exact role of these neurotransmitters is only at the beginning. Nevertheless it is evident that there is a number of redundancies in the system. For example, many substances can regulate neurohypophyseal function both at the perikaryon and at the axon terminal in the posterior pituitary (acetylcholine, dopamine, opiate peptides, etc.). The opioid peptides (e.g. dynorphin) are of special interest because of their co-localization with vasopressin in certain magnocellular neurons. Other substances, such as angiotensin II and atrial natriuretic factor, may regulate neurohypophyseal function through both hormone and neuro-transmitter mechanisms, thus providing the opportunity for a common recep-tive field to respond to regulatory substances generated at functionally related, but anatomically distant sites (Lichardus et al. 1977, Torda et al. 1978, Brooks et al. 1986, Sladek and Armstrong 1987).

Following stimulation of the AVP producing hypothalamic cells and sub-sequent depolarization of the nerve terminals a series of biochemical and morphological changes are triggered which result in the hormone release. Depolarization causes a brief influx of calcium which eventually leads to fusion of neurosecretory granules and the cell membrane with the consequent release of the entire neurosecretory granule content by exocytosis; the granule membrane is believed to be taken back within the terminal (see Fig. 4.1).

It is not fully clear whether vasopressin release into the systemic circulation is continuous or discontinuous (pulse-like). Blood samples withdrawn repe-atedly from adult individuals during osmotic stimulation showed a con-tinuous elevation of vasopressin levels in parallel to the increasing plasma osmolality (Robertson et al. 1976, Baylis 1987). On the other hand, marked and rapid fluctuations of the hormone plasma levels could be observed in blood withdrawn from experimental animals from sites closer to the site of the hormone secretion (i.e. from the right heart atrium or the jugular vein) (Weitzman et al. 1977). These fluctuations may actually reflect specific intrinsic characteristics of the neurosecretory cells themselves; however, they may also represent artifacts arising during the tests. The vasopressin secreting cell is one of the few neuron types within the mammalian brain which can be characterized by a specific intrinsic pattern of electric activity, typically involving periods of regular discharge interspaced by periods of silence. Stimulation of vasopressinergic cells modifies AVP release by altering the firing pattern in addition to simply initiating action potentials (Dutton and Dyball 1979, Day and Renaud 1984). Nevertheless, a relationship between this electric activity and the possible episodic fluctuations of plasma AVP levels is rather unlikely since changes in electric activity have a shorter periodicity and the duration of both the active and the quiescent phases is variable both for individual neurons and between neurons (Vincent et al. 1985).

5   REGULATION OF VASOPRESSIN SECRETION AND THIRST

The intensity of the neurohypophyseal secretion of AVP and also that of thirst may oscillate under the influence of various physiologic and pathophysiologic factors. Probably as a result of historical development in this field, commentaries on the regulation of AVP secretion and thirst have usually categorized the factors involved as being of osmotic or nonosmotic nature. Under normal conditions, the activities of both systems, the antidiuretic and the thirst-related, change mainly in dependence on alterations of plasma osmolality. The importance of the nonosmotic stimuli is in that they modify the activity of the osmoregulatory system according to actual needs of the organism. Under certain pathophysiologic conditions however, nonosmotic secretory stimuli can create a favorable background for the development of potential clinical disturbances of water metabolism (chapter 19).

5.1   OSMORECEPTOR MEDIATED REGULATION OF VASOPRESSIN AND THIRST

The concept concerning alterations of osmotic concentrations of body fluids as the primary control mechanism of vasopressin secretion and thirst originated with the pioneering studies of Verney and his coworkers (Verney 1947, Jewell and Verney 1957). In brief, these authors found that selective increasing of osmolality of blood perfusing the distribution area of the internal carotid artery in dogs can induce a rapid and considerable reduction of water diuresis. The osmoreceptor concept was proposed to explain this observation, i.e. cells localized in the anterior hypothalamic/preoptic areas which alter their volume in response to an osmotic challenge, thereby triggering or suppressing the release of an antidiuretic substance (vasopressin). This osmoreceptor concept was later extended to involve also the regulation of water intake (Andersson 1978). More recently, McKinley and his coworkers (1985, 1987) and Thrasher and Keil (1987) performing selective ablation experiments in animals identified the organum vasculosum of the lamina terminalis (OVLT), a part of the area composed of the anterior wall of the third cerebral ventricle (the anteroventral third ventricle region, AV3V), as at least one site of these osmoreceptors.

5.1.1 HYPOTHALAMIC OSMORECEPTORS AND/OR SODIUM SENSORS

The general validity of the classic osmoreceptor concept has been questioned by Andersson (1978) who observed alteration of AVP secretion and thirst as well natriuresis in response to intracerebroventricular administration of hypertonic NaCl solution into the anterior part of the third cerebral ventricle. Since no similar response could be observed on administration of other osmotically active agents (e.g. sucrose), or significantly weaker responses were recorded, it was postulated that the proposed receptors localized at the cerebroventricular side of the anterior third ventricle region (A3V) do not in fact respond to changes in effective plasma osmolality but rather to changes in sodium concentration in the extracellular fluid ("sodium receptors"). It seems however that these two models of sensors, the osmotic and the **sodium** model, are not necessarily mutually exclusive; rather, they may coexist as a dual system. The existence of independent intracerebral sodium sensors is highly provoking, mainly with respect to their relation to the atrial and brain natriuretic peptides (ANP and BNP) and to the postulated hypothalamic natriuretic hormone (endogenous inhibitor of $Na^+, K^+ - ATPase$) (chapter 1.3.3); yet so far, it remains but a subject of further investigation (Lichardus et al. 1987, Hansell et al. 1987). For practical reasons such a strict division between osmotic and sodium receptors seems substantially less significant, as an increase in effective osmolality in response to natural osmotic stimuli (e.g. after water deprivation) is determined mainly by an increased extracellular concentration of sodium and its anions (equations 1.1 and 1.2).

5.1.2 PERIPHERAL OSMORECEPTORS AND EXTEROCEPTIVE RECEPTORS (THE POTODIURETIC REFLEX)

Because water ingestion immediately triggers diuresis — the potodiuretic reflex — in addition to the central, cerebral sensors, the existence of accessory peripheral sensor area(s) was postulated (Tyriskina et al. 1981, Baertschi et al. 1985).

Recent studies have provided some clues to the nature of the potodiuretic reflex. In normal adults previously rendered hyperosmotic by infusion of hypertonic saline or dehydration, Thompson et al. (1987) observed an immediate decrease of plasma AVP and reduction of thirst in response to ad libitum water intake. An important point is that these changes were observed well before noticeable alterations in plasma osmolality could occur. It seems that the essential information to inhibit the secretion of vasopressin (and thirst) is nonosmotic in nature and comes from the oropharynx, since this phenomenon is still observed in animals where all absorption is bypassed. This view is further supported by the observation, that in dehydrated humans gargling with hypertonic fluid was also associated with a transient reduction of thirst and AVP secretion (Seckl et al. 1986). The physiologic importance of this potodiuretic reflex may be in prevention of the individual from hyperhydration, in particular of the brain (chapter 20.2). Indirect support for the homeostatic value of this mechanism comes from significantly less frequent development of convulsions in hypernatremic animals rehydrated by ad libitum oral fluid intake as compared to animals receiving intravenous rehydration fluids (Hogan et al. 1984). The involvement of peripheral (**exteroceptive**) receptors in rapid regulation of AVP secretion provides explanation for the widely known, though in clinical practice often underestimated, empirical observation that orally, dipsogenly administered fluid produces a more appropriate regulation of salt and water balance than does the same substance administered parenterally, bypassing the orogastrointestinal receptors.

5.1.3 FUNCTIONAL PROPERTIES OF THE OSMOREGULATORY SYSTEM OF VASOPRESSIN SECRETION

Over the next decade, the functional characteristics of osmoregulated vasopressin release were defined in healthy man (Robertson et al. 1976), data which confirmed Verney's original observations in the dog. In more recent years physiological and pathophysiological influences that alter osmoregulation have been investigated (Robertson 1987, Baylis 1987) and our understanding of the mechanisms responsible for a variety of clinical disorders of water metabolism has grown considerably.

5.1.3.1 Analytical models

The functional characteristics of the osmoregulatory system have been estimated from repeated determinations of plasma or urine vasopressin following intravenous administration of hypertonic solution of sodium chloride. The protocols employed are mostly modifications of the classic Hickey—Hare test (Vallotton et al. 1986a). In this regard, it is important to realize that plasma and urine vasopressin levels are qualitative rather than quantitative parameters. Consequently, the estimation of the activity of the osmoregulatory system is based on the evaluation of these parameters in relation to actual levels of plasma and/or urine osmolality.

The osmoregulatory system evaluated in this manner is of a threshold nature with a linear relationship between these variables (Fig. 5.1). This relationship can be described by a standard linear regression equation which, when transformed into a physiologically more acceptable form, reads $y = b(x - b/m)$, where [x] is plasma osmolality, [y] represents the dependent variable (plasma vasopressin), [b] is the regression coefficient, and the expression [b/m] determines the intercept of the regression line with x. In physiological terms, the correlation coefficient (r) of the curve can be considered an indicator of the precision of the system; the coefficient of regression (b), i.e. the slope of the curve, characterizes **sensitivity**, and the value of b/m determines the system **threshold**, i.e. the value of plasma osmolality that triggers the system, rendering it active upon increasing plasma osmolality or suppressing it upon decreasing plasma osmolality. Finally, the **specificity** of the system refers to its relative sensitivity to various solutes.

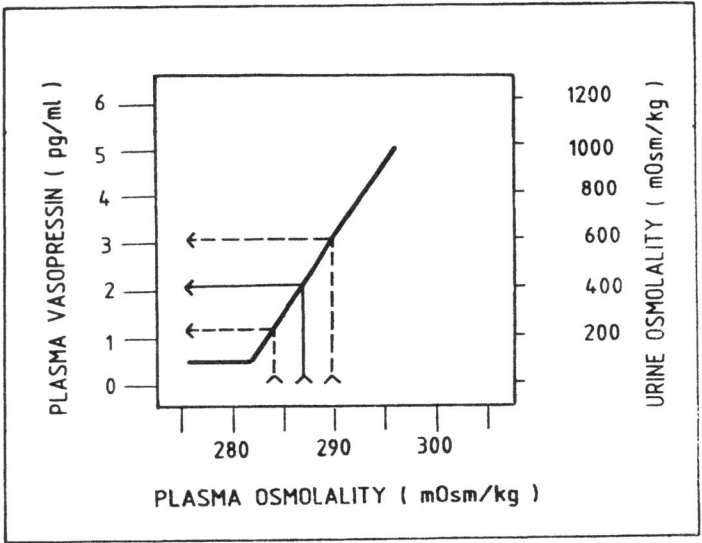

Fig. 5.1. Idealized relationships between plasma vasopressin, plasma osmolality and urine osmolality. The regression line was derived from data obtained in a group of healthy adults (from Robertson et al. 1976 with kind permisson).

The above defined major functional characteristics of the osmoregulatory system, i.e. sensitivity, threshold and specificity, very likely have different cellular or molecular basis. Each of them may therefore be subject to changes independent of other characteristics of the system. These changes and, more often, their various combinations, affect in a specific manner the state of water balance and help explain the heterogeneity of clinical manifestations of disturbances of AVP secretion.

This widely accepted, **discontinual, threshold model** still leaves a number of questions open. These can be summarized in two major problem areas. The first, and probably the most discussed problem concerns the question whether osmoregulation indeed is a discontinuous, threshold process as defined by the linear model, or rather a continuous process which can be better characterized by an exponential model assuming a weaker increase of vasopressin in response to lower, and a more pronounced increase in response to higher values of plasma osmolality. In experiments with acute alterations of plasma osmolality and vasopressin in sheep, Weitzman and Fisher (1977) observed a log-linear relationship between the two variables; however, reanalysis of their data by Rodbard and Munson (1978) showed that there was no significant difference between the exponential and the discontinual, linear model. An important consideration emphasized by Robertson et al. (1976) in their studies in man was that at high rates of changes in plasma solute concentrations (in excess of 2 per cent per hour) there was an exaggerated release of vasopressin. Analysis of data obtained under these experimental conditions would tend to fit the exponential model rather than the linear one. Thus current opinion favors the linear model in humans, provided that excessive rates of changes in plasma tonicity are avoided.

Another problem, more theoretical in nature, is related to the assumption that the osmoregulatory system might in fact be bimodal, i.e. include both stimulatory and inhibitory osmoreceptors. In this case they should have a common set point close to normal basal values of plasma osmolality (Robertson 1980). Elevation of plasma osmolality over this basal level (around 287 mOsm/kg in man) would then activate stimulatory, whereas decrease of P_{osm} below this level would stimulate inhbitory osmoreceptors. It has been proposed by Robertson (1987) that if the AVP-secreting cells are completely disconnected from their osmoreceptor influence, there is persistent release of vasopressin to give plasma concentrations about 1.0-1.5 pg/ml. According to this concept AVP secretion is increased from this "basal" rate by stimulation of a group of facilitory osmoreceptor cells but is decreased to minimal values by stimulation of inhibitory cells. Then however neither the continuo us nor the discontinuous model would characterize functions of one or the other group of receptors. Anyway, for practical reasons the linear model remains a pragmatic means to describe the functional properties of the osmoregulatory system as a unique entity, and to characterize the way how nonosmotic physiologic and/or pathophysiologic and pharmacologic factors can modify its activity.

5.1.3.2 Sensitivity of the osmoregulatory system

The sensitivity of the osmoregulatory system of AVP is determined by the slope or steepness of the regression line describing the relationship between plasma vasopressin levels and plasma osmolality. An analysis of pooled data obtained from a larger group of healthy adult persons allowed Robertson et al. (1976) to clearly demonstrate the extraordinary sensitivity of this system (see Fig. 5.1). As little as 1 per cent increase in plasma osmolality (2.9 mOsm/kg) is sufficient to elevate plasma vasopressin levels by 1 pg/ml, a change already detectable by radioimmunological methods. In addition, the linkage of the sensitive AVP-secretory response with the similarly sensitive renal antidiuretic mechanism grants that relatively small alterations of plasma osmolality can be transformed into relatively large changes in urine osmolality. The steepness of the regression line in Fig. 5.1 shows that an increase in urine osmolality by 250 mOsm/kg can be expected per each increment unit of plasma vasopressin. According to the above example, the original elevation of plasma osmolality (2.9 mOsm/kg) will be associated with an almost 100-fold change in urine osmolality. Consequently, these data show that under physiological conditions, the whole range of the renal osmoregulatory performance, from minimal to maximal urine osmolality (i.e. from 50 mOsm/kg to 1,200 mOsm/kg) is within the range of less than 10-fold changes in plasma vasopressin levels (from 0.5 pg/ml to 5 pg/ml).

Mediated through influence on the sensitivity of the osmoregulatory system, various factors are able to modify the intensity of vasopressin secretion (Fig. 5.2). In healthy adults the sensitivity exhibits considerable individual variations and may differ appreciably from the ideal relationship described above. Nevertheless, repeated studies on a group of healthy adults within 6 months have shown that the characteristics of the osmoregulatory regression line are remarkably constant for an individual person (Thompson and Baylis 1987), suggesting that the variation may be caused by genetic factors. Zerbe (1985) explored this possibility by studying mono- and dizygotic twins; his results clearly indicated a high concordance of both slope and threshold within the monozygotic but not dizygotic twins. For practical purposes, it is desirable to evaluate pooled data from a larger group of individuals in investigating effects of various factors on the functional characteristics of the osmoregulatory

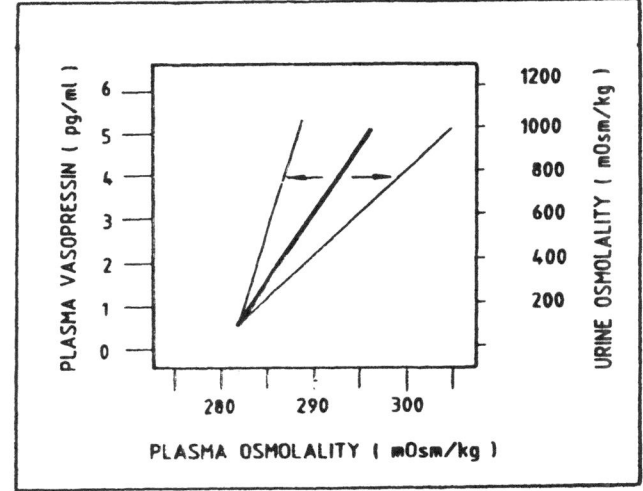

Fig. 5.2. Effect of changes in sensitivity of the AVP osmo-stat on the osmoregulatory function. The thick line illustrating the normal relationship was derived from Fig. 5.1.

system, or data obtained from the same individual before and during the action of nonosmotic stimuli. Another physiological determinant of the sensitivity of the osmoregulatory system of AVP secretion is the age of the individual. Available developmental evidence indicates that the slope of the osmoregulatory regression line gradually increases from fetal and neonatal life to the elderly (chapter 15.5). Regardless of possible causes and mechanisms underlying this age dependence, the existence of the phenomenon itself underlines the necessity of employing age-matched controls whenever investigating the function of the osmoregulatory system.

The sensitivity of the osmoregulatory system can be modified also by pathophysiological and pharmacological factors such as changes in the ionic composition of plasma or administration of drugs (see Fig. 5.2). For example, acute hypercalcemia and lithium administration raise the sensitivity of the AVP secretion system (and most likely also the sensation of thirst). On the contrary, carbamazepine, an antiepileptic drug, reduces the intensity of the vasopressin response to osmotic stimuli. Thus the known ability of carbamazepine to enhance antidiuresis in patients with partial central diabetes insipidus cannot be explained by its central action but rather by an increased sensitivity of the renal collecting tubuli to hydroosmotic effect of AVP. Such a reciprocal relationship between vasopressin secretion and its renal effects has been observed also in connection with factors raising the sensitivity of the osmoregulatory system and simultaneously decreasing the renal effect of AVP, such as lithium therapy and ageing. The consistency of this reciprocal relationship speaks against the random nature of this phenomenon and suggests the existence of some so far unknown feedback mechanism which may represent a connecting link between processes of vasopressin secretion and its renal effects (Robertson 1987).

5.1.3.3 Threshold (set point)

The abscissal intercept of the osmoregulatory regression line indicates the threshold for AVP release which must remain a theoretical concept as even the most sensitive RIA methods preclude measurement of AVP below its plasma values of 0.3—0.5 pg/ml. Nevertheless, plasma AVP concentrations as low as that are as a rule associated with maximum water diuresis suggesting minimal biological activity of vasopressin. For healthy adult persons under basal conditions threshold values of 280 mOsm/kg are usually measured (see Fig. 5.1). Obviously, individual variations of this parameter are significantly less determined genetically as compared with the sensitivity of the osmoregulatory system (Zerbe 1985).

An important characteristic of many nonosmotic stimuli of AVP secretion is their ability to shift the system threshold towards lower values of P_{osm}, i.e. to induce a condition during which water load results in maximal osmotic suppression of AVP, but only upon reaching extremely low values of plasma osmolality. In addition, downward resetting of the osmostat at the simultaneously unchanged sensitivity of the osmoregulatory mechanism means higher vasopressin plasma levels at any given values of plasma osmolality as compared to normal conditions (Fig. 5.3). Maybe the most frequent cause of downward resetting represents acute reduction of the circulating blood volume and decrease of blood pressure. The remarkable osmostat downward resetting seen in patients with edematous diseases (congestive heart failure, liver cirrhosis, nephrotic syndrome) is also explained by a reduction of the "effective" circulating blood volume. Many other physiological and pathophysiological stimuli (such as hypoglycemia, emesis, hypoxia, stress and others) can enhance AVP secretion, probably by shifting the set of the osmostat to abnormally low values of plasma osmolality. Distinct osmostat downward resetting is a typical phenomenon in the development of physiological conditions such as pregnancy and the luteal phase of the menstrual cycle.

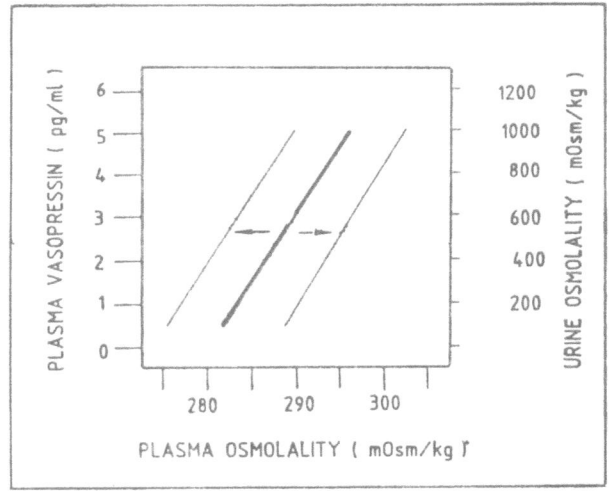

Fig. 5.3. Effect of alterations in threshold of the AVP osmostat on the osmoregulatory function. The normal relationship indicated by thick line was derived from Fig. 5.1.

Shift of the osmotic threshold for AVP secretion to higher values of plasma osmolality (above 280 mOsm/kg) (upward resetting of the osmostat) are less frequent. An example are patients with primary hyperaldosteronism characterized by moderate hypernatremia, in whom correction of chronic hypervolemia by diuretic treatment results in the osmostat threshold returning to normal values (Ganguly and Robertson 1980). The set of the osmoregulatory system can also be altered pharmacologically. Opiates like morphine and butorphanol transiently inhibit vasopressin secretion by raising the set of the osmostat (Kamoi and Robertson 1985).

5.1.3.4 Specificity

The relative sensitivity of the osmoreceptors to various solutes, i.e. the specificity of the osmoregulatory system, is usually characterized by the steepness of the regression line describing the dependence between plasma osmolality and plasma vasopressin measured during infusion of hypertonic solutions (Fig. 5.4). The different sensitivity to individual solutes can also supply some clues to the understanding of the mechanism whereby the osmoreceptor senses alterations of the composition of the internal environment. It has been postulated that "impermeable" solutes which do not penetrate readily cell membranes (e.g. sodium and mannitol) induce osmotic water flux from the intracellular into the extracellular space. The resulting cell shrinkage in turn stimulates vasopressin secretion (and thirst sensation). Conversely, solutes which freely penetrate cell membranes (e.g. urea) will not generate an osmotic gradient. Consequently, there is no shift in intracellular water, the cell volume remains constant, and AVP is not released. Thus, one

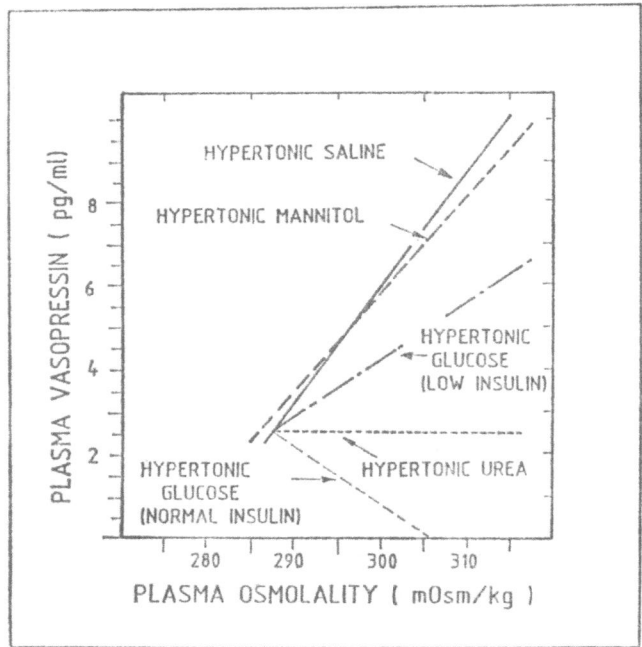

Fig. 5.4. The relationship of plasma vasopressin to plasma osmolality in healthy adults during the infusion of hypertonic solutions of various solutes. Note that the rise in plasma osmolality produced by infusion of hypertonic glucose is associated with a fall in plasma vasopressin in healthy subjects with normal insulin secretion, but a rise in plasma AVP in insulin-dependent state (i.e. in patients with type I diabetes mellitus) (from Zerbe and Robertson 1983 with kind permission).

may deduce from these observations that the osmoreceptor probably acts by changing its cellular volume (Zerbe and Robertson 1983).

With regard to its osmoregulatory influence, glucose is in special situation. Its stimulatory potential depends a great deal on the presence or absence of insulin. Infusion of hypertonic glucose to normal individuals is associated with a paradoxical reduction of vasopressin secretion most likely resulting from redistributon of body water from intra- to extracellular spaces with a subsequent decrease of sodium plasma concentrations (i.e. pseudohyponatremia; chapter 20.1.1). On the contrary, identical elevation of plasma glucose levels in uncontrolled insulin-dependent diabetic patients stimulates AVP secretion (see Fig. 5.4), a phenomenon which can completely be abolished by low insulin doses. The influence of insulin on the vasopressin response to hyperglycemia indicates that glucose uptake by the osmoreceptor is insulin dependent. In this case insulin deficiency decreases the rate of glucose penetration into the osmoreceptor neurons thus generating sufficient transmembrane osmotic concentration gradient capable of triggering the osmoregulatory system of AVP secretion (Vokes et al. 1987).

5.2 FUNCTIONAL PROPERTIES OF THE OSMOREGULATORY SYSTEM REGULATING THIRST

Water ingestion and its regulation are important components of the control of body fluid osmolality. Appreciation of thirst — defined in humans as a "generalized deep seated feeling of a desire for water" — is the sensation that motivates humans to seek and ingest water. Quantitation of this sensation has long been hindered by considerable methodological problems; recently a visual analog scale has been proposed for estimating acute changes in thirst at least in controlled, experimental conditions (Robertson 1984).

In healthy individuals, thirst is regulated mainly by changes in plasma osmolality. Osmoreceptors that control thirst are located in the hypothalamus close to the osmoreceptors that control AVP release (see Fig. 3.3); brain lesions associated with disturbances of thirst osmoregulation are almost without exception also coupled with a simultaneous defect of AVP osmoregulation (chapter 17.3). Yet experimental studies and unique clinical disorders (Hammond et al. 1986) demonstrating a partial anatomical dissociation of thirst and AVP regulatory areas indicate that the two functions are supported by separate sets of osmoreceptor neurons.

The two osmoreceptors for thirst and vasopressin release share remarkable similar functional characteristics. For practical purposes both systems can be described in terms of a threshold receptor (naturally, with theoretical limitations discussed in chapter 5.1.3.1) with similar sensitivity and specificity. The only difference seems to be that the osmotic threshold for thirst sensation is appreciably higher than that for AVP release (Fig. 5.5). Vasopressin secretion starts increasing as early as the average plasma osmolality of 280 mOsm/kg is reached whereas thirst starts being perceived at values of plasma osmolality exceeding 290 mOsm/kg. In other words, within a certain final physiological range of plasma osmolality values, determined by osmotic thresholds of both AVP secretion and thirst, termed the threshold gap, the standard composition of the body fluid is maintained mainly by vasopressin-mediated renal water conservation. The thirst mechanism becomes activated at the plasma osmolality level, which stimulates sufficient vasopressin to cause maximum antidiuresis (see Fig. 5.1), i.e. when no further rise of urine osmolality would be possible by additional AVP secretion. The significance of such a stepwise arrangement of osmoregulatory systems of AVP secretion and thirst is not difficult to appreciate. An osmoregulatory system arranged in this manner allows maximum employment of the renal concentrating capacity. At the same time, it prevents inconvenience which might arise if osmoregulation were purely dependent on sustained thirst even in the physiological range of plasma osmolality.

Similarly as the AVP secretion threshold, also the thirst threshold shows considerable individual variations. At the extremes, thirst threshold in certain individuals may be at lower plasma osmolality values than the value of Posm characterizing the treshold for AVP secretion in another subject (Robertson 1984).

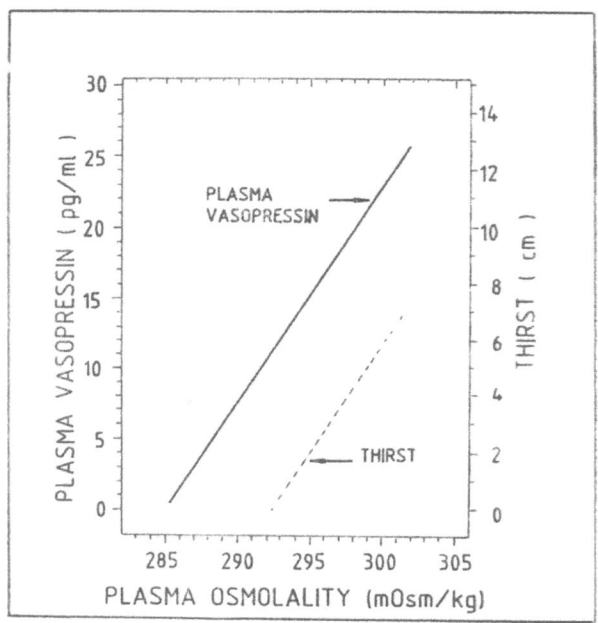

Fig. 5.5. Thirst and plasma vasopressin as an idealized function of plasma osmolality in healthy adults. Plasma vasopressin was determined by radioimmunoassay and thirst by an analog rating scale during an infusion of hypertonic saline (from Robertson 1984 with kind permission).

5.3 FUNCTIONAL RELATIONSHIP BETWEEN OSMOTICALLY STIMULATED VASOPRESSIN SECRETION AND THIRST

The individual functional characteristics of the osmoregulatory system of both AVP secretion and thirst are subject to physiologic and pathophysiologic alterations induced by nonosmotic stimuli (Robertson 1985b). It may be therefore of interest to understand ways whereby these changes, and in particular their combinations, can influence the water turnover of an individual and result in various different disturbances of water metabolism.

5.3.1 CHANGES IN OSMOTIC THRESHOLDS FOR VASOPRESSIN SECRETION AND THIRST

The most pronounced alterations are induced by factors which act by modifying thresholds of AVP secretion and/or thirst (Fig. 5.6). Perhaps most frequently both thresholds are reset in parallel, with the threshold gap remaining unchanged. Parallel downward resetting of the osmostat occurs for example in hypovolemic patients, in pregnant women, etc., while parallel upward resetting may be demonstrated in patients with hyperaldosteronism (see Fig. 5.6, panels 2 and 3).

Another type of disturbances arises from widening of the threshold gap, or even by effective loss of one or both osmoregulatory functions. An example of conditions of this kind may be patients with adipsia who display fluctuations of plasma osmolality over extreme ranges towards the lost function (see Fig. 5.6, panel 4). As a rule, parallel resetting of both osmostats, with or without widening of the threshold gap, are not associated with polyuria, whereas the latter frequently develops due to narrowed threshold gap. Such a narrowing of the threshold gap can occur in patients with hypercalcemia or hyperkalemia as well as in many subjects treated with lithium salts (see Fig. 5.6, panel 5). In these cases characterized by isolated downward resetting of the thirst threshold, the thirst sensation is stimulated "prematurely", i.e. thirst makes the person ingest fluids already at relatively low values of plasma osmolality at which osmotically induced AVP secretion could not yet have reached the level required to induce maximal antidiuresis. In practical terms this means that water ingestion is being stimulated as early as at relatively low values of urine osmolality resulting in slight to moderate polyuria and polydipsia. If these alterations are accompanied by simultaneously developing renal resistance to hydroosmotic effect of vasopressin (as it is the case in hypercalcemic and/or hypokalemic patients as well as in those receiving lithium for therapeutical reasons) a slight narrowing of the threshold gap can already become manifest by clinically significant polyuria and polydispia (chapter 17.2.2).

49

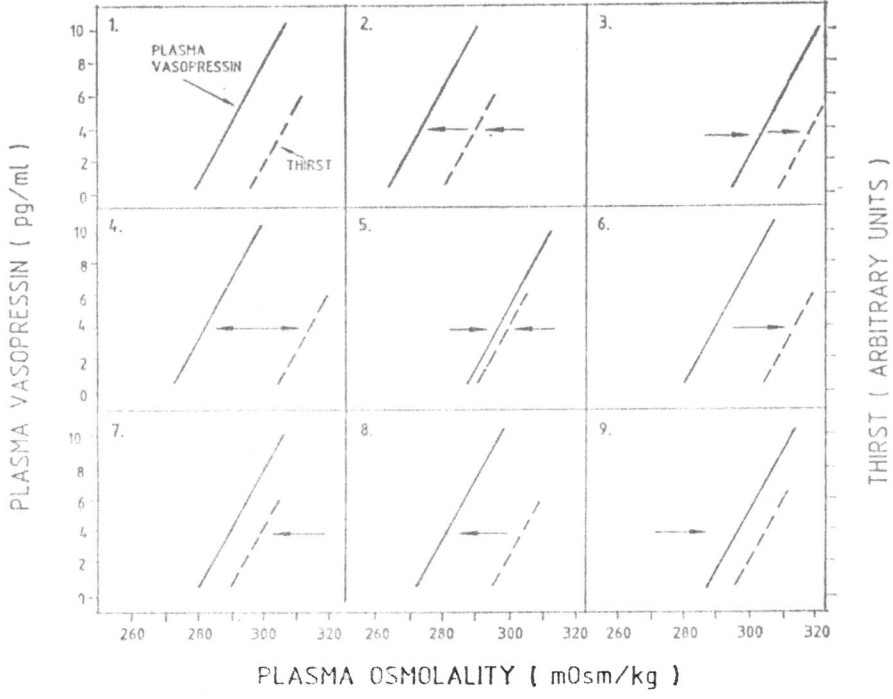

PLASMA VASOPRESSIN (pg/ml)

THIRST (ARBITRARY UNITS)

PLASMA OSMOLALITY (mOsm/kg)

Fig. 5.6. The effects on plasma vasopressin of resetting the osmostats for thirst and vasopressin secretion. Panel 1 taken from Fig. 5.5 exemplifies the typical relationships in a healthy adult. The remaining panels show how various changes in the set of osmostat for thirst or vasopressin affect mean plasma osmolality and the normal range of P_{osm} (i.e. the threshold gap). Note that when the thresholds are lowered (2) or raised (3) in parallel mean plasma osmolality is also lowered or raised but the threshold gap remains unchanged. If the thresholds were reset away from (4) or toward (5) each other, mean basal plasma osmolality would be unchanged, but fluctuations in Posm should increase (4) or decrease (5). Resetting one of the thresholds away from (6 and 8) or toward (7 and 9) the other one should alter the fluctuations in plasma osmolality in the same way as moving them together or apart, but in addition would bias mean plasma osmolality in the direction of the resetting.

5.3.2 CHANGES IN SENSITIVITY OF THE OSMOREGULATORY SYSTEM OF VASOPRESSIN SECRETION AND THIRST

The way, whereby changes in the osmostat sensitivity can modify water turnover perhaps most easily can be illustrated on the example of central diabetes insipidus. Fig. 5.7 outlines changes in vasopressin plasma levels, urine osmolality and thirst intensity as a function of plasma osmolality following different degrees of destruction of the neurohypophysis. Progressive reduction of the neurohypophyseal secretory capacity is reflected by decreased amounts of vasopressin released at each respective level of plasma osmolality.

However, the degree of impairment of AVP secretory capacity that is required to produce significant polyuria (> 2 l/day) depends on the threshold of the thirst mechanism. If it is normal, polyuria does not begin until AVP secretory capacity falls to 25% of normal. If the thirst threshold is "set" higher, ((+) in Fig. 5.7), or there is a widened threshold gap (as observed in some patients with simultaneous damage to thirst osmoreceptors), significant polyuria can occur at more pronounced AVP deficiency only, i.e. not until the sensitivity of the vasopressin response drops below 10—15% of initial levels. Conversely, if the thirst threshold is "set" lower than normal (as observed in some healthy individuals), significant polyuria can be induced by a considerably weaker, approximately 50%, reduction of sensitivity of the system. Finally, if the thirst threshold is "set" close to or even equal to that of

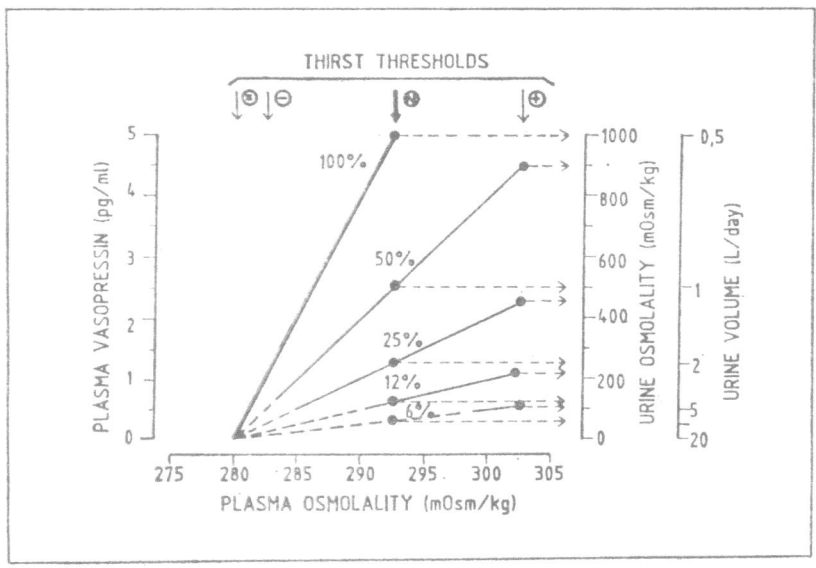

Fig. 5.7. Plasma AVP, urine osmolality and urine volume as a function of thirst and AVP secretory capacity (from Robertson 1985 with permission). The figure assumes normal renal solute load (600 mOsm/die) and normal renal sensitivity to AVP. Each oblique line depicts schematically the relationship between plasma vasopressin and plasma osmolality when secretory capacity is reduced to a specific percentage of normal. Each vertical arrow indicates the osmotic threshold for thirst as it occurs normally (N) or when it is abnormally high (+), low (—) or very low (=). The closed circles on each oblique line indicate the highest level to which plasma osmolality and AVP are normally allowed to rise at each thirst setting. The broken horizontal arrows indicate the daily urine osmolalities and volumes that result when plasma AVP is limited to the specified levels.

AVP secretion ((=) in Fig. 5.7), clinically significant polyuria and polydipsia can occur even at entirely normal secretory capacity of the neurohypophysis.

The above considerations suggest that — provided normal setting of the AVP secretion and thirst thresholds, adequate renal response to vasopressin, and free ingestion of hypotonic fluid — alterations of the sensitivity of vasopressin response to osmotic stimuli have only very limited effect on plasma osmolality levels (Robertson 1985a).

5.4 NONOSMOTIC REGULATION OF VASOPRESSIN SECRETION

While the beginning of the "vasopressin-story" passed in the spirit of studies of osmoregulation, the period since the introduction of radioimmunoassay methods is characterized by a burst of new knowledge concerning the nonosmotic secretory stimuli (Schrier and Berl 1975, Robertson et al. 1982, Baylis 1987). Now it is generally appreciated that hemodynamic factors — alterations in blood volume and/or pressure — constitute the second major stimulus for vasopressin secretion and are the main cause of nonosmotic release of the nonapeptide. Although osmotic and hemodynamic stimuli to vasopressin release do not act independently of each other, the precise subtle interactions between them and other nonosmotic stimuli (Table 5.1) remain to be clarified. Moreover, the release of vasopressin can be altered by hypnotically induced thirst or water intake (Zikmund and Lichardus 1962).

Table 5.1. Factors influencing vasopressin secretion

Stimuli	Inhibitors
Hyperosmolality	Hypoosmolality
Hypovolemia	Hypervolemia
Arterial hypotension	Ethanol
Emesis	
Glycopenia	
Age	
Pregnancy and menstrual cycle	
Hypoxia and hypercapnia	
Intracranial hypertension	
Ambient temperature	
Stress	
Endotoxin	
Pharmacological agents (nicotine, anesthetics, alpha adrenergic agents, clofibrate, etc.)	

5.4.1 HEMODYNAMIC REGULATION OF AVP SECRETION

If Verney (1947) is considered the father of the concept of osmoregulation of AVP secretion, then Gauer and Henry (1963, 1970) deserve a similar appreciation concerning baroreceptor regulation of AVP secretion. Although it has been known for long that isoosmotic ECF volume depletion is associated with an appreciable reduction of urine flow (Leaf and Mamby 1952), these authors were, who discovered the reflex control mechanism of volume-mediated AVP secretion and renal water excretion (chapter 1.3).

5.4.1.1 Receptors and the reflex arc

The localization of cardiovascular receptors which detect the volume of the circulating blood through changes in blood pressure has been clearly demonstrated by a series of experimental manipulations aimed at inducing blood volume redistribution either to the central vascular bed or to the periphery without concomitant changes in absolute blood volume. When the intrathoracic volume is expanded by blood redistribution, the kidneys respond by increasing urine volume as if the volume of the entire extracellular fluid were expanded. This occurs for example in a hydrated man upon changing from standing to recumbent position, during negative pressure breathing, upon immersion of the body up to the neck into water (with a temperature of 34°C — Fig. 5.8)

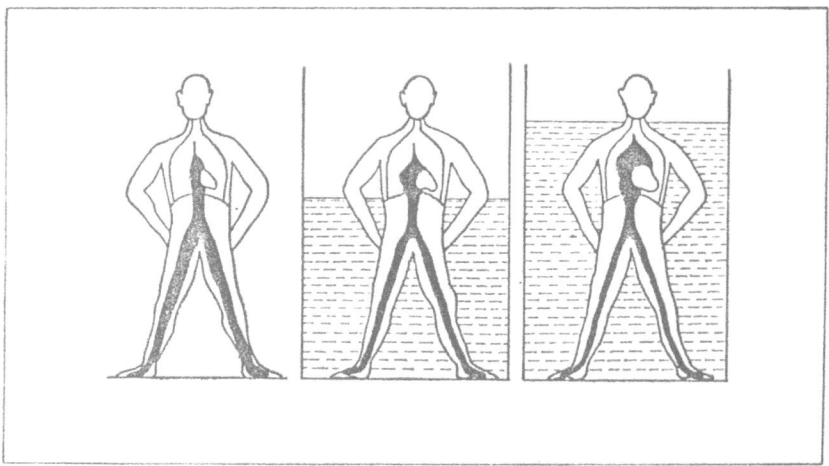

Fig. 5.8. Schematic representation of the effect of head-out water immersion (WI) on blood volume distribution. WI causes redistribution of blood volume from the peripheral to central (intrathoracic) circulation. This is sensed by intrathoracic volume-receptors as hypervolemia and results in decreased AVP secretion with subsequently enhanced diuresis (Gauer-Henry reflex).

or due to the application of positive pressure to the lower body. The same is observed in astronauts known to have an engorgement of the central circulation as long as they are in space (Epstein 1978, Grigoriev et al. 1983, Kovács et al. 1988). Also, upon expanding the volume of extracellular fluid by infusions of various isoosmotic and/or isooncotic solutions, the major volume increment concerns the central vascular bed in the chest due to its greatest distensibility. On the contrary, reduced filling of the intrathoracic vascular bed (for example during positive pressure breathing, following application of negative pressure to the lower body or caused by transition from recumbency to upright position) tends to induce reflex antidiuresis by a reduction of intrathoracic blood volume.

From the point of view of anatomical localization and functional significance, there are two groups of cardiovascular receptors recording changes in blood volume and/or pressure. The first group includes cardiopulmonary barore-

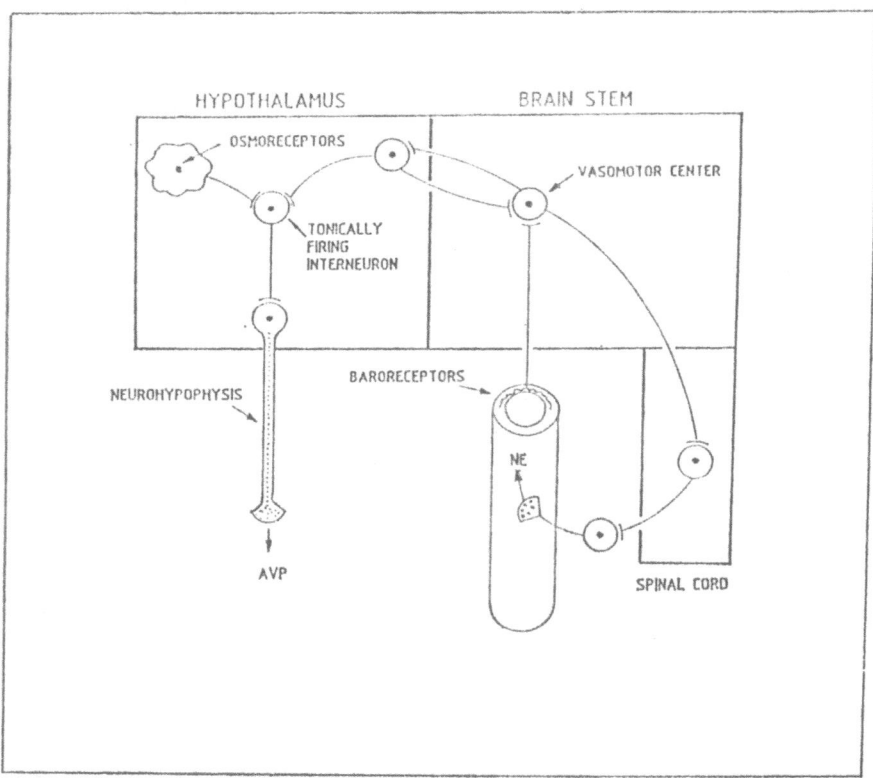

Fig. 5.9. The regulation of AVP secretion by osmoreceptor and baroreceptor inputs. Afferent baroreceptor input to the hypothalamus from the great vessels travels via the vasomotor center. Baroreceptor and osmoreceptor inputs interact on a hypothesized, tonically firing interneuron before AVP release (by Rowe et al. 1979 with kind permission).

ceptors located in the low-pressure part of the circulation (in particular in the wall of both the left and the right heart atrium and in the pulmonary vessels), whereas the second one concerns sinoaortal baroreceptors located in the high-pressure part of the circulation, in the aortic arch and extrathoracically in the carotic sinus and in the renal juxtaglomerular apparatus.

Afferent projections run from both groups of baroreceptors bilaterally via the n.vagus and n.glossopharyngeus to the reticular formation in the brainstem where they terminate by synapses, in particular on noradrenergic neurons involved in the regulation of cardiovascular functions (Figs. 3.4 and 5.9). Postsynaptic catecholaminergic (predominantly noradrenergic) pathways begin on neurons of the A1 cell group of the ventral medulla and after meeting fibers from the A2 cell group they project to the hypothalamus (chapter 3.1.3.2). The baroreceptor afferents normally maintain a tonic suppressive influence on AVP secretion; baroreceptor denervation causes an increase in AVP secretion.

Observations in AV3V-lesioned animals as well as in humans with selective loss of the osmoreceptor function (chapter 17.3) suggest that baroregulation of AVP secretion does not require the presence of osmoreceptor element since hemodynamic stimuli are able to influence AVP levels even in the absence of hypothalamic osmoreceptors. This conclusion, however, might seem to contradict the conclusion that hemodynamic stimuli act in such a way as to reset the osmoregulation of AVP (chapter 5.1.3.3). In fact, these two seemingly contradictory observations can be reconciled by postulating the existence of a tonically firing hypothalamic interneuron, as a site of the convergence of osmotic and hemodynamic, and possibly also of some other nonosmotic, secretory stimuli (see Fig. 5.9). The interneuron activation level would then determine the actual intensity of AVP secretion. The last synapse of the ascendent pathway runs from the interneuron to the cell bodies and to the dendritic zones of magnocellular neurons.

5.4.1.2 Functional properties of the baroregulatory system of vasopressin secretion

In the presence of normal ECF volume and osmolality, studies in the dog demonstrated cooperation of cardiac receptors with carotic and aortic baroreceptors. Although simultaneous denervation of all three receptor areas caused profound increases in plasma AVP, denervation of any single area was inconsequential (Bishop et al. 1984). Findings in primates and in humans have been somewhat different from those made in dog. In these studies upright posture appeared to be associated with a hierarchy of the receptor function that ranks arterial baroreceptors highest. Thus, in humans the cardiopulmonary baroreceptors appear to registrate mild changes in blood volume or pressure (Leimbach et al. 1984, Goldsmith et al. 1987). However, as soon as the hemodynamic alteration is sufficient to affect cardiac output or peripheral vascular resistance (e.g. during hemorrhage) also high-pressure baroreceptors are "turned on". Then, their activation is accompanied by a dramatic elevation of plasma AVP reaching values exceeding 10 to 100-fold the hormone concentrations required to induce maximal antidiuresis.

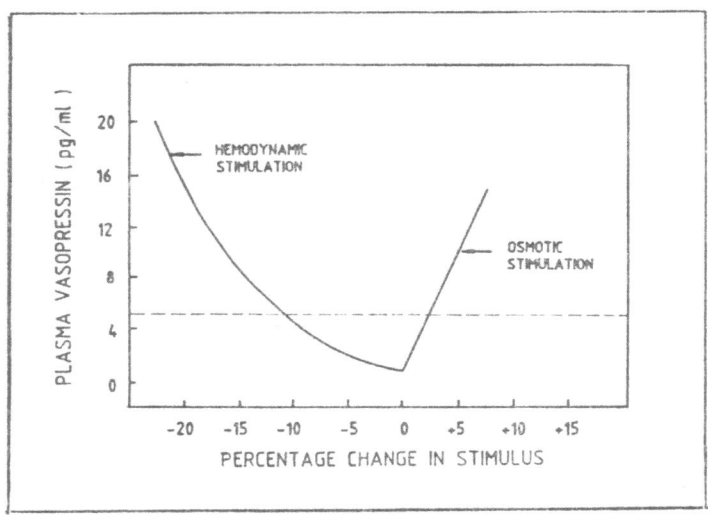

Fig. 5.10. Schematic comparison of the response of plasma AVP to hemodynamic (decline in blood pressure by graded trimephan infusion) and osmotic (hypertonic saline infusion) stimulation in healthy adults. The area below the broken line represents the reference range of plasma AVP under normal conditions of hydration with plasma osmolality varying from 284 to 293 mOsm/kg (by Baylis 1987 with kind permission).

This implies that the functional properties of the baroregulatory system differ from those of the osmoregulatory system (Fig. 5.10). The relationship of plasma osmolality and vasopressin appears to be linear, whereas that of blood volume or pressure and plasma AVP is distinctly curvilinear (Dunn et al. 1973, Baylis 1983). Usually it is thought that little or no increase in plasma vasopressin occurs until blood pressure or volume changes by at least 5 to 10 per cent. However, careful examination of the data illustrated in Fig. 5.10 suggests that significant changes in plasma vasopressin concentration (about 1 pg/ml) may occur with a drop of blood pressure of less than 5 per cent, within a range that influences urinary concentration (i.e. below 5 pg/ml). Although the sensitivity of the baroregulatory system within this segment of the exponential curve is considerably lower than that of the osmoregulatory system, an argument can be advanced based on the above data that small variations of blood pressure and/or volume may affect moment-to-moment regulation of AVP secretion and renal water excretion. Certainly, fluctuations in blood pressure of the order of 5 to 10 per cent have been reported in healthy adults performing normal activities throughout the day and these changes in cardiovascular parameters have been associated with significant increases in plasma and urinary vasopressin levels as compared to the night period or to the values during 24 hours of recumbancy (Kovács, 1985, Baylis, 1987).

5.4.1.3 Interactions between hemodynamic and osmotic stimuli for vasopressin secretion

It has become evident during the past decade that osmocontrol and volume control cannot be strictly separated from each other. Since they converge on the AVP secretory mechanism (see Fig. 5.9), they should work hand in hand. The constancy of the osmotic concentration is vital for the cells, but it is also self evident that the survival of the organism as a whole depends on the integrity of the circulation, i.e. on the fullness of the bloodstream. Indeed, neither of these systems has a dominant effect on AVP release. Compromise solutions, as generally typical of biological systems, occur upon conflict situations associated with simultaneous alterations of both the osmotic and the hemodynamic homeostasis (a good example is hypovolemia with concomitant hyperosmolality of the plasma).

Acute hemodynamic stimuli appear to act by producing upward or downward adjustments of the threshold of the osmoregulatory system (see Fig. 5.6, panels 2 and 3). As a consequence of these shifts, the amount of vasopressin secreted in response to a given level of plasma osmolality increases or decreases by amounts proportional to the magnitude of the disturbance in blood volume and/or pressure. However, secretion of the hormone still remains fully responsive to osmotic influences. Consequently, if plasma osmolality falls, vasopressin secretion can still be suppressed to levels that permit the development of maximum water diuresis. The only difference is that this protective limit is lower when blood pressure or blood volume is reduced, and is higher when blood pressure or volume increases (Robertson 1983).

When substantial hypovolemia and/or hypotension develop, the hemo-dynamically stimulated AVP secretion may be of benefit for the body. In these situations the potent vasoconstrictor effect of the hormone helps to maintain blood pressure (chapter 9.4.1), while the antidiuresis caused by this increased AVP acts to restore blood volume. However, downward resetting accompanied by sustained AVP secretion can also result in the development of hyponatremia provided there is a continuing supply of water which can be retained in the body (chapter 19). Taking together, the homeostatic reason of enhanced vasopressin release in hypovolemic states can be well expressed by the often quoted remark of Leaf and Frazier (1961), namely that "teleologically, hyponatremia is a lesser evil than circulatory collapse".

5.4.2 EMETIC REGULATION OF VASOPRESSIN SECRETION

Nausea with or without emesis is one of the most potent known stimuli to AVP secretion in primates and humans (Rowe et al. 1979, Verbalis et al. 1987). The stimulus for AVP release appears to be nausea per se since an increase in AVP was observed even in subjects who did not vomit, while vomiting that occurred in the absence of nausea, e.g. that induced by stimulation of the posterior pharynx, did not induce vasopressin release. Plasma vasopressin levels increase as much as 100 to 1,000-fold in response to nausea producing agents (apomorphine, nicotine, alcohol, cholecystokinin). Even water loading grossly elevates AVP levels if associated with the subjective sensation of nausea. Although transient vasovagal hypotension frequently accompanies vomiting, the increase in plasma vasopressin levels in humans appears to be much larger than could be produced by such hemodynamic changes alone. Furthermore, nausea-induced stimulation of vasopressin can be blocked by various antiemetic agents in doses sufficient to prevent subjective sensation of nausea. Consequently, it is clear that nausea with or without emesis is capable of stimulating AVP secretion in humans independently of classical osmo- or volume-regulatory mechanisms. This pattern of stimulation along with the known location of the nausea/emetic centers in the area postrema of the brainstem support activation of central pathways. Although there are uncertainties as to the potential homeostatic function of AVP secreted in response to nausea (Verbalis et al. 1987), it is a variable that must be considered in all clinical studies investigating the secretion of AVP.

5.4.3 GLYCOPENIC REGULATION OF VASOPRESSIN SECRETION

Acute hypoglycemia stimulates the release of ACTH, GH and prolactin from the anterior pituitary gland and thus supplies the basis for a test of adenohypophyseal function in humans. Insulin-induced hypoglycemia is also a stimulus, albeit a relatively weak one, to vasopressin and oxytocin release from the posterior pituitary (Baylis et al. 1981, Fisher et al. 1987). There is a three- to fourfold increase in human plasma vasopressin as blood glucose falls below 2.2 mmol/l (40 mg/dl) with substantial individual and age-related variations in this response (Seckl et al. 1987). It seems, however, that acute hypoglycemia does not disrupt the function of the osmoregulatory system, but rather augments the response to osmotic stimuli (Baylis and Robertson 1980). The most plausible explanation for the effect of hypoglycemia is intracellular neuroglycopenia. Both vasopressin and thirst increased in a comparable manner when 2-deoxy-D-glucose, a competitive inhibitor of the intracellular glycolytic enzyme hexokinase, was administered instead of insulin to healthy human volunteers (Thompson et al. 1981). The physiologic significance of this vasopressin response to neuroglycopenia is unclear. Although vasopressin is currently not regarded as a major counter-regulatory hormone, it may have a minor role in glucose homeostasis and directly or indirectly (by promoting the release of GH, ACTH and glucagon) contribute to the restoration of normoglycemia and to the regulation of glucoprivic feeding behavior (chapter 13).

5.4.4 MENSTRUAL CYCLE AND NORMAL PREGNANCY

Osmoregulation is markedly altered during pregnancy. Pregnant women have decreased plasma osmolality of 8—10 mOsm/kg below that of non-pregnant state. The change in osmolality occurs early in gestation and continues throughout gestation. A parallel fall in the osmotic thresholds for both vaso-pressin secretion and thirst appears to be responsible for this decrement, while no significant change in the slope of the osmoregulatory line could be demonstrated (Davidson et al. 1984) (see Fig. 5.6, panel 2). A similar, albeit modest, resetting of the osmostat coincides also with the ovulatory luteal phase in healthy young women (Forsling et al. 1982, Spruce et al. 1985a). Accordingly, osmoregulation in pregnant women and during the luteal phase of the menstrual cycle is similar to that observed otherwise except that it occurs around a new set point below the one in the nonpregnant state or during the follicular phase.

Both the reason and the mechanism responsible for the downward resetting of the osmostat in pregnancy and during the luteal phase of the menstrual cycle have yet to be clarified, but several possible explanations have been proposed. Obviously, this change in osmoregulation is not attributable to volume depletion since the extracellular (and probably also the intravascular) volume in pregnancy is substantially increased and, in theory, should suppress AVP secretion. In an attempt to overcome this evident controversy the "dilated" vasculature in pregnant women and the subsequent state of effective volume depletion have been suggested to cause relative hypovolemia which eventually should lead to resetting of the osmostat (Barron et al. 1984). Another attractive hypothesis assumes that products of the corpus luteum and/or the fetoplacental unit lower the set of the osmostat, but none of the many potential hormones examined so far has totally accounted for the observation (Lindheimer et al. 1985). In addition the blood of pregnant women contains large amounts of cystine aminopeptidase, an enzyme of placental origin, which is capable of destroying in vitro nanogram quantities of AVP per minute by cleaving bonds between amino acid 1 and 2, and those between amino acid 2 and 3 in the nonapeptide molecule (Viinamaki et al. 1986). However, since in vivo physiological levels of AVP appear protected from the action of this enzyme, the true biological importance of aminopepti-dase and its role in the pregnancy-induced osmoregulatory changes remain to be established.

5.4.5 PHARMACOLOGIC AGENTS AND ENDOTOXIN

Several pharmacologic agents can directly or indirectly affect vasopressin secretion; some of them stimulate while other block AVP release. Some drugs that stimulate AVP release (such as carbamazepine and clofibrate) became useful agents in the treatment of partial forms of central diabetes insipidus (chapter 17.1.4.2). On the other hand, the AVP-stimulatory effect of these drugs and that of some others (e.g. vincristine and cyclophosphamide) may contribute to the development of the syndrome of inappropriate secretion of antidiuretic hormone (chapter 20.3.1.10).

Ethanol inhibits the release of vasopressin, an effect likely to be mediated by the endogenous opioids (Oiso and Robertson 1985). On the contrary, alcoholics in withdrawal exhibit an antidiuretic state, which at least partly, can be attributed to concurrent elevation of plasma AVP, probably due to downward resetting of the AVP-osmostat. This change from diminished to increased AVP secretion when alcoholics discontinue drinking and develop withdraval symptoms might be explained by the occurrence of an augmented. rebound phenomenon. In concise terms, contemporary views hold that alcohol addiction is basically an expression of adaptation to the depressant effect of alcohol on neural function and that the condition of withdrawal may be the result of returning to the original drug-free state so rapidly, that re-adaptation cannot take place. This evidence of an antidiuretic state in alcohol withdrawal leads to the question, whether the practice of fluid supplementation in management of the withdrawal syndrome may not be potentially hazardous (Emsley et al. 1987). It is also possible that hypersecretion of AVP after discontinuation of drinking may be a factor that predisposes to enhanced water retention and more frequent development of hyponatremia in alcoholics treated in hospitals for severe underlying disorders.

Nicotine is a classic drug that causes antidiuresis by stimulating AVP release. Originally, this effect was attributed to a direct action of circulating nicotine on the hypothalamus via cholinergic receptors believed to be involved in the control of AVP release. However the effect may actually be more indirect since the doses required to release AVP almost always induce nausea or hypotension. More recent data indicate that the vasopressin response elicited by smoking is not due to emetic or hypotensive stimuli, but rather to an airways-specific mechanism (Rowe et al. 1980).

Anesthetics are known to elevate plasma AVP levels. Their effect is thought to be caused by suppression of autonomic influences (chapter 5.4.1.1) that exert tonic inhibition on AVP release (Ohilbin and Coggins 1978, Forsling et al. 1980).

Catecholamines have been known for many years to influence renal water excretion. Alpha-adrenergic stimulation by administration of intravenous norepinephrine to humans caused water diuresis, whereas beta-adrenergic stimulation produced antidiuresis. Following a series of studies by Schrier and his coworkers (Schrier and Kim 1987) it is now apparent that alpha- and beta-adrenergic effects on renal water excretion are mediated mainly by alterations in the secretion of vasopressin, a mechanism depending on the baroreceptor pathways. In addition, catecholamines also have distinct central effects, since catecholaminergic connections arise from the midbrain which mediate autonomic influences to the AVP secretory magnocellular neurons (Sladek and Armstrong 1987).

The administration of endotoxin to experimental animals was reported to be associated with very high plasma vasopressin levels, and it was suggested that circulating vasopressin plays a primary role in the maintenance of cardiovascular function during the development of endotoxin shock (Brackett et al. 1983).

5.4.6 HYPOXIA AND HYPERCAPNIA

Respiratory disorders are frequently complicated by impairment of renal water excretion. Substantial laboratory and clinical data suggest that both hypoxemia and acidosis are able to diminish the ability to osmotically suppress AVP release. The effect of both conditions on AVP secretion seems stronger during the intrauterine period (Rose et al. 1981, Szatalowicz et al. 1982, Daniel et al. 1982, 1984).

5.4.7 INTRACRANIAL HYPERTENSION

Speculation often ascribed nonosmotically elevated AVP secretion — seen in many neurological and neurosurgical disorders (Lester and Nelson 1981) as well as in fetuses during vaginal delivery (Hadeed et al. 1979) — to the common etiology of increased intracranial pressure (ICP). Probably the best data in support of this relationship involve work with monkeys. Gauflin et al. (1977) demonstrated increased vasopressin levels when they rapidly inflated subdural baloon catheters placed over the temporal lobes of monkeys. The amount of vasopressin released varied directly with the ICP increase, and the release was not suppressed by infusion of hypotonic solutions.

5.4.8 STRESS

The data obtained so far on the effect of stress upon the release of vasopressin are variable and sometimes also controversial. One of the first indirect, but convincing, reports on the increased release of AVP under stress was published by O'Connor and Verney (1942) who found a remarkable inhibition of water diuresis due to antidiuretic effect of stress in dogs, but after the removal of posterior pituitary in the same dogs such antidiuretic effect was not observed. In later experiments based on in vivo rat bioassay of antidiuretic activity, the exposure of laborary animals to several types of stress (ether, noise, pain, etc.) has fully confirmed the stress induced increase in plasma antidiuretic activity accompanied by a decreased urine flow as nicely expressed by the humorous saying: "You can hardly run away with a full bladder". The idea of stress stimulated release of AVP persisted for a long time until the unspecificity of AVP bioassay was uncovered. The more recent studies based on highly specific radioimmunoassay of AVP showed that only under some kinds of stress the plasma AVP level was truly elevated e.g. due to electric shock, traumatization, surgery and immobilization. Under some other kinds of stress the levels of plasma AVP remained unchanged, e.g. due to exercise, swimming, noise or cold. The level of plasma AVP may even decrease, namely if it had been elevated by dehydration prior to the start of stress evoked by ether or acceleration. The exact pathways whereby the above stimuli cause vasopressin release, remain to be defined (see Michajlovskij et al. 1988).

5.4.9 AMBIENT TEMPERATURE

Cold diuresis may be the result of decreased AVP levels, while inreased ambient temperature is known to stimulate AVP secretion (Segar and Moore 1968). On teleological grounds it would seem advantageous for the conservation of body fluid volumes, because the recognition of raised temperature would be an "early warning" of the evaporative losses which result from compensatory cooling mechanisms such as sweating and panting. It has been suggested that changes in vascular tone accompanying decrease or increase in body temperature may influence the baroreceptor pathways involved in AVP secretion. Exposure to high temperatures does increase also brain AVP levels and a role for centrally released AVP as an endogenous antipyretic agent has been proposed (Veale et al. 1984, Kasting 1986).

6 VASOPRESSIN ASSAYS

Progress in characterization of the functional aspects of AVP secretion was hampered by the lack of sensitive and reproducible assays to measure circulating hormone. Until the early 70s only bioassays were available; but the major advance in our understanding of AVP secretion was heralded by the development of specific radioimmunoassays able to detect vasopressin at the extremely low concentrations found in the body fluids of mammals.

6.1 BIOASSAYS

Standard bioassays have remained the basic techniques for pharmacological characterization of new analogs and methods for estimating antagonistic activities (Manning et al. 1987, Kinter et al. 1988). Vasopressor activity is estimated by intravenous injection of agonist analogs to anesthetized rats pretreated with an alpha-adrenergic or ganglion blocker or after pithing. Vasopressor responses to an unknown agent are compared with those to a reference standard; natural vasopressin possesses 0.380 µU vasopressor activity per pg. Antidiuretic activity is usually tested in assays involving intravenous administration of analogs to ethanol-anesthetized water loaded rats (Heller et al. 1959). The sensitivity of the techniques oscillates between 5 and 10 µU, arginine vasopressin possesses 0.330 µU antidiuretic activity per pg.

6.2 RADIOIMMUNOASSAYS (RIA)

Roth et al. already described radioimmunoassay for AVP in 1966, but it took several years before a clinically usable method for measuring AVP in urine (Oyama et al. 1971) and plasma (Robertson et al. 1973) was developed. Several general principles should be followed when performing any clinical study of vasopressin function: 1. Since many drugs influence vasopressin secretion and/or action they should be discontinued, if possible. Smoking and caffeine-containing fluids should not be allowed for 24 hours beforehand the study. 2. The study should be provided in a sitting or recumbent position. During the study the patient should be observed carefully for vasovagal reactions, nausea and/or hypotension, since these represent potent nonosmotic stimuli for AVP release. 3. For the interpretation of the results, normal values as well as results obtained in previously studied patients and healthy volunteers should be requested from the same laboratory, since laboratories differ in their reference standards (Vokes and Robertson 1988).

6.2.1   VASOPRESSIN IN PLASMA

Plasma AVP of normally hydrated subjects with samples obtained after overnight fasting have been typically observed to range from 2 to 5 pg per ml. Water deprivation for 24 to 36 hours in healthy humans results in plasma levels of about 10 to 20 pg/ml. On the other hand, standard water load suppresses immunoreactive AVP to unmeasurable levels, i.e. to levels below 0.5 pg/ml (Fig. 6.1). Hypertonic saline infusion (3 per cent saline given for 1 to 2 hours at a rate of 0.1 ml/kg/min) is somewhat cumbersome, but more reliable method for examining osmoregulatory function at low physiologic levels of P_{AVP}. More stressful events, such as minor or major surgery and hypovolemia, result in large elevations of plasma AVP. The most dramatic elevations of P_{AVP} have been observed with syncope, nausea, traumatic surgical procedures and delivery which may increase plasma AVP concentrations to levels ranging from 100 to 500 pg/ml (Šrámková et al. 1979, DeVane and Porter 1980, Horký et al. 1981, Vallotton et al. 1986a).

However, one should realize that the absolute concentrations of plasma vasopressin, which might oscillate from "very high" to "very low" values even in healthy individuals, are not decisive for estimating the osmoregulatory function. Therefore vasopressin levels should always be interpreted in view of concurrent plasma and urine osmolality. Also precise measurement of plasma osmolality is very important. A potential error of as much as 10 mOsm/kg can arise if the blood specimen is stored at room temperature for 1 to 4 hours after it was obtained. In this setting, persistent glycolytic activity in erythrocytes and leucocytes results in production of lactic acid and its release into the plasma. This problem can be prevented if the plasma is separated from the cells within 20 minutes (Radetzki et al. 1972). If the accuracy of the technique is poor or in doubt, measurements of plasma sodium should be used (equation 1.2).

Fig. 6.1. Changes of plasma and urine osmolality, plasma vasopressin as well as urinary vasopressin concentration and excretion during 36 hours of water deprivation in healthy adults (upper panel). Influence of orally administered standard water load (20 ml/kg) on plasma and urinary AVP, plasma and urine osmolality and on urine volume is illustrated on the lower panel. Results are means ± SEM (by Horký et al. 1981 with kind permission).

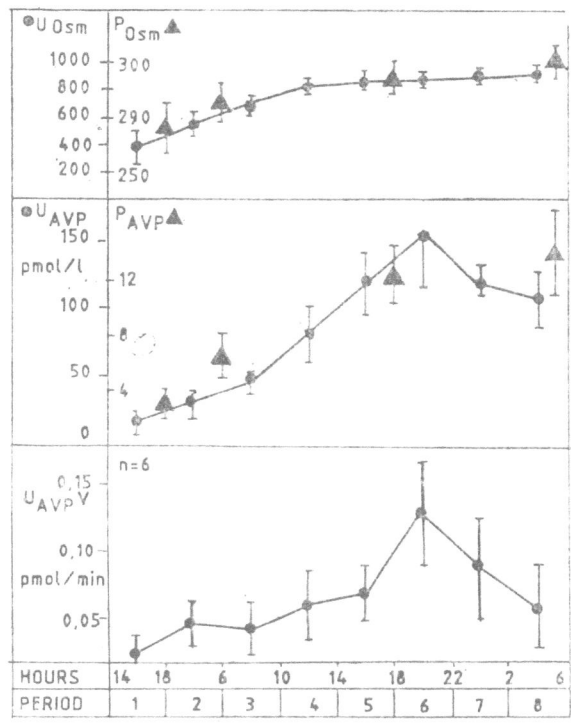

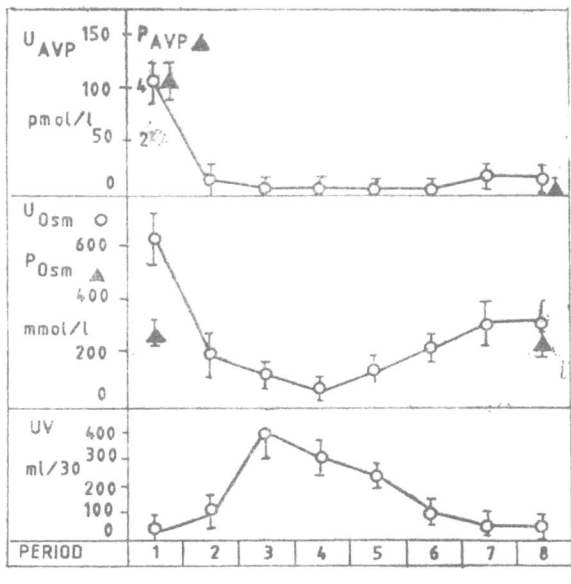

6.2.2 VASOPRESSIN IN URINE

Specific and highly sensitive antisera to detect the small physiological amounts of AVP present in circulation are still very rare, which imposes limitations on their clinical usefulness. To overcome this problem some workers developed radioimmunoassay techniques for the estimation of AVP in human urine. There are several advantages of urinary AVP measurements. AVP in urine is present in higher concentrations than in plasma; samples are easy to obtain; the hormone in urine is more stable than in plasma; urine samples do not have to be processed immediately. Since plasma AVP may vary rapidly in response to test stimuli providing only an instantaneous reflection of AVP secretion, the measurement of urinary AVP may provide a more accurate indication of small sustained changes in AVP secretion integrated over a period of time. Moreover, RIA AVP in plasma require relative large sample volume which is a particular problem in newborns and small infants. Some caution is needed to be exercised in the interpretation of urine AVP as there is evidence that large changes in solute excretion may influence fractional AVP clearance (Robertson 1977), and AVP estimation in urine by RIA may not entirely represent authentic AVP (Claybaugh and Sato 1985). Nevertheless, convincing evidence indicate that both urinary excretion (Miller and Moses 1972, Fressinaud et al. 1974, Khokhar et al. 1978) and urinary concentration of AVP (Thomas and Lee 1976, Horký et al. 1981, Tausch et al. 1983, Rees et al. 1983, Dunger et al. 1988) closely reflect changes in secretion and plasma levels of the hormone in adults as well as in infants, provided there are no major perturbations in glomerular filtration and solute excretion rates (see Fig. 6.1).

6.2.3 VASOPRESSIN IN CEREBROSPINAL FLUID

AVP is present in the CSF of normally hydrated human subjects in concentrations lower (0.6 to 2.2 pg/ml) than the corresponding plasma values. There is little or no rostrocaudal gradient of AVP in CSF, and the concentration seems to be fairly constant during the diurnal cycle (Luerssen and Robertson 1980, Sørensen 1986).

7 RECEPTORS AND SYNTHETIC ANALOGS OF VASOPRESSIN

One of the most vital properties of organ and organism function is that hormones acting on their cells are able to induce physiological responses. The hormone itself which evokes cellular response is the "first messenger". However, the hormone-induced activation of cellular response is not direct but mediated through the intracellular "second messenger". The latter is produced as a result of the interaction of the hormone with its specific cell receptor, and plays the key role in the expression of hormonal activation. The two most significant second messenger systems known in the physiology of hormones are the cyclic adenosine monophosphate (cAMP) and the calcium $[Ca^{++}]$ system; vasopressin exerts its hormonal effect using both these pathways.

7.1 VASOPRESSIN RECEPTORS

The effects of AVP are mediated by the activation of specific vasopressin receptors which have been classified by Mitchell et al. (1979) into V1 and V2 receptors, the designation being derived as functional analogy to alpha and beta adrenergic, or H1 and H2 histamine, receptors. The two major biologic actions of vasopressin correspond exactly to the two main subtypes of the receptor, each of them being coupled with a different second messenger system on the membrane of the target cells. Consequently, V1 and V2 receptors may be defined operationally in terms of the second messenger involved. They are also characterized pharmacologically as V1 and V2 receptors, depending on the relative potency of a series of natural agonists (see Fig. 2.1) and synthetic analogs with agonist and antagonist activities (Fig. 7.3).

7.1.1 V1 (PRESSOR) RECEPTORS

The V1 subtype (often also called pressor subtype) receptors are located in selected vascular beds and on specific cell types of several organs including the liver, brain and platelets. In the kidney V1 receptors are present at least at three different sites: the glomerular mesangial cell, the vascular smooth muscle cell, and the renomedullary interstitial cell. Activation of the V1 receptors is linked with changes in intracellular free calcium, [Ca⁺⁺], as the cellular signal. Briefly, occupancy of V1 receptors by vasopressin activates the breakdown of membrane phosphoinositols with the formation of two intracellular signals: diacylglycerol and 1,4,5-inositol monophosphate, the latter releasing calcium from its intracellular stores (Fig. 7.1, right side). Diacylglycerol, and perhaps

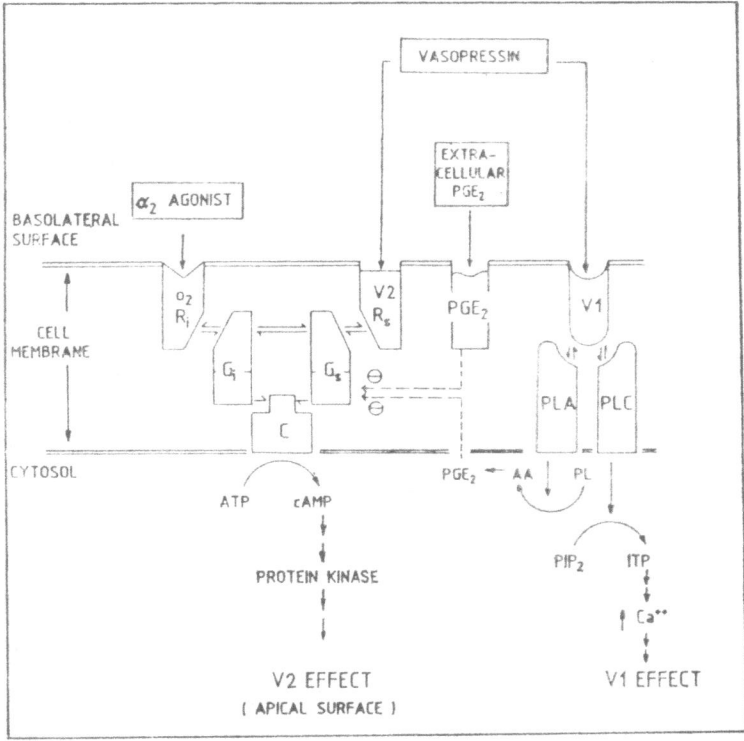

Fig. 7.1. Schematic representation of vasopressin effect on its target cells (for details see text).
Abbrevations used: V1 and V2: vasopressin receptor subtypes; R_s and R_i: receptors for stimulatory and inhibitory agents acting on adenylate cyclase; G_s and G_i: stimulatory and inhibitory guanine regulatory unit; C: catalytic unit; cAMP: cyclic adenosine monophosphate; ATP: adenosine triphosphate; PGE_2: prostaglandin E_2; PL: phospholipid pool; AA: arachnoid acid; PLA: phospholipase A; PLC: phospholipase C; PIP_2: phosphatidylinositol-4,5-biphosphate; ITP: inositol triphosphate; Ca⁺⁺: cytosolic free calcium (by Kinter et al. 1988 slightly modified with permission).

released calcium, are thought to activate protein kinase C; the latter then leads to the final biologic response mediated by V1 receptors (e.g. vascular contraction, platelet aggregation, glycogenolysis, CNS action, etc.).

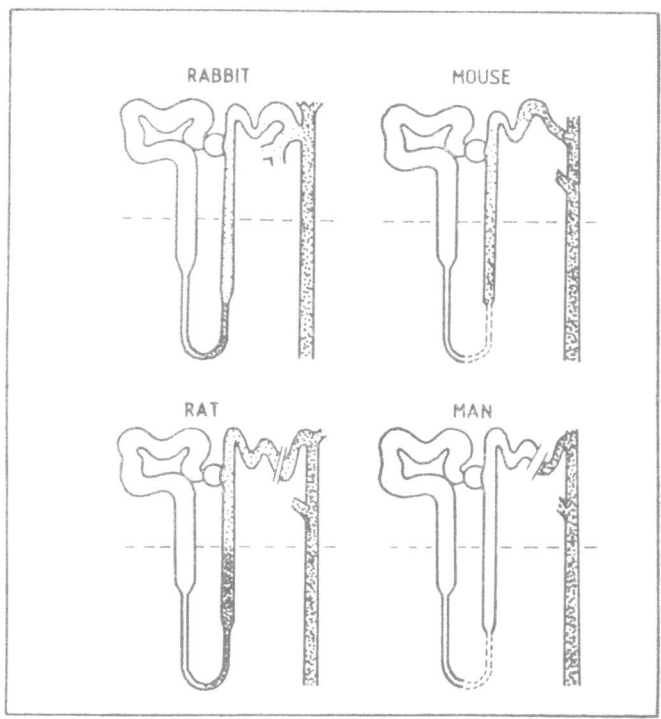

Fig. 7.2. The pattern of renal tubular receptors for AVP in four different species. The dot density in this diagram of a renal tubule is proportional to the increase in adenylate cyclase activity induced by AVP. The effect of AVP on the thin ascending limb was not tested in the mouse and human kidney (by Morel et al. 1981 with permission).

7.1.2 V2 (ANTIDIURETIC) RECEPTORS

Vasopressin acts on its target cells also via V2 subtype receptors (i.e. anti-diuretic as opposed to V1, pressor, receptors). V2 receptors, coupled to cAMP generation as the intracellular signal, are located not only in the cells of cortical and medullary collecting ducts as expected, but also in other epithelial cell types of the nephron, including those in the thin ascending limb, in the medullary and cortical portions of the thick ascending limb, and in the early distal convoluted tubule with striking differences in their distribution in various species (Fig. 7.2). As far as these receptor-holding segments corres-pond to physiological target sites for AVP in the nephron, the biological response induced by the hormone is expected to be different in each segment depending on the transport properties specific for the cell type itself (Morel et al. 1987).

Recently progress has been made concerning the mechanism of modulation at the transduction step between V2 receptor occupancy and the activation of adenylate cyclase (Orloff and Handler 1962, Kinter et al. 1988). It has become clear that adenylate cyclase (the enzyme that catalyzes the production of cAMP from adenosine triphosphate) is a part of a complex regulatory system consisting of at least three functionally different subunits for hormonal activation: the receptor (R), the guanine nucleotide regulatory protein (G), and the catalytic unit (C) (see Fig. 7.1). According to a model proposed by Rodbell (1980), adenylate cyclase is linked to two receptors of opposite nature: one of them (R_s) stimulates, whereas the other one (R_i) inhibits its activity through guanine nucleotide regulatory units of G proteins (G_s and G_i, respectively). They either activate (G_s) or inhibit (G_i) adenylate cyclase when, respectively, the activating or the inhibiting receptor is occupied. Vasopressin uses the stimulatory pathway (V2 receptor) while, for example, alpha-2-adrenergic agents, are expected to act as inhibitors when they occupy their receptor (R_i coupled to G_i, Fig 7.1) (Abramow et al. 1987).

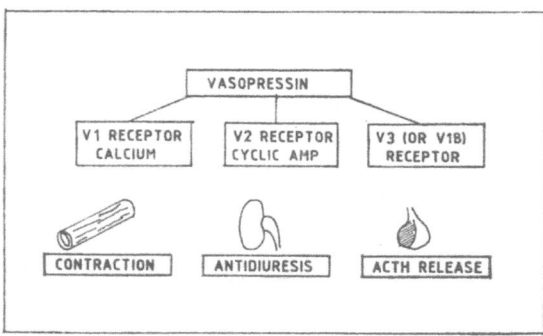

Fig. 7.3. Established AVP-receptor subtypes.

7.1.3 NOVEL VASOPRESSIN RECEPTORS

The number of organs where vasopressin receptors and binding sites have been disclosed increases rapidly (Jard 1983a, b). However, there is increasing evidence that not all receptors mediating the effects of AVP can be accommodated in the V1/V2 classification.

In the past few years a new type of AVP receptors was described on anterior pituitary corticotrophs, where AVP acts as a promotor of ACTH release or modulator of CRF-induced ACTH secretion (chapter 11.1). This novel subtype has been designated V3 or V1b, as distinct from the vascular and hepatic receptors which have been termed V1a receptors. Although not thoroughly characterized, this new receptor type has some attributes of both

70

the V1 (pressor) and V2 (antidiuretic) receptor. V1 (or V1a) or V2 agonists of AVP bind and induce release of ACTH from anterior pituitary cells in vitro, but V1 antagonists have no inhibitory effect. Moreover, vasopressin-induced secretion of ACTH was reported to be mediated by cAMP, a characteristic of V2 receptors (Antoni et al. 1984, Jard et al. 1986).

In addition to the well characterized renal V2 receptors, V2-like receptors may be present on vascular endothelium in view of V2 agonist's ability to stimulate circulating factor VIII levels (chapter 10). Furthermore, at this time one cannot exclude the existence of specific V2-like target sites located in peripheral vasculature or in some brain areas, which under specific conditions (high circulating levels of selective V2 agonists and/or selective blockade of V1 receptors) might mediate some rather unexpected cardiovascular effects of the hormone, which are opposite to its well appreciated V1 effects (Liard 1986, (chapter 9). Finally, AVP has been implicated in the pathogenesis of brain edema and a central V2-like receptor subtype has been postulated (Rosenberg et al.1986).

Also the receptors mediating the behavioral effects of AVP show a specificity different from that of "classical" V1 or V2 receptor. Burbach et al. (1983) showed that AVP undergoes proteolysis (in vitro) yielding the metabolite [pGlu4, Cyt6] VP - (4—9), a fragment that lacks antidiuretic, pressor and uterus-stimulating activities, but has a much more potent effect on memory processes than does the parent hormone (chapter 12.2.3).

It cannot be excluded that depending on the organ or tissue studied additional subtypes of receptors for vasopressin and/or its biologically active fragments will be disclosed in future (Constantini and Pearlmutter 1984). It can be hoped that synthesis of new and more selectively acting AVP agonists and antagonists will help to elucidate their nature.

7.2 REGULATION OF VASOPRESSIN RECEPTORS

Although the regulation of plasma vasopressin levels is clearly a primary determinant of water homeostasis, recent data suggest that physiological down- and upregulation of V2 receptors, circulating hormones, local modulator substance(s) (e.g. prostaglandins), and possibly of V1 receptors may also play a significant role in net hormonal response (Ausiello et al. 1987, Kinter et al. 1988).

7.2.1 RECEPTOR DOWN- AND UPREGULATION

It has been established for many hormones that the number of free receptors in target cell membranes as well as stimulation of adenylate cyclase activity coupled to the occupancy of these receptors may be reduced when the tissue was previously exposed to a high concentration of the corresponding hormone. This phenomenon, called downregulation or desensitization, results from an increased rate of receptor internalization, when the hormone concentration has been greatly enhanced, i.e. when the fractional occupancy of receptors is high. On the other hand, the total number of V2 receptors found on the vasopressin-sensitive renal epithelial cells is increased (upregulation) in situations when the blood levels of endogenous vasopressin are reduced or even lacking (e.g. rats receiving repeated gastric water load or Brattleboro rats lacking circulating AVP) (Morel et al. 1987). The vasopreussin pregulation may have some physiological relevance in patients with untreated neurogenic diabetes insipidus who are extremely sensitive to exogenous vasopressin (Block et al. 1981). These changes in vasopressin receptor number are associated with parallel changes in maximal adenylate cyclase activation by the hormone. Although an abundance of "spare" vasopressin receptors is present in the kidney (i.e. the occupation of but a small percentage of the total receptor population by vasopressin is sufficient to produce maximal response), down- and upregulation of the receptors might contribute to a modulation of kidney responsiveness to vasopressin stimulation. Indeed, for any value of free vasopressin concentration the number of occupied receptors is directly proportional to the total number of receptors (Rajerison et al. 1977). Down- and upregulation of V1 receptors could also be demonstrated (St. Louis et al. 1986).

7.2.2 MULTIHORMONAL CONTROL OF ADENYLATE CYCLASE

It should be mentioned that hormones other than AVP may also stimulate adenylate cyclase in different nephron segments. This is particularly striking for the medullary and cortical portions of the thick ascending limbs in the rat: vasopressin, glucagon, calcitonin and, to a lesser extent, beta-adrenergic agonists stimulate a common pool of adenylate cyclase in this structue. Some hormones, e.g. gluco- and mineralocorticoids, increase the hydroosmotic effect of AVP on the epithelial cells of the collecting duct, while other agents, such as alpha 2 adrenergic agonists or bradykinin, have inhibitory activity. However, the exact role played by them in the overall functioning of the renal urine concentrating and diluting mechanism is still poorly understood (de Rouffignac et al. 1987).

7.2.3 INTERACTIONS BETWEEN V1 AND V2 RECEPTOR SIGNALS; THE ROLE OF ENDOGENOUS PROSTAGLANDINS

During the last several years it has become increasingly apparent that the majority of hormone-stimulated transport events involve interactions between the two major second messenger systems, the cAMP and the $[Ca^{++}]$ system.

These interactions can occur at the level of the production of the second messengers themselves, or at a variety of steps leading to the physiologic response to the hormone. Thus rather than functioning in a single stereotyped fashion, the interactions between these two systems display an amazing plasticity. As a consequence, the nature of the interactions vary from tissue to tissue (Rasmussen et al. 1986).

The modulatory role of prostaglandins may serve as a physiological example of such an interaction. Within the kidney various epithelial and nonepithelial cells represent targets for AVP and also synthesize prostaglandins. Prostaglandins (principally PGE_2) in turn antagonize the AVP-mediated pressor or antidiuretic effects (Raymond and Lifschitz 1986). AVP-induced prostaglandin synthesis in vascular smooth muscle cells, particularly in those in the renal medullary microcirculation, is related to a "pressor" or V1 type receptor. Also the effect of AVP on the release of PGE_2 from epithelial cells of the medullary collecting duct is mediated by activation of a V1 subtype receptor; this stimulation occurs independently of the activation of adenylate cyclase, being coupled to a V2 subtype receptor (Vallotton et al. 1986b) (see Fig. 7.1). The possibility that the same tubular cells harbor both V1 and V2 receptors is strongly supported by recent reports (Garcia-Perez and Smith 1984). Hence, the V1-stimulated prostaglandin synthesis could alter the V2-mediated effect of the hormone in the same cell and thus probably represent a part of a feedback mechanism which would buffer excessive variations in hormone-induced water permeability. The role prostaglandins play in the urine concentrating defects in a variety of pathologic conditions (such as hypokalemia or hypercalcemia), however, remains controversial and awaits further clarification.

7.3 SYNTHETIC ANALOGS OF VASOPRESSIN

The relatively easy synthesis of small molecules of the neurohypophyseal hormones has allowed to prepare hundreds of analogs of the natural AVP by modifying the vasopressin molecule. The aim was to prepare analogs with prolonged or otherwise clinically advantageous activities. One of the goals derived from in vivo bioassays of structural analogs of vasopressin and oxytocin was to design agonists that selectively activate a given receptor subtype (e.g. V1, V2, or uterine oxytocin receptors). A well known example of a potent V2-selective agonist is [1-deamino-8-D-arginine] vasopressin (dDAVP, desmopressin) synthesized in Prague by Zaoral et al. (1967) (Fig. 7.4). Another, more difficult goal was to design antagonists selective for each receptor type, i.e. peptides that would bind to, but not activate, a given receptor type and thus competitively antagonize the agonistic responses at these receptors. Several V1 and V1/V2 antagonists have recently become powerful probes of the physiological, biochemical, and pharmacological actions of the parent peptide. These receptor antagonists also offer promise as long-sought drugs for the therapy of a variety of conditions due to excessive secretion of AVP (Manning and Sawyer 1986, Kinter et al. 1988).

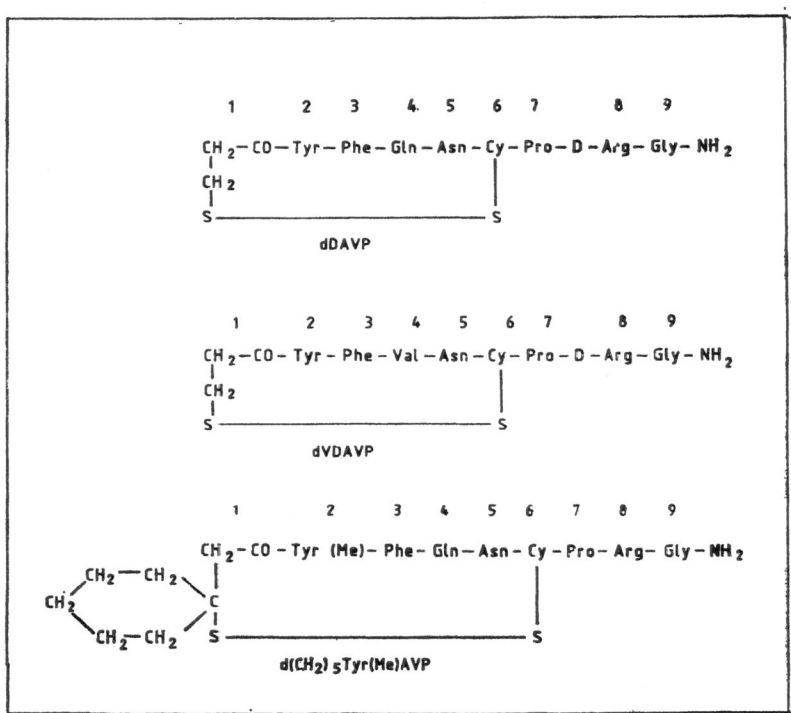

Fig. 7.4. Structure of V2 agonists dDAVP and dVDAVP and the V1 antagonist d(CH2)5 Tyr(Me)AVP.

7.3.1 SELECTIVE V2 (ANTIDIURETIC) AGONISTS

During the 20 years which have elapsed since the synthesis of dDAVP (see Fig. 7.4), this analog has become a generally employed V2 agonist both in clinical practice and under experimental conditions in studying physiological effects of the hormone vasopressin (Vávra et al. 1968; Oravec and Lichardus, 1972; Némethová et al. 1979; Némethová and Lichardus 1974; Marek et al. 1978, Bakoš et al. 1984, Richardson and Robinson 1985). In contrast to the natural hormone, the synthetic analog acquired a substantially more protracted antidiuretic effect (it undergoes a much slower enzymatic cleavage; even the cystine-aminopeptidase of human pregnancy does not degrade desmopressin), and lost almost entirely vasopressor activity. As compared to natural AVP with antidiuretic and pressor activity in an approximately 1 : 1 ratio, desmopressin has an A/P ratio of about 2,000—3,000 : 1. In addition, dDAVP is a 1—3-times more potent stimulator of renal medullary adenylate cyclase than natural vasopressin (Pliska 1985). Increasing the hydrophobic character of the residue in position 4 of dDAVP molecule gave an even more potent and specific antidiuretic peptide, 1-deamino, 4-valine, 8D-arginine vasopressin (dVDAVP) (see Fig. 7.4). It exhibits an even more pronounced antidiuretic activity than does dDAVP, and is also in fact a V1 antagonist, albeit a rather weak one.

dDAVP is now available for clinical use and can be administered by intravenous, subcutaneous and intranasal routes. Intravenous injection of 2 to 20 µg of dDAVP produces antidiuresis for 12—24 hours, and has virtually no pressor or uterotonic effects (warranting safety in patients with heart disease and in pregnant women) (Oravec and Lichardus 1972). Half-life estimations have been highly variable, apparently due to individual differences in the metabolism of dDAVP. After i.v. injections of 2 to 20 µg dDAVP disappeared from the plasma with a second exponential phase of 50 to 158 minutes. This finding can be compared with the half-lives of AVP and LVP (3 to 24 minutes). Most frequently, the peptide is administered by the noninvasive route (intranasall y in doses of 5—20 µg. It is estimated that 4—20% of the desmopressin applied to the nasal mucosa is absorbed; however, this proportion may be substantially lower in patients with rhinitis or coryza. In studies using intranasal administration of desmopressin, half life estimations give highly variable results ranging from 24 to 240 minutes with a mean of 90 minutes, probably reflecting variable nasal absorption of the peptide. Intranasal doses greater than 40 µg seem inefficient, possibly because the volume of fluid (0.4 ml) is more than can be handled by the nose, and excess fluid escapes into the nasopharynx (Richardson and Robinson 1985). The peptide is absorbed also from the mucosa of the oral cavity as well as from the intestinal tract; a reliable dose-dependent diuresis for up to 12 hours can be achieved after sublingual and/or oral administration (Fjellestad and Czernichow 1986). A major disadvantage of oral administration lies in the economic aspect: 10—40-fold larger doses of desmopressin are required by this route to achieve comparable levels of antidiuresis.

The liver and kidneys are the chief sites of metabolic inactivation of arginine-vasopressin. Both organs metabolize desmopressin slower than vasopressin; the liver approximately 66 per cent slower and the kidney more than 90 per cent slower. Renal metabolism includes cleavage of the peptide bond between proline(7) and arginine(8) and it has been proposed that substitutions of D- for L-arginine may retard this cleavage. The lack of the usual enzymatic destruction allows 40 per cent of an injected dose of desmopressin to appear intact in the urine within 6 hours of administration and as much as 60 per cent of the peptide is excreted in this fashion (Richardson and Robinson 1985).

Desmopressin has been remarkably free from adverse effects, especially when given intranasally for diabetes insipidus. Only very rarely headache, abdominal pain or profound sweating have been reported requiring withdrawal of the drug. Initial facial flushing can occasionally be observed after intravenous administration of dDAVP. There is a notable lack of decreased response to desmopressin during chronic therapy compared with lysine-vasopressin, although an increased dose has been required to maintain antidiuresis in a few patients. Yet probably the most surprising is the scarcity of induced hyponatremia during acute or chronic administration of desmopressin. The safety of this peptide can, at least partially, be related to the relatively high level of the osmotic threshold for thirst in humans. As thirst in humans becomes symptomatic above a plasma osmolality of about 290 mOsm/kg (see Fig. 5.5), the patient is not thirsty until all excess water is excreted. However, when desmopressin is given simultaneously with a nondipsogenic supply of fluids an increased risk of excessive fluid retention with subsequent hyponatremia should be considered (Némethová et al. 1977, 1979).

Because of its favorable pharmacologic characteristics and virtually no adverse effects, desmopressin has become the drug of choice in the treatment of patients with both partial and complete forms of central diabetes insipidus (chapter 17.1.4.2). Other diagnostic and/or therapeutic applications of dDAVP are possibly less known but not less important. The use of dDAVP in a test of urinary concentration (the rapid dDAVP concentration test) avoids inconveniences associated with the classic approach to the testing of renal concentrating capacity and its disturbances of various origin (chapter 8.4.1.3), including the differential diagnosis of polyuric states (chapter 17.5.2.2). Several clinical trials have demonstrated the value of desmopressin in diminishing bedwetting in otherwise normal children and adults (chapter 15.6.1). Some rather unexpected effects of dDAVP on blood clotting processes and the levels of both factor VIII and von Willebrand factor were reported by Mannucci et al. (1975). This finding was subsequently confirmed and extended, and for hemophilia A and Willebrand's disease of mild to medium severity desmopressin has become a widespread agent for the control of blood clotting (chapter 10.4). dDAVP was also reported to enhance some aspects of memory (chapter 12.2.4). Finally, desmopressin-induced controlled hyponatremia appears effective in the prevention and shortening of painful crises of sickle cell disease (chapter 17.2.2.8).

7.3.2 SELECTIVE V1 (PRESSOR) AGONISTS

Of the many synthetic vasopressin analogs 2-phenylalanine, 3-isoleucine, 8-ornithine vasopressin is the most selective V1 agonist known to date. However, its pressor/antidiuretic (P/A) ratio of 218 "pales" by comparison with the A/P ratio of dDAVP, dVDAVP and numerous other selective V2 agonists.

In clinical conditions usually included in the indications of V1 agonist administration (hemorrhage and/or hypotension) a residual V2 effect may even be advantageous. Therefore, substantially less selective vasopressin analogs, such as ornipressin (8-ornithine vasopressin) which has a P/A ratio of 4, or glypressin (Na-triglycyl-8-lysine vasopressin) which is converted to lysine-vasopressin in the body, are used in similar conditions. Locally administered vasopressin and/or its V1 analogs effectively diminish bleeding during stomatological, gynecological or surgical interventions. The vasoconstrictor effect of intravenously or intraarterially administered vasopressin (or its V1 analogs) has been used in the treatment of life-threatening hemoptysis (Magee and Wiliams 1982) and for the cessation of gastrointestinal bleeding from esophageal varices (chapter 9.4.2).

7.3.3 SELECTIVE V1 (PRESSOR) ANTAGONISTS

A number of potent and highly selective V1 antagonists are now available. Virtually all these peptides also exhibit varying degrees of oxytocin and antidiuretic antagonism. $d(CH_2)_5Tyr(Me)AVP$ possesses only about $1 : 1,000$ of the antidiuretic activity of the natural nonapeptide; this peptide is in fact one of the most potent and selective antivasopressor peptides known to date (see Fig. 7.4). Not surprisingly, it has become the most widely used V1 antagonist as a pharmacologic tool in studies of the central and peripheral role of AVP in cardiovascular regulation and in studies of AVP receptor subtypes (Manning et al. 1987).

This V1 antagonist has been recently used in healthy volunteers and in patients with hypertension and/or congestive heart failure (Weaber et al. 1986). The data obtained point to an active role of circulating AVP in cardiovascular regulation in man, in particular on markedly elevated plasma concentrations such as in patients with severe congestive heart failure. However, it is not known to date whether such patients would benefit from V1 receptor blockade. It is conceivable that AVP release is stimulated when the other two major pressor systems (the sympathetic nervous system and the renin-angiotensin system) are not sufficient to maintain blood pressure under the given conditions. Thus if the vasoconstrictor effects of AVP are blocked, circulatory failure may ensue. However, the possibility cannot be excluded that in patients with normal or moderately raised AVP, V1 antagonists might have interesting and so far unexplored therapeutic effects if they are administered on a long-term basis (Hofbauer and Seng Chin Mah 1987).

7.3.4 SELECTIVE V2 (ANTIDIURETIC) ANTAGONISTS- "AQUARETICS"

The case for the development of therapeutically useful antagonists of the antidiuretic (V2) response to vasopressin is much more compelling. In addition to serving as useful pharmacologic tools for studying the contribution of vasopressin to water retention in normal and pathologic states, there is obvious need for V2 receptor antagonists for the treatment of hyponatremia secondary to the syndrome of inappropriate secretion of antidiuretic hormone (SIADH). It is expected that these compounds (also termed "aquaretic agents" to distinguish their pharmacology and potential therapeutic utility from conventional saluretics which cause both salt and water diuresis) would make it possible to treat disorders of water homeostasis without affecting the electrolyte balance.

Unfortunately, no truly selective V2 antagonists could be synthesized so far. All known inhibitory compounds which bind to V2 receptors retain at least some degree of affinity for V1 receptors (therefore they are usually termed V1/V2 antagonists). In addition, they are also partial V2 agonists in that they induce a transient antidiuretic response followed by a longer period of inhibition of antidiuretic responses to exogenous AVP. Nevertheless, recent animal models support the hypothesis that available aquaretic V1/V2 antagonists, e.g. $[d(CH_2)_5'D\text{-}Tyr(Et)_2Val4desGly9]$ AVP which is one of the most effective compounds of this kind, make possible an effective therapy to selectively remove excessively accumulated body water in the presence of inappropriately elevated circulating levels of vasopressin (László and Baláspiri 1986, Kinter et al. 1988).

8 VASOPRESSIN AND RENAL REGULATION OF WATER HOMEOSTASIS

Besides the role of fluid intake in osmoregulation — which normally depends mainly on our will and of course on the access to water and our physical ability to ingest it — the most important effector of the regulation of body water are the kidneys. The ability of mammals to excrete urine either more or less concentrated than plasma, permits them to maintain the osmolality of body fluids within a remarkably narrow physiological range (280—300 mOsm/kg) compatible with normal cellular function in the face of wide variations in salt and water intake. This homeostatic process which protects body fluids from life-threatening deviations in osmolality involves 1. a complex cascade of processes of generation and maintenance of a renal cortico-medullary osmotic gradient, and 2. processes connected with utilization of this gradient supposing normal regulation of vasopressin secretion and the presence of the collecting duct epithelia responsive to the hydroosmotic effect of AVP. Vasopressin which acts predominantly on the most terminal segment of the nephron, is doubtlessly the principal, although not the only, factor involved in regulation of renal water excretion. The effect of this hormone no longer can be described by the simplified scheme: "vasopressin = urine concentration". AVP is a factor, whose action depends on the effectivity of the preceeding, "preparatory" phases of urine generation. Thus any discussion about the various means whereby vasopressin might affect the renal osmoregulatory function must be based on the understanding of the nature of these "preparatory" phases. In the following section presenting first the definition of the free water concept, a brief description will be given of the mechanisms of renal concentration and dilution along with an analysis of the role of AVP in these processes.

8.1 RENAL OSMOREGULATORY PERFORMANCE — THE OSMOTICALLY FREE WATER CONCEPT

Functional separation of water excretion from solute excretion by the kidney is vital to homeostasis, specifically with regard to maintenance of constancy of body fluid osmolality and extracellular fluid volume. For many years it has been appreciated that to concentrate urine it is necessary to reabsorb relatively more water than salts from the glomerular filtrate. Conversely, dilution of urine has supposed reabsorption of salts in excess to water.

Idealized quantitative relationships between osmotic concentrations of plasma and urine, the amount of ingested water and the volume of excreted urine in typical healthy adults are schematically shown in Fig. 8.1. These relationships stress the fact that processes of urine "concentration" and "dilution" are not separated phenomena; rather they represent two aspects of the same continuous process of the formation of definitive urine. Although it is the importance of the "concentration" aspect of this process that is usually being emphasized, only a relatively minor volume of water saved for the body can be expected to ensue from the processes of raising urine osmolality from isotonicity to maximal hypertonicity (U_{osm} max $= 1,200$ mOsm/kg), associated with a reduction of daily urine flow from 2 to 3 liters to about 0.5 l (see Fig. 8.1). In contrast, significantly greater changes in absolute urine volume occur in the "diluting sector", where a decrease of urine osmolality from isotonicity to maximal hypotonicity (U_{osm} min $= 50$ mOsm/kg) causes an increment of daily urine flow from 2 to 3 liters up to 15 to 20 liters. Conversely, decrease of urine osmolality from isotonicity down to maximal hypotonicity

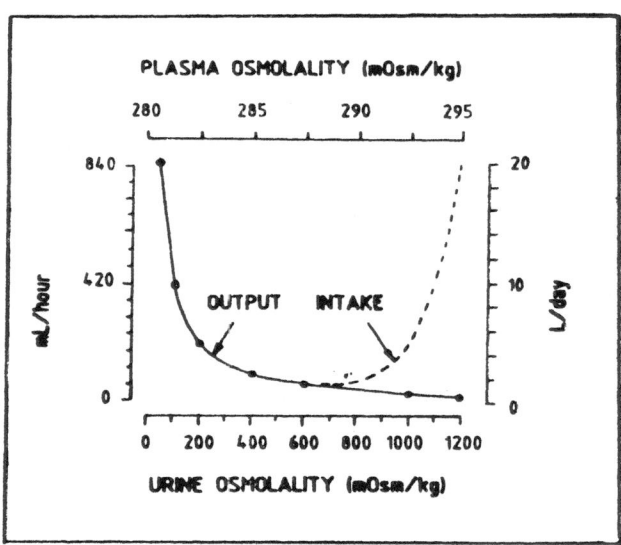

Fig. 8.1. The calculated rate of water intake and excretion as a function of plasma osmolality in a typical healthy adult assuming a solute excretion rate of 600 mOsm/day and both extrarenal water loss and incidental water intake of 1 l/day (by Robertson 1981 with kind permission). The point at which output and intake lines cross indicates the level at which balance state is achieved. Note that in a typical healthy adult it occurs at a point where water turnover is minimal and plasma osmolality is about halfway between the osmotic thresholds for vasopressin secretion and thirst.

(urine dilution) allows thereby urine volume increases so that the organism can handle all but the most pathologically excessive rates of water intake without any disturbances occurring in the composition of body fluids.

The level of urine osmolality reflects the actual concentrating and/or diluting capacity of the kidneys, but is far from being a sufficiently exact parameter allowing to estimate effectivity of the osmoregulatory performance of the kidneys; the latter depends, to a significant degree, also on the intensity of urine solute excretion.

It was Homer Smith (1951) who introduced the free water clearance for the quantitation of renal osmoregulatory performance. Free water clearance can be most easily conceptualized by dividing the urine volume into two fractions (Fig. 8.2). One fraction, the osmolal clearance (C_{osm}) represents that volume of urine (liters per day) that is necessary to excrete all of the solutes contained in it at an osmolality equivalent to plasma. The other fraction, the free water clearance (C_{H_2O}) represents the difference between the total urine volume (in liters per day) and the osmolal clearance ($V - C_{osm}$). In reality, this is not a true clearance value; instead, the difference $V - C_{osm}$ indicates that volume of urine from which solute has been completely removed during the formation of diluted urine, or that volume of solute-free water which has been "saved" by the organism during the formation of concentrated urine. Thus when urine flow (V) is greater than the osmolal clearance, urine is hypotonic, i.e. free water clearance is positive (see Fig. 8.2, A). Conversely, when urine flow is less than osmolal clearance, the kidneys produce hypertonic urine, i.e. C_{H_2O} is

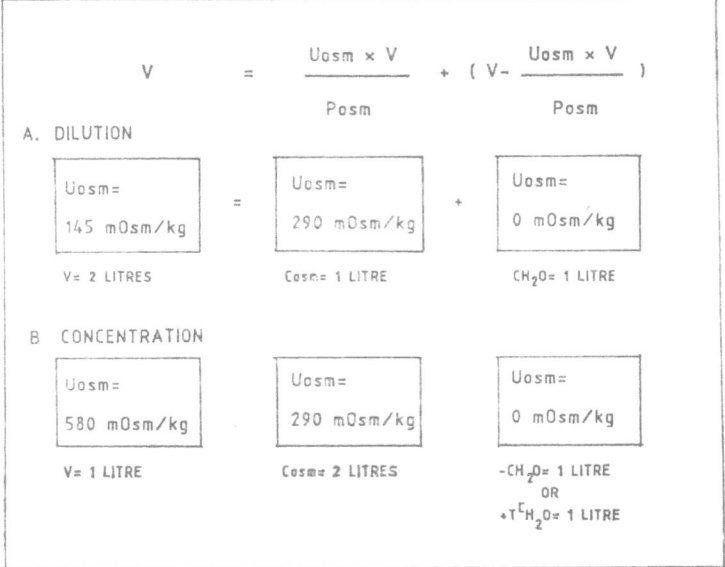

Fig. 8.2. Schematic illustration of the free-water concept during production of diluted (A) and concentrated (B) urine.

negative ($-C_{H_2O}$ or $+ T^c_{H_2O}$ i.e. tubular reabsorption of water) (see Fig. 8.2, B). For practical purposes, C_{H_2O} is often related to glomerular filtration rate (GFR) and expressed as percentage: $C_{H_2O}/GFR \times 100$ (in this case it represents filtered water that is excreted into the definitive urine).

8.1.1 GENERATION AND MAINTENANCE OF A RENAL CORTICO-MEDULLARY OSMOTIC GRADIENT

The generation and maintenance of cortico-medullary osmotic gradient, which is a prerequisite for the hydroosmotic effect of AVP, is brought about by a coordinated function of nephrons and the renal microcirculation. Each kidney contains more than one million nephrons. This functional unit of the kidney is composed of the glomerulus and the tubule, the latter being roughly subdivided in one proximal segment, the descending and the ascending limb of the Henle's loop, and the distal tubule. The distal tubule then continues to form collecting ducts which unite and mouth at the top of the papillae into the renal calices. Mammalian kidneys have major zones including the cortex, the medulla (outer and inner) and the inner medulla's tip called the papilla (Fig.

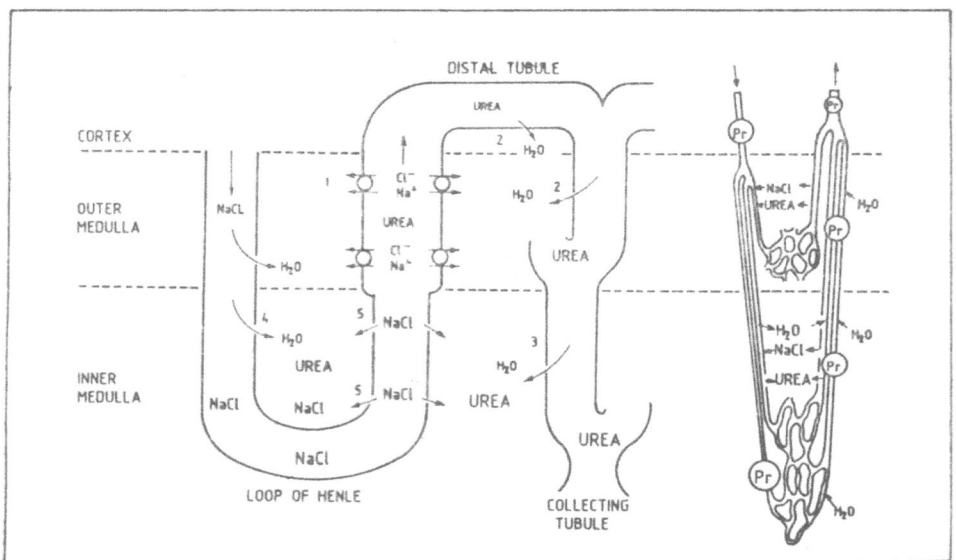

Fig. 8.3. Schematic illustration of processes involved in the "passive" concentrating mechanism (left side) and in vasa recta function (right side). The encircled Pr denotes plasma protein. The size of type indicates the relative concentration of each solute with respect to its localization in the medulla but not necessarily with respect to the concentrations of other solutes. For details see text. (From Kokko and Rector 1976 and Jamison and Kriz 1982 with kind permission.)

8.3). Nephron heterogeneity is determined, at least partially, by the length of the Henle's loop. One, outer cortical, subpopulation of nephrons has relatively short loops reaching up to the limit of the outer and inner medulla, whereas the thin segment of another, juxtamedullary, nephron subpopulation (in humans making up some 15% of the nephrons) immerses deep into the inner medulla.

The process of urine formation starts by plasma ultrafiltration in the glomerules. Active and passive mechanisms operative in the proximal tubuli of the nephron then act to resorb roughly two thirds of the total filtered load of water and salts present in the lumen. Thanks to the permeability characteristics of the tubular wall this proximal resorption is isoosmotic. Consequently the osmotic concentration of the tubular contents leaving this segment remains identical with that of the plasma. However, this does not mean that these processes are insignificant from the viewpoint of the renal osmoregulatory activity. Alterations of glomerular filtration rate and/or of intensity of proximal isotonic tubular absorption of water and salts can significantly affect the tubular fluid load shifted to more distal nephron segments, and thereby alter the volume of the potentially producible solute-free water (Berliner and Davidson 1957, Valtin and Edwards 1987).

8.1.2 PROCESSES OF GENERATION OF SOLUTE-FREE WATER AND OF CORTICO-MEDULLARY OSMOTIC GRADIENT (COUNTERCURRENT MULTIPLIER)

Kuhn and collaborators were by no means the first to relate the loop of Henle to the process of urine concentration (Kuhn and Ryffel 1942, Wirz et al. 1951). They postulated that the loop of Henle can operate as a countercurrent multiplier, i.e. that under conditions of 1. countercurrent flow, 2. different permeability characteristics of the loop limbs, and 3. in the presence of energy source for the separation of water and salts ("single effect") the loop is able to augment relatively small "horizontal" transtubular differences in osmotic concentration to a large "vertical" osmotic gradient between the renal cortex and the top of the papilla. The short loops of Henle indeed seem to meet all the three above principal criteria for the function of a countercurrent multiplier. Nevertheless, this concept could not explain the nature of the concentration process in the inner medulla, where the most pronounced rise of interstitial osmolality occurs. The inner medulla contains only the thin segments of the long loops of Henle, whereas their thick segments responsible for the "single effect" (active transport of chlorides) are localized in the outer medulla. An elegant solution to this contradiction is offered by the "passive model" of the concentrating mechanism proposed simultaneously by Stephenson (1972) and Kokko and Rector (1972). According to this model, countercurrent multiplication associated with the generation of the intramedullary osmotic gradient is due to the transport of two instead of one solute: sodium chloride and urea (see Fig. 8.3). The extent to which this model has been verified has been discussed in recent papers (Jamison 1987, Stephenson 1987). Existing uncertainties by no means impair the applicability of Stephenson's general model which still serves as an etalon for estimating the validity of any other model of the concentrating mechanism.

Details of the "passive model" are illustrated in Fig. 8.3. The energy source, active chloride reabsorption accompanied passively by sodium (the "chloride pump") is confined to water impermeable thick ascending limb of the Henle loop (see Fig. 8.3 (1)). Salt and water separation generates free water, the latter remaining in the lumen of the tubule renders the lumen hypoosmotic and the surrounding outer medullary interstitium hyperosmotic. Since urea permeability in this segment is low, urea remains in the tubule fluid. As tubule fluid flows into the distal nephron in the presence of vasopressin water is being reabsorbed in the cortex and the outer medulla. As a result, the concentration of urea in the collecting duct increases sharply by the time the tubular fluid reaches the inner medulla (see Fig. 8.3 (2)). There in the presence of vasopressin urea is reabsorbed and trapped in the inner medulla (see Fig. 8.3 (3)). The high concentrations of urea in the inner medulla extract water from the descending limb of the Henle's loop (see Fig. 8.3 (4)) and establish a transepithelial gradient for passive reabsorption of sodium chloride through the salt-permeable, water impermeable thin ascending limb (see Fig. 8.3 (5)). The osmotic gradient thus generated between the cortical and the inner-

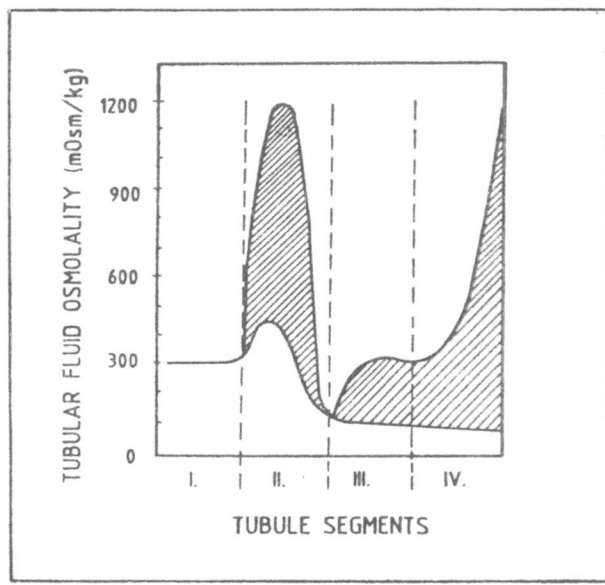

Fig. 8.4. Changes in tubular fluid composition in different nephron segments during maximal water diuresis (lower line) and maximal antidiuresis (upper line). (I-proximal tubule; II-Henle's loop; III-distal tubule and cortical collecting duct; IV-medullary collecting duct.)

84

medullary interstitium by sodium chloride and urea serves then as the driving force for passive water reabsorption during the process of urine concentration (see Fig. 8.3 (2)).

Due to specific permeability characteristics of the individual segments of the tubular wall, the osmotic concentration of the tubular contents gradually changes along the nephron (Fig. 8.4). Due to isolated passive reabsorption of water (and possibly also to urea recirculation) in the descendent limb of the Henle's loop, the osmolality of the tubular contents increases, reaching its maximum at the top of the loop. The value of tubular fluid osmolality at this locality indicates the magnitude of the medullary osmotic gradient, and thus also the value of the maximally attainable osmotic concentration of definitive urine. In the ascending limb, thanks to passive (the thin segment) and active (the thick segment) NaCl reabsorption, the osmolality of the tubular contents markedly decreases. In the beginning of the distal tubule, the tubular fluid is always hypotonic to the plasma, regardless of whether the body is set to diuresis or to antidiuresis. It is significant that more than four fifths of the glomerular filtrate are reabsorbed between the proximal and the distal tubule, and only the rest gets into the collecting ducts, where the osmotic concentration of urine is definitely adjusted in dependence on the measure of the cortico-medullary osmotic gradient and on the actual level of circulating vasopressin.

8.1.3 PROCESSES INVOLVED IN THE MAINTENANCE OF THE CORTICO-MEDULLARY OSMOTIC GRADIENT (MEDULLARY MICROCIRCULATION)

Under normal conditions, the volume of the definitive urine reaches not more than 1—3% of the total volume of about 150 l filtered daily in the glomerules, whereby most of the glomerular filtrate gets reabsorbed into the renal interstitium. Such a significant medullary fluid load requires the existence of some mechanism capable of meeting dual function: 1. to eliminate reabsorbed water and 2. to trap solutes in the medulla to maintain the cortico-medullary osmotic gradient. Owing to the absence of lymphatic vessels in the renal medulla, these tasks are met by the medullary microcirculation (vasa recta) derived from the efferent arterioles of the juxtamedullary glomeruli. Since vasa recta are permeable to both solutes and water, they reach near osmotic equilibrium with the surrounding interstitium. In the descending limb of capillary (see Fig. 8.3 right side) solute enters and water leaves its lumen as the plasma osmolality reaches 1,200 mOsm/kg at the papillary tip (under the conditions of maximal urine concentration). If the vasa recta left the kidney at this point, the combination of solute removal and water addition would reduce medullary osmolality. However, medullary osmolality is maintained, because the vasa recta, like the loops of Henle, turn around at the papillary tip and return to the cortex. The solute removed from the interstitium in the descending limb is returned to the interstitium, i.e. exchanged, in the ascending limb down a concentration gradient from the lumen to the interstitium. Similarly water added to the interstitium in the descending limb reenters the capillary in the ascending limb. Allowing for a lag in equilibration, the blood returning to the cortex **remains** slightly hyperosmotic to plasma (Zimmerhackl et al. 1986).

The low rate of medullary blood flow (6 to 10 per cent of renal blood flow) also contributes to the maintenance of interstitial hyperosmolality. If medullary blood flow is increased, more blood which is slightly hypertonic to plasma in general circulation will leave the medulla, and a significant washout of medullary solute can occur with reduction in interstitial osmolality. The latter effect will also diminish water reabsorption in the descending limb of the loop of Henle since there will be a **weaker** osmotic gradient between the tubular fluid and the interstitium. A clinical example where each of these changes occurs is osmotic diuresis in which a large amount of non-reabsorbed solute is present in the urine. This may be seen in glycosuria in uncontrolled diabetes mellitus or after an intravenous infusion of hypertonic mannitol. In these settings medullary blood flow is enhanced by an unknown mechanism, resulting in a decrease in papillary osmolality and an elevation in urine output, primarily due to a fall in descending limb water reabsorption. Another example is that seen in patients with free-water diuresis. Water diuresis of any etiology diminishes maximal renal concentrating ability primarily due to washout of the medullary osmotic gradient. This effect is a usual source of considerable diagnostic uncertainties in differentiating polyuric syndromes (chapter 17.5.2.2).

8.1.4 UTILIZATION OF THE CORTICO-MEDULLARY OSMOTIC GRADIENT — THE ROLE OF THE COLLECTING DUCTS

The processes of the generation and conservation of the cortico-medullary osmotic gradient are a prerequisite for the resorption of solute-free water in the collecting duct in a manner dependent on AVP. The effect of vasopressin is of permissive nature; changing the permeability properties of this particular nephron segment the hormone allows the osmotic equlibration of the tubular fluid with the interstitial tissue. In the presence of AVP, the transepithelial osmotic gradient enables water to be reabsorbed in the cortical collecting duct; this results in an increase of tubular fluid osmolality to isotonicity and markedly decreases the delivery of water to the medullary collecting duct. Even if the renal medulla were not hyperosmotic, the most important effect of AVP on conservation of body water has already occurred in the cortex. In an adult man, this means the difference between excreting 15 to 20 liters and 2 to 3 liters per day (see Fig. 8.1). Conversely, in absence of AVP, the hyperosmotic urine leaving the loop of Henle does not equilibrate with the interstitium, and diluted urine is excreted (Kokko 1987).

8.2 RENAL ACTIONS BY WHICH VASOPRESSIN MAY AFFECT THE CONCENTRATION OF URINE

The role of vasopressin in the kidneys has classically been considered to result solely from its ability to increase water permeability in the collecting duct, the hydroosmotic effect of the hormone. Recent evidence for the presence of vasopressin receptors also in other nephron segments in addition to the collecting ducts (see Fig. 7.2) and also in renal vessels suggest that AVP is able to stimulate the production of its intracellular messenger (cAMP or calcium) at these sites as well. Owing to this, the renal action of the hormone may be of a more comprehensive nature. Indeed, the hormone may also play an active role in determining the other major components of the concentrating process, i.e. the generation and the maintenance of interstitial tonicity (Table 8.1) (Valtin 1984, Anger and Berl 1986). These recently discovered effects, however, are probably only adjuncts (at least in man and dog) to the main hydroosmotic effect of AVP. They make the urine more concentrated than it otherwise would be, but are not essential to forming urine with an osmolality greater than that of plasma.

Table 8.1. Renal effects by which vasopressin may affect the concentration of urine

---

Increased permeability of the collecting duct to water
Increased sodium reabsorption in the medullary thick ascending loop of Henle
Increased permeability of the inner medullary collecting tubule to urea
Increased glomerular filtration rate
Decreased inner medullary blood flow

8.2.1 HYDROOSMOTIC ACTION OF VASOPRESSIN

The most important physiologic effect of AVP undoubtedly is its hydroosmotic action on epithelial cells of the collecting duct. These AVP-responsive structures are characterized by an extremely low permeability for water in the resting state, which is by all means necessary for the excretion of a diluted urine by the kidney. Under the action of vasopressin (and its V2 agonists) the water permeability of the rate limiting barrier, the apical (luminal) epithelial membrane, is brought to values approaching those of most plasma membranes, including the basolateral membrane of the epithelial cells (De Sousa 1986).

The first steps of the hydroosmotic response to AVP are relatively well-known (see Fig. 7.1). The binding of the hormone to its V2 receptors at the basolateral cell membrane generates cAMP in these cells, which in turn activates a cAMP dependent protein kinase. Beyond this step however, there is a chain of events that is still incompletely understood. For many years, a pore or channel has been proposed as the simplest biophysical model to account for passive water transport across biological membranes. The crucial question remained: by which mechanism, then, does AVP bring about an increase in the number of these narrow water channels in the luminal apical membrane?

Ultrastructural observations carried out in recent years led to a major break-through in this field. By using the technique of freeze-fracture on the toad urinary bladder (which is an amphibian analog of the mammalian collecting duct) Chevalier et al. (1974) were the first to report the appearence of distinctively organized clusters or aggregates in the apical membrane after vasopressin stimulation, whereas nonstimulated epithelia were devoid of such particles. Later similar structures could be demonstrated also in the collecting duct of the mammalian kidney; the number of intramembrane clusters increased as a function of AVP dose, and correlated with the value of urine osmolality

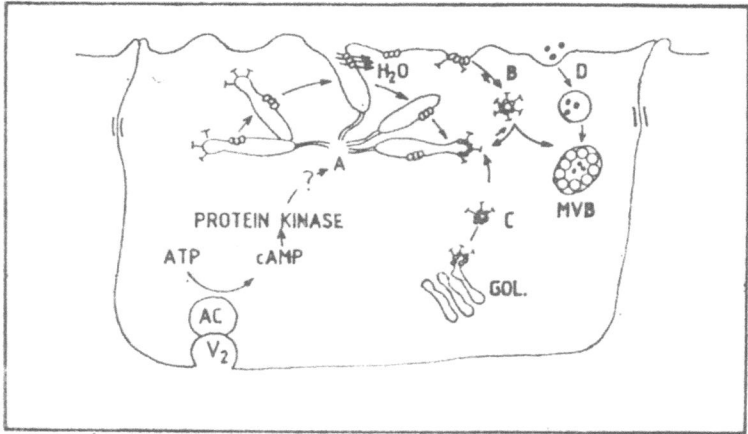

Fig. 8.5. Schematic view of some possible relationships of the aggrophores with vesicular traffic in the cell. In (A) — left to right — the aggrophores are shown in their horizontal position in the unstimulated cell; angulated after stimulation by AVP; fused and delivering particles to the luminal membrane; detached; and again horizontal after withdrawal of hormonal stimulation. (B) and (C) show two possible pathways by which coated vesicles bring aggregates to or from the membrane (B) or the Golgi (C). In (D) the pinocytic pathway for membrane recovery is shown, involving an endosome and a multivesicular body (MVB). For further details see text. Modified from Hays et al. 1987 with kind permission.

achieved under this hormonal action (Harmanci et al. 1980). Although the function of these aggregates has not been proved directly, the conviction has grown very strong that these structures represent the water channels themselves, or at least contain them. In this respect it may be interesting that no clusters could be found after vasopressin stimulation in mice with severe form of hereditary nephrogenic diabetes insipidus (the DI $+/+$ Severe strain), but clusters were detected in mice with an intermediate deficiency of urinary concentration (the DI $+/+$ Non Severe animals), although the cluster frequency was less than that found in control mice (Brown et al. 1985).

After years of focusing on the apical membrane it was recognized that the aggregates in fact exist even in cells unstimulated by AVP. These aggregates, however, are not present in the apical membrane, but subapically in the cytoplasm, where they occur in distinctive aggregate-containing tubular membrane structures, called aggrophores (Fig. 8.5). One end of the tubule is often spherical. The spherical ends of the aggrophores may be clathrin-coated vesicles indicating that the aggrophores are docking points for aggregate-containing vesicles that possibly originate from the Golgi complex. Filaments run from the sides and ends of the tubules to the surrounding cytoskeleton. Their primary function may be to anchor and to position tubules within the cytoskeleton; some of these filaments may be responsible for tubular motility. In the resting state the tubules are virtually parallel to the luminal membrane; some message convened by AVP causes their angulation. Subsequently, the intramembrane structures carried by the aggrophores are inserted into the apical membrane by an exocytosis-like process.

Thus it now appears that an important final step in the action of vasopressin involves the fusion of tubular membrane structures with the apical membrane and the insertion into this membrane of organized arrays of water channels. Conversely, after AVP removal the tubules return to their initial horizontal "resting" position, becoming available for subsequent fusions. It appears that the recovery of the vesicular membrane from the fusion with aggrophores is through some endocytosis-like process (see Fig. 8.5). In addition, evidence has accumulated indicating that the mechanism controlling membrane transport rates by an "exocytosis-like" insertion of transport units and by their subsequent "endocytosis-like" removal back to the cytoplasm is not unique property of AVP-sensitive cells, but rather represents the first example of a very general intracellular mechanism for controlling both passive permeability and active transport processes (Stenton 1984, De Sousa 1986).

8.2.2 EFFECTS OF VASOPRESSIN ON THE MEDULLARY THICK ASCENDING LIMB

Vasopressin is known to produce two effects on the amphibian urinary bladder: it increases the osmotic permeability to water and stimulates active sodium transport. In contrast, in the mammalian kidney, the active chloride (or rather sodium chloride) transport and the segment where AVP controls water reabsorption are clearly separated. In view of these anatomical differences it has been suggested that AVP might stimulate both salt and water reabsorption in the mammalian kidneys, each effect being separated in a different nephron segment, i.e. the collecting duct for the effect on water and the thick ascending limb for that on sodium chloride transport. The demonstration of vasopressin receptors in both these nephron segments (at least in rodents, see Fig. 7.2) provided some support to this hypothesis (Morel et al. 1987). Since AVP receptors are primarily located in the medullary as opposed to the cortical thick ascending limb, the effect of the hormone is to add sodium chloride to the medullary interstitium and thereby to enhance the cortico-medullary osmotic gradient. It is tempting to postulate that the greater ability of rodents to concentrate urine is dependent on this mechanism, which may be absent in the rabbit and in humans. Adenylate cyclase in the thick ascending limb however, is an order of magnitude less sensitive to AVP than that in the collecting duct, possibly reflecting the primacy of the latter effect (de Rouffignac at al. 1987).

There is another effect of AVP on the medullary thick ascending limb that results from chronic rather than acute administration of the peptide. As Trinh-Trang-Tan et al. (1987) have recently reviewed, chronic administration of dDAVP to rats with hereditary central diabetes insipidus (the Brattleboro strain) was associated with a marked increase in diameter and cellular thickness in the epithelium of the thick ascending limb. These data indicate that the presence of a normal level of AVP in blood plasma is required not only to regulate the permeability of the collecting duct to water, but also to ensure, by its trophic effect, the full morphological and functional development of the medullary thick ascending limb.

8.2.3 EFFECT OF VASOPRESSIN ON UREA PERMEABILITY IN THE INNER MEDULLARY COLLECTING TUBULE AND ON MEDULLARY RECYCLING OF UREA

Recent evidence seems to support the premise that the collecting duct does not represent a single renal tubule segment with homogenous properties, but it rather consists of at least two morphologically and functionally distinct subsegments (Kokko 1987, Sands et al. 1987). In the cortical and the outer medullary parts of the collecting duct the differential effects of vasopressin on the permeabilities to urea and water allow the concentration of urea to rise in these nephron segments as water but not urea is reabsorbed. Thus tubular fluid entering the inner medulla is very rich in urea. On the contrary, the inner medullary collecting duct and mainly its terminal part resembles, as for its permeability properties, the amphibian urinary bladder, in that in this subsegment vasopressin increases both the urea and water permeability. Vasopressin-mediated urea reabsorption in this segment provides an additional driving force to generate inner medullary hypertonicity, and serves to remove water from the urea impermeable descending limb of Henle loop.

8.2.4 EFFECT OF VASOPRESSIN ON THE GLOMERULAR FILTRATION RATE (GFR)

The delivery of tubular fluid to the diluting segment of the nephron (the ascending limb of the Henle loop) is an important determinant of interstitial tonicity (Berliner and Davidson 1957, Valtin and Edwards 1987). Evidence obtained in experiments with Brattleboro rats suggests that chronic, but not acute, administration of AVP to these animals increases the glomerular filtration rate of juxtamedullary nephrons, not influencing GFR of superficial nephrons. This effect, however, is probably not due to direct action of the hormone on the glomerular vessels; rather, it is the consequence of either a structural or functional alteration caused by its administration (Gellai et al. 1984).

8.2.5 EFFECT OF VASOPRESSIN ON INNER MEDULLARY BLOOD FLOW

Vasopressin reduces the inner medullary blood flow, both indirectly by its antidiuretic (V2 receptor mediated) action and directly by its vasoconstrictor (V1 receptor mediated) effect (chapter 9.1).

8.3 URINARY CONCENTRATION

The development of the countercurrent multiplication system and the emergence of the antidiuretic action of vasopressin were key events in vertebrate evolution contributing to the colonization of the terrestrial and even the desert environment (Smith 1959). The maximally attainable osmotic concentration of urine is limited, and is different for various animal species. For example, several species inhabiting desert areas (jerboa, pocket mouse, a.o.) are capable of raising urine osmolality to reach values as high as 4,000 mOsm/kg or even higher (Jamison 1987).

8.3.1 URINARY CONCENTRATING CAPACITY AND ITS DISTURBANCES

In healthy adults dehydration causes a rise of urine osmolality to maximal values of approximately 1,200 mOsm/kg, when the osmotic concentration index (R; urine to plasma osmolality ratio) reaches a value of about 4.

$$R = \frac{U_{osm}}{P_{osm}} \qquad \text{(equation 8.1)}$$

With regard to the renal osmoregulatory function, this index describes in fact the magnitude of the cortico-medullary osmotic gradient (i.e. the relationship between osmotic concentration at the top of the renal papilla and that at the cortico-medullary junction, see Fig. 8.4), provided the secretion of AVP is normal and the collecting tubule is sensitive to the hormone.

Stephenson (1987) performed a more detailed analysis to describe the major factors involved in processes of conservation of solute and water in the medulla in normal and pathological conditions. Straightforwardly analysing the mass balance in the medulla he arrived at an expression of the concentration ratio of urine to plasma osmolality (R) by the following dimensionless equation:

$$R = \frac{1}{(1-f_T) \times (1-f_U) \times (1-f_W)} \qquad \text{(equation 8.2)}$$

The validity of the above equation is restricted exclusively to values of $R > 1$, considering that the equation applies only to concentrating (nondiuretic) kidney. The terms on the right side of the equation describe the three major factors involved in urine concentration in terms of solute balance. The term f_T stands for the fractional solute transport out of the ascending limb of Henle loop to be added to the medullary interstitium. f_U is an index of the trend toward depletion of the medullary interstitium of solute due to urinary losses of the latter. Finally, f_W describes fractional solute dissipation from the medulla due to blood flow or, as usually called, the vascular washout of the medullary osmotic gradient.

The concentrating mechanism is complex and vulnerable to interference in many ways. It is obvious that anything that lowers the solute supply to the medulla (f_T) or enhances urinary (f_U) or vascular (f_T) solute losses, is expected to diminish the cortico-medullary osmotic gradient and thus the overall concentrating ability of the kidney. Obviously, substantial changes in each variable alone are necessary to significantly reduce (R). In a given clinical disturbance, however, usually more than one variable is affected; this is especially true for diseases that distort or destroy the medullary architecture. Anyhow, a similar approach (equation 8.2, see Table 8.2) can serve as a useful guide in pathogenetical classification of clinical disturbances of renal water conservation (Jamison and Oliver 1982).

Table 8.2. Disorders of urinary concentration (by Jamison and Oliver 1982)

1. Conditions decreasing fractional solute reabsorption by ascending limb of Henle's loop (fT)
   — loop diuretic administration
   — protein malnutrition
   — urinary tract obstruction

2. Conditions increasing urinary fractional solute excretion (fU)
   — chronic renal failure
   — diuretic administration
   — osmotic diuresis (glucose, mannitol, salt, urea)

3. Conditions increasing vascular fractional solute loss from the renal medulla (fW)
   — polydipsia
   — potassium depletion
   — acute pyelonephritis
   — hyperviscosity syndromes
   — sickle cell anemia

4. Disorders of medullary architecture that involve all three elements (fT, fU, fW)
   — advanced chronic renal failure,
   — medullary cystic disease
   — chronic interstitial obstruction
   — chronic interstitial inflammation
   — reflux nephropathy
   — uric acid nephropathy
   — analgesic abuse
   — advanced sickle cell disease

5. Conditions associated with disturbed secretion of AVP or increased tubular resistance to the hydroosmotic action of the hormone (Table 17.4)

8.4 CLINICAL EVALUATION OF RENAL CONCENTRATING PERFORMANCE

Clinical tests of renal concentrating performance were introduced into clinical routine by Korányi in 1897. His observation that patients with chronic renal disorders cannot produce urine with osmotic concentration as high as do healthy individuals, stimulated clinical interest in functional investigation of the kidneys. Unfortunately, the kryoscopic measurement of the osmotic concentration of biological fluids by freezing point depression, as he recommended, was not an easy method suitable for everyday use until the recent development of more advanced osmometers. Because of this, the freezing point measurements have been substituted, for a long time, by the simple estimation of specific gravity of urine. There is a simple linear relationship between osmolality and specific gravity if only one substance is dissolved in water. However, urine is a complex solution of many substances, and therefore the relationship between urinary osmolality and specific gravity can be taken only as a useful approximation of urine osmolality, but this substitution is not acceptable for exact studies.

8.4.1 MAXIMAL RENAL CONCENTRATING ABILITY

Under clinical conditions there are principally three ways how to test the renal concentrating ability. Approximate data can be obtained 1. by measuring osmolality of a morning urine sample, but a more exact evaluation requires standard procedures such as 2. the classic dehydration test or 3. the shortened desmopressin test. Because the renal concentrating ability depends on the age of the subject (chapters 15 and 16), the results obtained should be interpreted with respect to this age-dependency.

8.4.1.1 Evaluation of osmolality in the first morning urine sample

It is generally accepted that morning urine is relatively more concentrated, mainly due to lower fluid intake during the night hours. The age-dependent variations of morning urine osmolality are shown in Table 8.3. The relatively low mean values found in newborns and small infants (who are normally on nocturnal water supply) rapidly increase after 4 to 6 months of life to reach values typical of childhood and adult age (about 900 mOsm/kg) with a new tendency to decline after the age of 50. When a patient's morning urine osmol-

Table 8.3. Osmolality of morning urine samples (mean ± SD) (Lehotská et al. 1981b, Schück 1984)

Age (months)	Mean	SD	Age (years)	Mean	SD
− 1	227	92	15 − 20	980	107
− 2	247	97	21 − 30	988	94
− 3	239	95	31 − 40	857	210
− 4	386	165	41 − 50	860	262
− 5	513	316	51 − 60	814	200
− 6	788	440	61 − 70	703	196
− 7	847	227	71 − 80	689	150
− 8	865	279			
− 9	781	152			
− 10	759	301			
− 11	1,103	110			
− 12	1,074	267			
12 − 24	884	307			

ality on repeated examinations lags behind these informatory mean values, disturbed renal concentrating capacity should be suspected and standard concentration tests should be provided.

8.4.1.2 The classic dehydration test

In healthy subjects, urine osmolality reaches maximum values only after a prolonged period (24 to 36 hours) of strict water restriction. However, this procedure, which is greatly inconvenient for the patient is not an unavoidable attribute of clinical evaluation. Major disturbances of renal concentrating ability can be excluded, and fluid restriction discontinued already after a substantially shorter period of water deprivation if urine osmolality during the test reaches age-dependent mean values shown in Table 8.3.

The basic requirement in carrying out the water deprivation test is the certainty that the patient has no access to water. Intake of larger amounts of water during days preceding the test substantially decreases the maximal renal concentrating capacity, most likely by washout of the medullary osmotic gradient (deWardener and Herxheimer 1956). Obviously, a similar mechanism is operative in patients with polydipsic diabetes insipidus, who often show slight disturbances of maximal renal concentration capacity. However, this kind of disturbance is only transient in nature and spontaneously improves after fluid intake has normalized (chapter 17.5.2.2). Since the renal concentrating capacity is dependent also on the intensity of urine solute excretion, the content of proteins and salts in the diet should also be controlled during the test.

The examination usually begins in the evening; at 6 : 00 p.m. fluid intake is cut off. The next morning, after 12 hours of water restriction, the subject is weighted and after spontaneous voiding the first collection period begins. When on the basis of repeatedly low morning urine osmolalities a serious disturbance of the renal concentration capacity is supposed with a possible rapid development of circulatory collapse during dehydration, the test should better be started in the morning to grant a better follow-up of the clinical condition.

Urine is collected spontaneously in 4 h intervals at the beginning of the test and more frequenty, hourly, with advancing dehydration. If possible urine osmolality is measured immediately after each voiding. After each urine portion, or at least in 2 to 4 h intervals, the patient should be repeatedly weighed and pulse rate and blood pressure should be taken.

The test can be discontinued as soon as urine osmolality has reached the age-dependent mean values shown in Table 8.3 and no further testing is necessary to exclude major disturbances of the renal concentrating capacity. Otherwise, the test is terminated only after the urine osmolality has reached a plateau, as evidenced by a change of less than 30 mOsm/kg in three consecutive hourly determinations. The test should be discontinued "prematurely" (i.e. even before a plateau has been reached) if patient's body weight markedly decreases (by > 5 per cent as compared to initial pretest values) and there is a risk of dehydration-induced circulation collapse.

Any limitation of water intake for dehydration test is contraindicated in patients with advanced chronic renal disease as well as in those with chronic renal failure. As a rule, no tests are indicated in subjects showing values of endogenous creatinine clearance above 200 µmol/l. Reduction of fluid intake is also contraindicated in volume depleted and/or hypernatremic subjects; in these cases osmolality values of spontaneously voided or catheterized urine are sufficient to provide the information required. No dehydration test should be performed in patients with edematous diseases and in persons with acute infections of the urinary tract and urolithiasis. Reduction of fluid intake may provoke painful crisis in patients with sickle cell anemia. Neither newborns and infants below 4 months of age are subjected to concentration test; if unavoidable, specific pediatric modifications of the test should be employed (Poláček et al. 1965). Finally, dehydration test is potentially hazardous in patients who are not able to report thirst.

8.4.1.3 The shortened desmopressin (dDAVP) concentration test

Prolonged fluid deprivation is unpleasant for the patients and is often contraindicated. A modification of this test employing exogenous vasopressin (pitressin tannate in oil) has not found broader clinical application mainly due to the hormone's potentional V1 receptor mediated side effects (vasoconstriction, enhanced small bowel motility, etc). To circumvent these shortcomings desmopressin, a selective V2 agonist of AVP, has been introduced to test renal concentrating ability (Némethová et al. 1974, 1977, Aronson and Svenningsen 1974, Svenningsen and Aronson 1976).

Doses of 20 µg desmopressin are administered intranasally (or 1 µg subcutaneously) to both children and adults, as a rule in the morning after overnight fluid deprivation. This period of fluid restriction is usually sufficient to generate a statisfactory cortico-medullary osmotic gradient. Lower doses (10 µg intranasally) without preceding fluid restriction have been suggested for newborns and young infants. In the latter cases, only a half-amount of dietary milk should be given during the test period (Lehotská et al. 1981b).

After desmopressin administration the patients do not receive any fluids during the subsequent 4 h (with the exception of newborns and small infants). Spontaneously voided urine samples are collected in 1 h intervals during the test. The highest value of U_{osm} is taken as an index of maximal concentrating ability. As a rule, this value is reached in the 3rd or 4th urine sample. The values of urine osmolality achieved in healthy subjects of various age are given in Table 8.4. These values are usually slightly lower than those observed after prolonged (24 or 36 hours) water deprivation (Fig. 8.6); these differences probably are due to additional changes in renal hemodynamics and medullary osmolality caused by prolonged thirsting (Némethová et al. 1977, Schück 1984).

Table 8.4. Maximal urine osmolality ($\pm$ SD) after dDAVP administration (Lehotská et al. 1981b, Schück 1984)

Age (months)	Mean	SD	Age (years)	Mean	SD
—1	671	160	15—20	1,037	63
—2	742	167	21—30	1,020	120
—3	899	118	31—40	1,029	103
—4	896	213	41—50	1,026	87
—5	979	164	51—60	971	140
—6	990	223	61—70	857	72
6—12	934	178	71—80	858	79

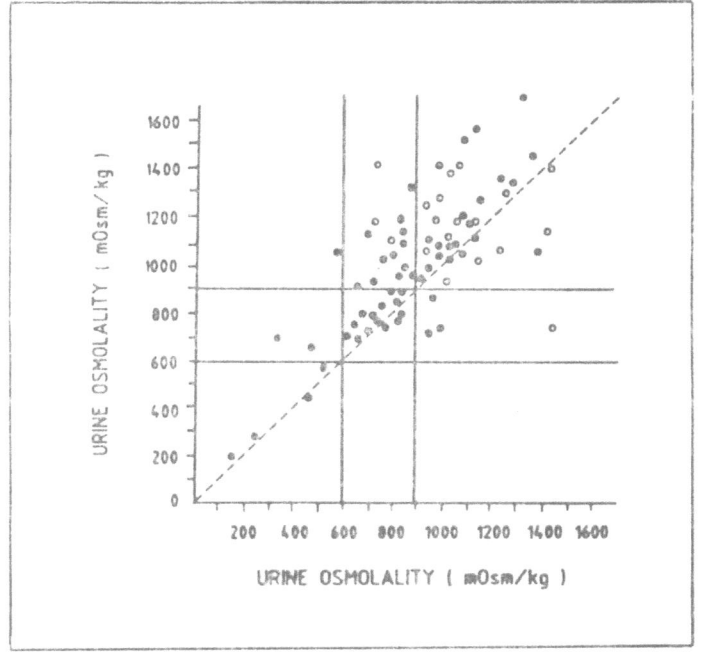

Fig. 8.6. Relationship of maximal urinary osmolality obtained during concentrating test with dDAVP (horizontal axis) and after 24 hours of thirsting (vertical axis) in children with diseases of the vesicoureteral tract (•) and in healthy children (o). If the maximal urine osmolality falls following dDAVP administration into the interval between 600 and 900 mOsm/kg, the renal concentrating ability must be reexamined also by the classic concentrating test, i.e. after 24 to 36 hours of thirsting (by Némethová et al. 1977).

For differential diagnostic purposes in patients with polyuria, the desmopressin test is usually performed after completion of the the classic dehydration test (chapter 17.5.2.2).

8.4.2 EVALUATION OF PATIENTS WITH DISTURBED RENAL CONCENTRATING ABILITY

In patients with disturbed concentrating ability additional information about the nature of the concentrating defect can be obtained by determining the relationship of urine osmolality to other indices of water and salt homeostasis and renal function (Schück 1984).

Parallel determinations of urinary and plasma osmolality (U_{osm}/P_{osm}, the osmotic concentration index) should be routinely employed to estimate the appropriateness of the renal concentrating performance on the given level of hydration of the body. The distinction between polyuric states may be ambiguous if the levels of plasma osmolality and sodium achieved during dehydration do not exceed 295 mOsm/kg and 145 mmol/l respectively, i.e. when AVP secretion was stimulated insufficiently. On the other hand, low levels of urine osmolality at abnormally high values of plasma concentrations of osmotically active substances unambiguously suggest a severely reduced renal osmoregulatory capacity (chapter 12.5.2.3).

8.4.2.1 Solute excretion rate

Although the role of solute excretion may at first look appear to be of interest only to the physiologists, it becomes clinically important in several situations, particularly in disorders in which the rate of AVP secretion is relatively constant, as it is in patients with diabetes insipidus. If, for example, solute excretion is 600 mOsm/day, but urine is persistently diluted at 60 mOsm/kg, the daily urine output will be 10 liters. One way how to treat this disorder is to reduce solute excretion by limiting dietary salt and protein, thereby reducing water excretion: in a case as mentioned above, for example by reducing daily solute excretion to only 300 mOsm a reduction of daily urine flow to 5 liters would be achieved.

Another aspect how solute excretion rate may influence the renal concentrating peformance is illustrated in Fig. 8.7. It shows that, in spite of maximal levels of circulating AVP, urinary osmolality in normal man progressively diminishes as solute excretion increases. At high rates of solute excretion urinary osmolality asymptotically approximates isotonicity even though submaximal doses of AVP are infused. Yet, with the infusion of submaximal doses of AVP in patients with central diabetes insipidus an increase in solute excretion may be associated with production of hypotonic urine (see Fig. 8.7).

It follows that measurement of the urinary excretion of osmotically active solutes is an important component of the investigation of both the concentrating and the diluting function of the kidney. The intensity of excretion of osmotically active agents is expressed in terms of the osmotic clearance (C_{osm}, chapter 8.1). In healthy adults on normal diet containing about 600 mOsm of solutes per day, the value of the osmotic clearance usually varies between 2 and 3 ml/min; any value above 4 ml/min is abnormal.

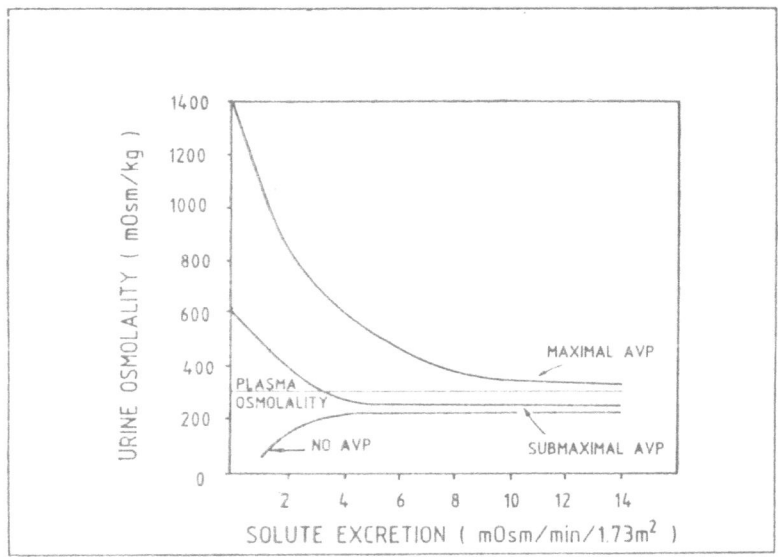

Fig. 8.7. Effect of solute exretion on renal concentrating and diluting mechanisms. Submaximal response to AVP may be due to presence of submaximal amounts of AVP or diminished response of collecting duct to maximal amounts of AVP (by Schrier and Berl 1980 with kind permission).

The part of the osmotically active solutes which were filtered in the glomeruli, but which escaped tubular reabsorption and thus were excreted into the definitive urine (fractional excretion of osmotically active solutes, FE_{osm}) can be then expressed as the ratio of C_{osm} to glomerular filration rate (GFR):

$$FE_{osm}\,(\%) = \frac{C_{osm}}{GFR} \times 100 = \frac{U_{osm}/P_{osm}}{U_{creat}/P_{creat}} \times 100 \quad \text{(equation 8.3)}$$

Because osmotic diuresis most often occurs due to sodium salts (chapter 12.5.1), in these cases it may be useful to determine the excretory fraction of sodium, FE_{Na}, representing the fraction of the filtered sodium load which is excreted in the final urine:

$$FE_{Na} (\%) = \frac{C_{Na}}{GFR} \times 100 = \frac{U_{Na}/P_{Na}}{U_{creat}/P_{creat}} \times 100 \quad \text{(equation 8.4)}$$

Calculation of FE_{osm} enables to estimate whether or not osmotic diuresis exists in the subject investigated. Mean values of FE_{osm} for healthy adults are about 2%, with 3 per cent considered the upper limit of normal. FE_{Na} in healthy volunteers on normal diet has a value of < 1 per cent; as a rule values exceeding 2 per cent are considered abnormal.

Finally, to estimate the portion of water filtered in the glomerules and reabsorbed along the nephron we need the value of the excretory fraction of water (FE_{H_2O}), or the concentration index of endogenous creatinine (P_{creat}/U_{creat}):

$$FE_{H_2O} (\%) = \frac{V}{GFR} \times 100 = \frac{P_{creat}}{U_{creat}} \times 100 \quad \text{(equation 8.5)}$$

Healthy adults on normal diet and free access to fluids show FE_{H_2O} values of about 1 per cent. With low water intake this parameter can decrease; any calculated value exceeding 2 per cent is considered abnormal. With renal disease associated with decreased GFR and osmotic diuresis, the fractional water excretion increases (Schück 1984).

8.4.2.2 Localization of the primary site of the concentrating defect along the nephron

Because solute excretion rate also determines the amount of water excreted, the quantity of free water reabsorbed is best measured directly as $-C_{H_2O}$ or $+T^c_{H_2O}$ (see chapter 8.1 for definitions), rather than being inferred solely from the urine osmolality. In humans on regular diet, the maximal $T^c_{H_2O}$ is 2 to 2.5 liters/day, while the maximum of $+C_{H_2O}$ is 10 to 20 liters/day. As water is reabsorbed along the entire collecting duct and in concentrating kidneys the hypoosmotic tubular fluid becomes isoosmotic at the cortico-medullary junction (see Fig. 8.4) maximal $+C_{H_2O}$ approximates the potential volume of water reabsorbed by the cortical collecting duct, while $T^c_{H_2O}$ represents the potential conservation of water along the medullary collecting duct (Jamison and Oliver 1982).

As it was already mentioned, reabsorption of osmotically active solutes and thus generation of solute-free water and the cortico-medullary osmotic gradient is quantitatively due mainly to reabsorption of sodium and accompanying anions in the distal diluting sites of the nephron (loop segment and early distal tubule). According to Smith's (1951) postulates, namely that 1. no further reabsorption of osmotically active solutes occurs in more distal nephron segments and 2. in the absence of vasopressin the collecting tubules are entirely impermeable to water, clearance measurements may be of value in approximating the localization of the primary site of the renal concentrating defect (nephrogenic diabetes insipidus) along the nephron. Decreased loop solute reabsorption contributes to polyuria by overwhelming the rather limited reabsorptive capacity of more distal portions of the nephron. The adequacy of loop solute transport in these cases is generally evaluated in an indirect fashion by measuring 1. negative solute-free water clearance ($-C_{H_2O}$ or $T^c_{H_2O}$) during the infusion of hypertonic saline and AVP and 2. solute-free water clearance (C_{H_2O}) and minimal urine osmolality (U_{osm} min) during maintained, steady-state water diuresis (see also chapter 8.5.2.2).

Agents that decrease C_{H_2O} (and have no effect on GFR) and increase U_{osm} min are presumed to act by inhibiting NaCl reabsorption in the ascending limb of Henle's loop. Since $T^c_{H_2O}$ is a measure of overall renal concentrating capacity (and as such is affected by defects in either cortico-medullary osmotic gradient generation or gradient utilization), it would be expected to be decreased in such circumstances. Conversely, if $T^c_{H_2O}$ is decreased, but C_{H_2O} and U_{osm} min are normal, electrolyte (and urea) delivery and transport are assumed to be adequate to allow for the generation of the osmotic gradient. Therefore an isolated abnormality in $T^c_{H_2O}$ is presumed to be due to a defect in the response of the collecting duct to vasopressin (Braden et al. 1985).

8.5 URINE DILUTION AND ITS DISTURBANCES

The organism of terrestrial animals and humans is most usually in a state requiring water conservation by forming hypertonic urine. Under certain conditions (after excessive water ingestion or following nondipsogenically administered hypotonic solutions), however water excess must be excreted by diluting urine. This is possible thanks to the fact that mammalian (and also human) kidneys have preserved during evolution the ability of their provertebrate ancestors to excrete appreciable amounts of water excess by forming urine with lower osmotic concentration than that of the plasma.

8.5.1 THE RENAL DILUTING CAPACITY AND ITS DISTURBANCES

The fact that processes of opposite direction, urine dilution and concentration, are brought about by the same renal mechanism, is a clear demonstration of the general economy of physiological processes. Urine dilution is a natural process associated with the production of solute-free water along the distal diluting sites of the nephron (the thick ascending and early distal tubule).

Simplistically, the ability to generate and excrete free water and thus produce maximally diluted urine depends on three major factors (Fig. 8.8) : 1. there must be adequate delivery of solute to the distal diluting sites of the nephron, whereby the amount of the solute delivered depends on the actual level of renal blood flow (RBF), glomerular filtration rate (GFR), as well as on the intensity of isotonic proximal water and salt resorption (see Fig. 8.8.

Table 8.5. Disorders of urinary dilution

1. Conditions decreasing solute delivery to ascending limb of Henle's loop
   — ECF volume depletion (extrarenal or renal sodium losses)
   — edematous disorders (congestive heart failure, liver cirrhosis, nephrotic syndrome)
   — chronic renal insufficiency
   — myxedema
2. Conditions decreasing solute reabsorption by ascending limb
   — loop diuretic administration
   — thiazide diuretic administration
   — adrenal insufficiency
   — Bartter's syndrome
3. Conditions associated with increased water permeability of the collecting duct
   — ECF volume depletion
   — edematous disorders
   — syndrome of inappropriate secretion of AVP (Table 20.2)

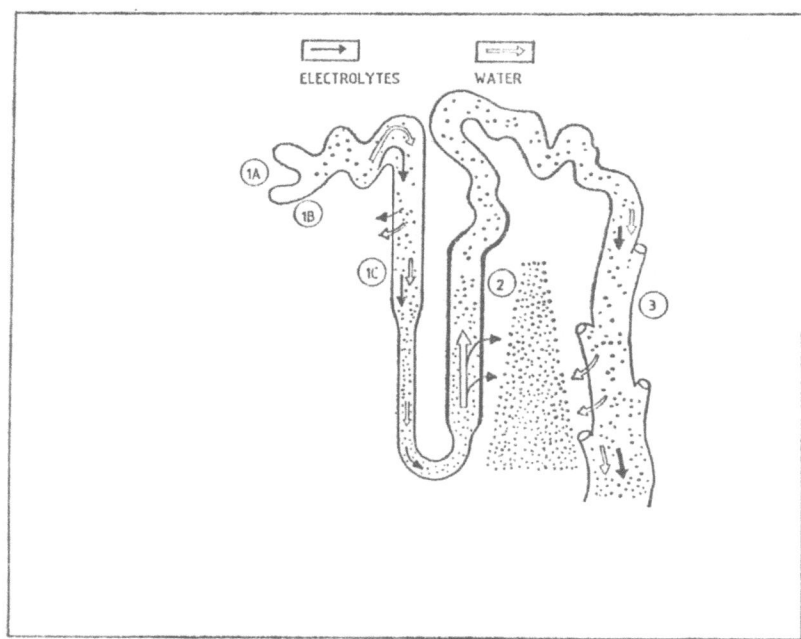

Fig. 8.8. Mechanisms of urine dilution. (1) tubular fluid delivery to the distal diluting sites — (1A) renal blood flow, (1B) glomerular filtration rate, (1C) proximal tubular reabsorption —; (2) free-water generation, (3) free-water reabsorption.

1A, 1B, 1C); 2. these distal diluting sites must be functionally intact to generate sufficient amounts of free water (see Fig. 8.8; 2). Anything that reduces fluid delivery to the collecting duct, whether diminished renal blood flow, diminished glomerular filtration rate, increased reabsorption of water by the proximal tubule, or an impaired function of the distal diluting sites, will impair urinary dilution even in the absence of AVP and, under certain conditions, completely abolish free water clearance (Berliner and Davidson 1957; Valtin and Edwards 1987). Finally, **3.** the free water generated must still escape reabsorption in the collecting duct; for this to occur there must be adequate osmotic suppression of AVP (see Fig. 8.8; 3). With this approach in mind the clinical disorders of diluting capacity can be analysed (Table 8.5); usually more than one of the above mechanisms are involved in the development of a particular clinical disorder.

8.5.2 CLINICAL EVALUATION OF RENAL DILUTING CAPACITY

The investigation of renal diluting capacity was introduced by Volhard (1910). In recent years, new interest has been growing in investigating renal diluting capacity, in particular owing to the raising frequencies of hyponatremic conditions in clinical practice.

Maximal water diuresis represents a minimal urine osmolality which an additional water load or a further decrease in P_{osm} will not further decrease. It has been assumed that this state represents the maximally attainable suppression of vasopressin release (see Fig. 5.1). The usual evaluation of the diluting capacity involves measurement of U_{osm}. Physiologically however, it would be more correct to evaluate U_{osm} in relation to P_{osm} (U_{osm}/P_{osm} ratio; osmotic concentration index). Since P_{osm} can vary only to a limited degree, the value of U_{osm} alone is usually also of clinical importance. The water excretory capacity of the kidney can be evaluated also by measuring maximal urine flow. Maximal urine flow per minute is determined as maximal level of FE_{H_2O} (equation 8.4), the value of which reaches approximately 15% during maximal water diuresis. In other words, under conditions of maximal water diuresis approximately one sixth of the total volume of fluid filtered in the glomeruli, is delivered to urine. It may be also useful to measure the time taken by the kidney to excrete some specified fraction of the administered water load. Under normal conditions, the total standard "bolus" water load (see below) is excreted within a period of 3 to 4 hours.

8.5.2.1 Maximal diluting capacity

Maximal water diuresis is usually induced by oral water load. The load can be a single "bolus" test after which the diuretic response reaches its peak for a short time only. Following bladder emptying tap water or unsweetened tea is given to drink by the subject (22 ml/kg within 30 min). Urine is collected at 30 min intervals for the next 3—4 hours. Usually, it is best to have the subject seated (except for micturition). The subject is weighed before and after the investigation. Each urine sample is measured for changes in osmolality or, for purposes of orientation only, in specific gravity. The peak urine flow rate and the minimal urine osmolality usually are observed in the third or fourth 30 min collecting period.

Once the peak is reached, a maximal diuretic state of long duration can be maintained by replacing the water losses as they occur (maintained maximal water diuresis). In this case, when urine volume is measured after the first and as many subsequent collecting periods as desired, the subject drinks the same volume as excreted plus 1 ml for each minute elapsed in the collecting period. This modification of diuretic investigation is of use in studying the action of various factors on tubular sodium reabsorption (vide infra).

Water diuresis can be induced also by infusion of hypotonic NaCl or dextrose solutions. The most frequently employed solution for these purposes is 1/2 normal (1/3 normal in infants) physiologic solution. In order to maximalize suppression of endogenous AVP secretion, a small amount of ethanol can be added. In adults the infusion rate can vary from 10 to 20 ml/min. An infusion rate of 4 ml/min/1.37 m² body surface area during 2 h has been suggested for newborns and infants (Rodriguez-Soriano 1983, Schück 1984).

Both oral and intravenous water loading is contraindicated in patients with cardiovascular disease and in patients with renal failure. Special supervision and frequent monitoring of the clinical condition and plasma sodium concentration is necessary in water load tests performed in patients with supposed marked disturbance of the renal diluting capacity (e.g. secondary to nonosmotic stimuli-induced hypervasopressinism).

8.5.2.2   Evaluation of loop solute transport

Estimates of the clearance of solute-free water, (C_{H_2O}), during induced water diuresis have become the basis of localization of the site of action of a number of substances on tubular transport of osmotically active solutes (in particular sodium) in the nephron. In agreement with Smith's views (1951) it can be assumed that during water diuresis in absence of vasopressin tubular reabsorption of water in the distal segment of the nephron (i.e. the segment distal to the diluting sites) is negligibly small. Although this point has been recently challenged (Jamison and Oliver 1982), the measurement of C_{H_2O} under conditions of maximal water diuresis has been and continues to be a useful estimate of the action of drugs on the kidney, and in studying detailed alterations in a number of pathological states (Schück 1984). During maximal diuresis C_{H_2O} approximates the reabsorption of NaCl at the distal diluting segments of the nephron and urine volume excreted (V) represents the fraction of filtrate that reaches the ascending loop of Henle. In such circumstances the sum of free water and sodium clearances, $(C_{H_2O} + C_{Na})$, provides an estimate of distal sodium chloride delivery. Finally, the percentual proportion of distal NaCl reabsorption is assessed by relating distal reabsorption to distal load $(C_{H_2O}/C_{H_2O} + C_{Na})$ (Rodriguez-Soriano et al. 1983, Schück 1984).

8.5.2.3 Solute excretion rate

The kidney's ability to excrete free water load, similarly as its concentrating capacity (chapter 8.4.2.1) depends on the rate of solute excretion. This is particularly important when there is a persistent AVP release, as with the syndrome of inappropriate secretion of AVP. If, for example, solute excretion is normal at 600 mOsm per day, but the minimum U_{osm} is 200 mOsm/kg, maximum water excretion is only 3 liters/day and water intake above this level will not be excreted. One way to enhance the excretory capacity is to increase the rate of solute excretion by using a high salt, high protein diet or by administering urea (Decaux et al. 1982). If solute excretion is increased by 50 per cent to 900 mOsm/day, water excretion will rise to 4.5 liters/day (i.e. 900 mOsm/day: 200 mOsm/kg = 4.5 l/day), thereby making water retention less likely.

Another clinical example how solute excretion rate can influence water excreting capacity is seen in some elderly patients, who are maintained on tea-and-toast diet or in small infants who are given excessively diluted formula or pure water (chapter 20.3.1.6). This is because solute-free water cannot be excreted solely; even the production of maximally diluted urine requires a minimal amount of solutes (at least 50 mOsm per liter of urine) to be excreted along with water.

9 VASOPRESSIN IN CIRCULATORY CONTROL

For decades it has generally been accepted that in mammals the physiologic role of AVP is restricted to its antidiuretic properties, whereas its cardiovascular effects are merely of pharmacologic interest. This view was challenged only sporadically until the 70ies when a series of experimental findings provided convincing evidence that AVP may play a role in the control of cardiovascular function, even under physiologic conditions. The interest in the cardiovascular effects of vasopressin has grown considerably over the past few years as documented by numerous reviews devoted to different aspects of this subject (Cowley 1982, McNeil 1983, Share and Crofton 1984, Morton and Padfield 1986, Cowley and Liard 1987, Liard 1987). Now it is well established that AVP has multiple and diverse actions on the cardiovascular system (Table 9.1), including direct vasoconstriction, augmentation of peripheral vasoconstrictor effects of sympathetic nerves and circulating catecholamines, modulation of the baroreflex and central action on cardiovascular autonomic neural centers (Liard 1987, Kvetňanský et al. 1988, Lichardus et al. 1988). All this in concert with the sympathetic nervous system and the renin-angiotensin system (and very likely the atrial and brain natriuretic peptides as well) form the important part of an integrated neurohumoral system to maintain blood pressure. When one system is removed it can be partially and sometimes completely compensated for by increasing activity in the remaining systems (McNeil 1983).

Table 9.1 Cardiovascular actions of vasopressin

Vasoconstriction of arterial smooth muscle
Central nervous system actions
Modulation of baroreflex
Autonomic functions
Interaction with sympathetic nervous system
Interactions with renin-angiotensin system
Inhibition of renal renin release
Direct cardiac effects (chronotropic, inotropic)
Antidiuretic-volume effect

9.1 VASOPRESSIN-INDUCED PERIPHERAL VASOCONSTRICTION

The in vitro and in vivo studies have established that vasopressin, acting directly through its vascular, V1 receptors, is an extremely potent constrictor of arterial and arteriolar vascular smooth muscle. As a matter of fact, on molar basis it is more potent than any other known vasoconstrictor (Altura and Altura 1984, Liard 1987). The sensitivity to vasopressin increases progressively as the vessel size decreases. In addition, there are variations in sensitivity of different vascular beds. As a consequence, plasma AVP raised in conscious dogs as little as to approximately 10 pg/ml causes profound redistribution of systemic blood flow. The skeletal muscle, cutaneous, pancreatic, thyroid and adipose tissue circulation seem the most sensitive: perfusion of these tissues decreases by about 30%. The coronary, mesenteric, iliac and brain blood flow decreases by approximately 15%, while renal and liver blood flow seems to be the least affected by AVP (Iwamoto et al. 1979, Liard 1987). Skin and skeletal muscle can easily tolerate relative ischemia during emergency situations. On the other hand, a reduction in myocardial and cerebral blood flow with relatively low levels of circulating AVP is a less desirable component of the vascular action of the hormone.

Despite the fact that the kidneys are among organs with the smallest sensitivity to the vasoconstrictor effects of AVP, there has been much interest in the action of AVP on intrarenal hemodynamics because of its possible relationship to the antidiuretic effect of the hormone (chapter 8.2.5). The medullary plasma flow was found to be 40—70% higher in water diuresis than in antidiuresis. On the other hand, physiologically increased AVP concentrations during antidiuresis reduce vasa recta flow without changes in glomerular filtration rate. This effect could be prevented by the administration of an AVP vascular antagonist (Zimmerhackl et al. 1986). AVP may thus assume a role in the regulation of intrarenal hemodynamics and renal water excretion by controlling the vasa recta flow and consequently also the level of the cortico-medullary osmotic gradient, while no measurable changes in total renal blood flow occur. This might facilitate free water excretion in the absence, or potentiate free water reabsorption in the presence, of vasopressin.

9.2 BLOOD PRESSURE

In view of the demonstration that vasopressin is the most potent vasoconstrictor agent it seemed surprising that blood pressure did not increase significantly upon infusion of vasopressin into intact conscious dogs or humans unless extremely high plasma levels (exceeding 50 pg/ml) were produced (Cowley et al. 1980, Möhring et al. 1980a, b, Montani et al. 1980). This is because AVP interacts also with the nervous control of circulation and enhances or rather facilitates powerful buffering baroreceptor reflex mechanisms which limit rises in blood pressure despite increases in total peripheral vascular resistance. The baroreflex facilitation has two components: 1. marked bradycardia and decreased cardiac output, 2. inhibited peripheral sympathetic activity and activity of the renin-angiotensin system (Cowley et al. 1974, Patel and Schmid 1987).

The conclusion that AVP facilitates baroreflexes is based on the fact that sinoaortic denervation potentiates the pressor sensitivity to AVP. Another evidence for the requirement of AVP for normal baroreceptor function comes from increased activity of the sympathetic nervous system observed in hereditary diabetes insipidus rats of the Brattleboro strain suggesting a suppressed baroreceptor function which however is correctable by the administration of AVP in even lower doses than those required to produce maximal antidiuresis (Cowley et al. 1974, Montani et al. 1980). Similar observations (i.e. pronounced increase of blood pressure following AVP administration) have been reported in human subjects with chronic orthostatic hypotension due to inadequate baroreflex function (Möhrig et al. 1980 a, b; chapter 9.4.5). It is thus apparent that in the absence of autonomic reflex control of circulation changes in vasopressin plasma concentration that are well within the physiologic range can have positive influence on arterial pressure (Cowley 1982).

9.3 EFFECTS ON THE CENTRAL NERVOUS SYSTEM

The baroreflex-induced decrease in both heart rate and cardiac output observed with the administration of AVP is far greater than usually seen with other vasoconstrictor agents. Moreover, the exaggerated pressor sensitivity to vasopressin infused after baroreceptor denervation (50—100-fold) or CNS ablation (2,000—8,000-fold) exceeds by far the enhancement of the pressor responsiveness to either angiotensin II or norepinephrine (4—6-fold) (Cowley 1982).

It thus appears that the ability of plasma vasopressin to centrally "antagonize" its own vasoconstrictor effects is directly related to the magnitude of afferent nerve activity from cardiopulmonary and arterial baroreceptors. These effects are mediated via the peripheral and central nervous system (Patel and Schmid 1987). The increase or "upregulation" of central effects of AVP is manifested in the stimulation of the vagal nerve activity, in a decreased sympathetic tone (and secondarily of the renin-angiotensin system), bradycardia and a reduced cardiac output. Thus, the rise in arterial blood pressure initiated by the direct vasoconstrictor action of the hormone is greatly attenuated. Conversely, a decreased baroreceptor afferent neural activity characteristic of hypovolemic states such as during hemorrhages, diminishes or "down-regulates" central effects of AVP. Under these conditions the vasopressin-induced bradycardia and withdrawal of the sympathetic nerve activity will be minimal and the prevailing direct vasoconstrictor effects may contribute to restoration of blood pressure. In this way baroreceptor activity would serve as the mediator of neural actions of vasopressin and enhance the feedback gain of the autonomic reflexes to better control arterial blood pressure in a variety of situations (Cowley 1982).

The vascular sensitivity to vasopressin in the absence of CNS is appreciably higher than the AVP pressor activity after only baroreceptor deafferentation. This would suggest that even in the absence of baroreflexes AVP can act somewhere in the CNS to attenuate the rise in blood pressure expected from AVP vasoconstriction. The ways (other than the baroreflex pathway) whereby circulating AVP influences elements of the nervous system remains to be better determined. The circulating hormone can probably act on areas of the brain that lack the blood-brain barrier (e.g. the periventricular organs, the area postrema of the brainstem) or alternatively, peripheral receptors could transmit information to central structures when plasma levels of AVP increase (Applegate et al. 1987, Cowley and Liard 1987). Generally speaking, the facilitation of baroreflexes is probably mediated by the effect of AVP via specific central noradrenergic nuclei. Increased baroreceptor activity (e.g. due to blood volume expansion) is associated with decreased central noradrenergic function and vice versa (decrease of baroreceptor activity, e.g. due to hemorrhage, increases central noradrenergic function). Changes of noradrenaline turnover were found in the median preoptic nucleus, nucleus tractus solitarii (NTS) and the area postrema. It is however nucleus paraventricularis (PVN) which seems to be the key integral component in the baroreflex control of sympathetic nervous system activity. It has afferent noradrenergic projections from sites belonging to the baroreflex arc (e.g. NTS).

The central vasopressinergic pathways which originates in PVN and projects to the vasomotor centers in the brainstem (areas A1, A2 and A6; see Fig. 3.3) as well as to other extrahypothalamic sites (see chapter 12) are involved in the central vasopressin control of circulation and baroreflex function. According to the present view AVP effects are mediated by V1 type receptors in the brain which however also interact with V2 agonist dDAVP.

The neurally mediated responses to endogenous brain AVP or to AVP administered intracerebroventricularly or into the specific brain areas are complementary to the action of circulating AVP (Blessing and Willoughby 1987). Centrally administered AVP induces in conscious animals an elevation of blood pressure and tachycardia (in strict contrast to peripherally acting hormone, which causes bradycardia). Thus, activation of the CNS vasopressin system obviously increases central sympathetic drive and inhibits cardiac baroreceptor reflex. It will be of interest to reveal in future the exact relationship between circulating AVP and the intracerebral vasopressinergic network.

9.4 ROLE OF VASOPRESSIN IN BLOOD PRESSURE MAINTENANCE

During the past several years considerable attention has been given to evaluating the possible role of vasopressin in blood pressure maintenance in various pathophysiological conditions.

9.4.1 VOLUME DEPLETED STATES

Data on the role of AVP in the regulation of blood pressure in volume-depleted states are contradictory. During mild dehydration in rats plasma AVP increases due to increased osmolality rather than to the reduction of blood volume (Quillen and Cowley 1983, Fejes-Tóth et al. 1985). During pronounced dehydration plasma AVP may increase up to 30 pg/ml, and similar AVP concentrations may have more pronounced hemodynamic effects and may support blood pressure.

Also in mild nonhypotensive hypovolemia due to hemorrhage plasma AVP concentrations may reach approximately 10 pg/ml and they rise inversely proportional to the decrease of left atrial pressure. Similar AVP concentrations are nevertheless sufficient to induce blood volume redistribution by inducing vasoconstriction in skeletal muscle and skin without any impact on blood pressure. In hypotensive hemorrhage, however, the high-pressure sinoaortic baroreceptors stimulate enhanced AVP release and plasma AVP concentrations may reach values of approximately 50 pg/ml if blood pressure drops to about 75 mmHg (Cowley et al. 1984a, b). In the absence of AVP in diabetes insipidus animals or after blocking V1 receptors the decrease of blood pressure may be even more pronounced (Laycok et al. 1979, Cowley and Liard 1987). These data fit the concept that AVP is involved in blood pressure support during hemorrhage.

It is important to stress, however, that dogs may have a better chance to survive shock secondary to severe hemorrhage if deprived of AVP or its effects or if applied the converting enzyme inhibitor. This means that alleviation of vasoconstriction in shock may have a rather beneficial effect (Errington and Rocha e Silva 1974). In contrast, Altura (1976a, b) found, that Brattleboro rats with hereditary lack of circulating vasopressin are extremely sensitive to hemorrhagic shock as well as to bowel ischemic shock. Beneficial effect in these animals may have V1 receptor agonists with postarteriolar site of action (e.g. triglycyl-vasopressin) which have been shown to increase tissue perfusion and thus the chance to survive traumatic and hemorrhagic shock (Lichardus and Vigaš 1968, Altura 1976a, b). In addition Brackett et al. (1983) reported that Brattleboro rats showed a much larger blood pressure decrease in early endotoxin shock and did not recover, also suggesting a beneficial effect of vasopressin in this form of shock. This question is of clinical significance because vasopressin is often used in man in the treatment of gastrointestinal or bronchial bleeding, which represent states of hypovolemic hypotension (vide infra).

9.4.2 GASTROINTESTINAL BLEEDING

For the last 20 years, intravenously or intraarterially administered vasopressin has become an important agent for the emergency therapy of bleeding esophageal varices (Hussey 1985, Sherlock 1987, Snady 1987). Vasopressin by his constrictive effect on the splanchnic vessels reduces blood flow and pressure in the portal vein thereby diminishing or arresting bleeding from variceal sources (Ohnishi et al. 1987). It is also possible that some V2- effects of the hormone and its analogs also contribute to the hemostatic action (chapter 10.4.3). However, the effectiveness of the treatment remains controversial and, unfortunately, both systemic intravenous and superior mesenteric arterial infusion of V1 agonists are associated with multiple adverse hemodynamic effects on the heart and the systemic circulation. Myocardial ischemia, cardiac dysfunction, ventricular arrhythmia are the most frequent complications encountered with this therapy (Boyle and Segel 1986). The failure of vasopressin therapy to improve survival, despite the control of bleeding from esophageal varices, may be partly due to these undesired side effects. Recently, evidence has been presented that the addition of nitroglycerin to i.v. infusion of vasopressin reversed the detrimental side effects of the peptide with the beneficial effects being preserved (Groszmann et al. 1982).

9.4.3 ARTERIAL HYPERTENSION; SIADH

Slightly elevated AVP levels have been reported in both experimental hypertension (DOCA-salt or genetic hypertension in spontaneously hypertensive rats of the Okamoto strain but not of the New Zealand strain; in renal one-kidney-one-clip and two-kidney-one-clip hypertension) and human arterial hypertension. Nevertheless, the understanding of the role of AVP in the mechanism of chronic blood pressure elevation is by now inconclusive (Cowley and Liard 1987). The involvement of AVP in the pathomechanism of various forms of hypertension may be via its impact on body fluid volumes, on the distribution of effective blood volume in the organism, on the sensitivity of the vascular bed to other vasoconstrictor agents, or on the activity of the cerebral cardio-regulatory system (Gardiner and Bennett, 1983, Cowley and Liard 1987). Administration of AVP antagonists is associated with only a short-lived blood pressure decrease in any of the above types of hypertension.

Neither patients with the syndrome of inappropriate antidiuretic hormone secretion (SIADH) have elevated blood pressure (Morton and Padfield 1986).

It is obvious that the understanding of the role of AVP ir the pathomechanism of arterial hypertension is dependent on a more detailed than currently
knowledge of the entire mosaic of elements concerning the pathomechanism
of the disturbance.

9.4.4 CONGESTIVE HEART FAILURE

Congestive heart failure is characterized hemodynamically by a rised total
peripheral resistance which helps to maintain blood pressure, sometimes at the
expense of cardiac output. This increase in total peripheral resistance is due to
activation of both the sympathetic nervous system and the renin-angiotensin-
aldosterone system. The third major hormonal system, important in the
maintenance of blood pressure and water balance is vasopressin. Nonosmotically elevated AVP secretion, reported in patients with congestive heart failure
and in some experimental models of heart failure (Kortas et al. 1986) can lead
to water retention and contribute to the development of hyponatremia frequently seen in patients with this disorder (chapter 20.3.3.1). Small increases in
circulating arginine-vasopressin can also contribute to the raised peripheral
vascular resistance in heart failure, all the more because there may be an
increased sensitivity to vascular effects of AVP due to an abnormally attenuated baroreflex (Ferguson et al. 1984, Goldsmith et al. 1986a, b). On the basis
of these data it is possible that — similarly as with the renin-angiotensin-
aldosterone system and converting enzyme inhibiton — therapy targeted at
arginine-vasopressin mediated vasoconstriction might prove to be another
step in the rational design of specific vasodilator treatment for some patients
with this disease (Creager et al. 1986).

9.4.5 CHRONIC ORTHOSTATIC HYPOTENSION
(AUTONOMIC FAILURE)

Disruption of the afferent baroreceptor pathways or of their central connections
to the magnocellular neurons results in impaired hemodynamic stimulation
of vasopressin secretion. Such an association has already been demonstrated
in patients with some forms of chronic orthostatic hypotension (e.g. Shy-Drager
syndrome) as well as in otherwise healthy very old people (Rowe et al. 1982,
Zerbe et al. 1983). In addition to attenuated vasopressin response to hemodynamic changes these patients exhibit also an increased pressor sensitivity
to endogenous or exogenous AVP: increases in AVP levels within the physiologic range can raise blood pressure as much as by 40 mmHg (Möhring et al.
1980b, Williams et al. 1986). Fluid and electrolyte homeostasis are also disturbed in patients with autonomic insufficiency. They cannot concentrate urine

during overnight recumbent dehydration or produce diluted urine during upright rehydration. The nocturnal diuresis and natriuresis lead to extracellular fluid depletion and a profound intensification of orthostatic symptoms on rising in the morning. Sleeping with the head and trunk raised 20 per cent reduces nocturnal diuresis and tends to restore fluid volume and reduce orthostatic symptoms. This is a single most important measure in treating patients with chronic orthostatic hypotension secondary to autonomic insufficiency. Drug treatment may be necessary if tilting the bed at night does not produce improvement. Drugs that increase extracellular fluid volume (e.g. hydrocortisone) are those of choice. Recently the possibility of employing desmopressin for the treatment of these patients has also been investigated. In a short-term study, patients given dDAVP at night had less nocturnal diuresis and weight loss, and their daytime blood pressure improved. Unfortunately, water intoxication developed in a patient, resembling the syndrome of inappropriate secretion of vasopressin. Only long term studies using intranasal dDAVP administration will show whether this drug is useful for these purposes (Onrot et al. 1986).

10   VASOPRESSIN AND HEMOSTASIS

Some rather unexpected extrarenal efects of AVP to improve blood clotting processes have been reported by Mannucci et al. (1975, 1981). Also, it has been noted that the V2 agonist dDAVP has a similar activity (Table 10.1). As could be expected, these reports gave a major impetus to efforts to apply the hemostatic effects of vasopressin to the treatment of various bleeding disorders. Patients with significant coagulation defects need blood derivates rich in the respective factor they lack during bleeding episodes or, prophylactically, during surgery. The limited supply of blood products but mainly the risk of infection with transmissible agents such as non-A, non-B hepatitis and acquired immune deficiency syndrome (AIDS) made the search for reasonable alternatives to treatment with blood products imperative. As a result of this effort, dDAVP has now become a safe and effective alternative to the use of blood products for individuals with mild to moderate hemophilia A, in many subjects with von Willebrand's disease as well as in those with various forms of secondary bleeding disorders (Mannucci et al. 1977, Lusher and Warnier 1984, Kobrinsky et al. 1984).

Table 10.1 Hemostatic effects of vasopressin

Factor VIII release
VonWillebrand's factor release
Increased fibrinolysis
Platelet aggregation
Direct vasoconstriction

10.1   VASOPRESSIN AND FACTOR VIII COMPLEX

Vasopressin can affect hemostasis in several different ways (see Table 10.1). Probably the best characterized effect of the hormone concerns its ability to induce a dose-dependent short-lasting increase in all factor VIII-related activities in plasma, i.e. factor VIII (FVIII), a glycoprotein, which is deficient

114

in hemophilia A and von Willebrand's factor (VWF), a multimeric protein involved in platelet adhesion, which is either reduced or abnormal in von Willebrand's disease (VWD) (Nussey et al. 1986a, b). FVIII circulating in blood is in a non-covalently linked complex with multimeric VWF which has VWF:Ag (VWF:Antigen) and VWF:RCo (VWF:Ristocetin Cofactor) activities, the latter being related to bleeding time. Although it is known that VWF is synthesized in vascular endothelial cells, the site of FVIII synthesis is uncertain, though a hepatic source is likely (Peake 1984).

The physiologic processes controlling circulating levels of FVIII, VWF:Ag and VWF:RCo activities are uncertain. Increases in factor VIII-related activities occur at relatively high concentrations of AVP only (about 15 pg/ml) (Nussey et al. 1986a), i.e. at levels usually found in the plasma during hypotension, hypovolemia and/or nausea. Studies in healthy volunteers repeatedly confirmed that desmopressin (dDAVP) administered in a single intravenous dose also raises the activities of FVIII, VWF: Ag and VWF:RCo as rapidly as within 30 min, maximal values being achieved within 2 hours. When various doses were tried, i.v. dDAVP was found to produce maximal response in doses 0.3 µg/kg body weight; with this dose the individual activities were 3 to 5 times higher as compared to the respective initial values. When administered intranasally, approximately 10 times larger doses of dDAVP had to be given to obtain similar, albeit less consistent, effects. The maximum effect in each case lasted relatively short, the half disappearance time of these blood clotting factors was 5 to 8 hours. In order to study the effect of prolonged administration of dDAVP five daily infusions of this V2 analog were given to healthy volunteers (Mannucci et al. 1981). Following the second and third dose the responses were significantly reduced. There was, however a tendency to return to the initial response strength by the fourth day.

The above cited observations offer an insight as to the nature of the hormone's action as well. The rise of all components of the FVIII system produced by AVP or dDAVP occurs as rapidly that increased synthesis is unlikely to account for it; thus the release from endogenous sources seems more likely. Furthermore the high potency of dDAVP strongly suggests that V2 receptors are involved in both FVIII and VWF release. Indeed, studies in conscious dogs given various structural analogs of vasopressin failed so far to separate the FVIII-releasing and the antidiuretic activities of the peptide (Vilhardt 1988).

10.2 VASOPRESSIN AND FIBRINOLYSIS

Using dDAVP to release factor VIII there is always the risk of fibrinolytic degradation due to the concomitant release of plasminogen activator from the endogenous sources. The time course of the latter effect is however somewhat different. Following intravenous dDAVP the plasminogen activator reaches its maximum levels already within 10 min. The response of the fibrinolytic system to dDAVP is analogous to that occurring during venous occlusion or after physical exercise. Hence, desmopressin has been successfully administered to evaluate fibrinolytic capacity in patients with venous thrombosis (Brommer et al. 1982).

10.3 VASOPRESSIN AND PLATELET FUNCTION

Platelet-rich fractions of blood contain much of the circulating AVP. Platelet-associated AVP is taken up from the plasma and it originates in the hypothalamus. At high circulating levels the platelet-associated fraction of the hormone is clearly increased as compared to the platelet-poor fraction. Hence, platelets may play a role in the rapid clearance of vasopressin from the circulation. Single platelet AVP measurements could eventually provide some information about the long-term stimulation of the hypothalamo-neurohypophyseal AVP system (Bichet et al. 1987).

On the other hand, AVP taken up by the platelets may play a role in modulating platelet function. Platelets possess AVP receptors of the V1 type and undergo changes in cytosolic free calcium and inositol lipids in the presence of the peptide. However, in vitro concentrations of more than 2 ng/ml (such high levels are actually never seen in any pathophysiologic circumstances) are required to induce platelet aggregation or significant changes in platelet biochemistry (Nussey et al. 1986b). Nevertheless, further observations and experiments are required to determine the in vivo effects of the hormone when a "network" of different signals in the locality of an endothelial lesion might potentiate the platelet response to AVP (Nieuwenhuis and Sixma 1988).

10.4 CLINICAL EXPERIENCE WITH DESMOPRESSIN IN THE TREATMENT OF VARIOUS BLEEDING DISORDERS

In recent years desmopressin has been used in the treatment of various bleeding disorders. In order to prepare improved factor VIII concentrates dDAVP can be administered also to blood donors (Mikaelsson et al. 1984). This approach is valuable in reducing the quantity of blood products needed in the treatment of bleeding disorders and thus in reducing, but not eliminating, the risk of infections with transmissible agents. In an effort to eliminate this risk, it seems better to administer desmopressin directly to patients who respond to this drug. In view of the less predictable response to subsequent doses when the drug is given for several days in succession (Mannucci et al. 1981), it is wise to limit this form of treatment to situations in which a short-time increase in

FVIII complex is expected to be sufficient. These situations include early acute hemarthros in individuals with mild or moderate hemophilia A, and tonsillectomy, teeth extractions and other oral and nasal surgical interventions in individuals with mild to moderate hemophilia A and von Willebrand's disease. In the latter cases, the administration of dDAVP (0.3 µg/kg intravenously or the respective intranasal dose) should immediately be followed by epsilon-aminocapronic acid (EACA) or tranexamic acid to inhibit the enhanced fibrinolytic activity (Lusher and Warrnier 1984).

10.4.1   VON WILLEBRAND'S DISEASE

Probably the greatest attention has been paid to the therapeutic efficacy of dDAVP in von Willebrand's disease. This is a dominantly inherited disease characterized by prolonged bleeding time; at least three different variants of the disease are known. Approximately 70 per cent of the patients suffer from the classic (type I or quantitative type) variant with subnormal amounts of functionally normal FVIII complexes. A beneficial effect of desmopressin in these cases is likely. The drug causes transitorily shortened bleeding time, raises FVIII and VWF:RCo activities and the hemorrhage ceases (Mannucci et al. 1977, Ruggeri et al. 1982). However, in some severely affected subjects from this group (i.e. those with no detectable FVIII complex activity to start with), the storage sites are empty, and the drug will have no significant therapeutic effect. In another, less frequent variant (type IIA) the hemostatic defect is due to abnormal molecular forms of VWF. In these cases desmopressin may shorten but not normalize bleeding time (Ludlam et al. 1980). Finally, dDAVP is not indicated in von Willebrand's disease type IIB, as the drug may cause platelet aggregation and thrombocytopenia due to the release of a platelet aggregating factor (Holmberg et al. 1983).

Hence, prior to starting dDAVP administration for spontaneous bleeding or in surgical situations the type of the disease present in the patient should be determined. Similarly as in other hemostatic indications of desmopressin, the effectivity of the treatment should (if possible) be tested by giving a test dose during the resting phase or preoperatively to see if there is any correction of bleeding time after the drug. The disadvantages of intravenous administration might be avoided by the recently suggested possibility of oral administration of the drug. However, it should be remembered that the effect of oral administration can be expected to occur but after at least 5—10-fold peptide doses as compared to the intranasal route. This approach raises the costs of the therapy; nevertheless the costs still remain much lower than those of blood products used for the same purpose.

10.4.2 HEMOPHILIA A

In healthy volunteers the increase in FVIII complex activities depend on the subject's initial values (chapter 10.1), and the same is true for patients with hemophilia A. The clinical severity of this inherited disease mainly depends on the level of FVIII. In severe cases less than 1—2% of normal values are found whereas moderate and mild cases have 2—5% and 6—30% of normal activity respectively. Because dDAVP raises factor VIII concentrations 3—5 times (Mannucci et al. 1981), it can be expected to induce hemostatically effective levels mainly in patients with initial levels higher than 2 per cent. Traumatic and/or spontaneous bleedings in patients with hemophilia may often occur under conditions that do not enable immediate administration of kryoprecipitates (when out of home, during trips, etc.). Then desmopressin can be the drug of the first aid which attenuates, or even completely stops, bleeding thus decreasing the dependence of the patient on blood products.

The question of efficacy of dDAVP in patients with severe hemophilia A remains still open. The majority of investigators consider administration of dDAVP to these patients ineffective to elevate factor VIII level, although they admit that the drug favorably influences the bleeding intensity (Sutor 1978, Markwick 1983). A similar situation also occurs in patients with circulating inhibitor of factor VIII. Because hemorrhagic incidents are difficult to manage in such patients, the efficacy of dDAVP has been repetitively tried after failure of other therapeutic methods. In some patients the coagulation time in partially activated thromboplastin test temporarily shortened and bleeding stopped, although the inhibitor level stayed uninfluenced (Sutor 1980a, b, de la Fuente et al. 1985). Thus, the final evaluation concerning the efficacy of desmopressin therapy in patients with severe form of hemophilia A and with factors VIII inhibitor still awaits a new mode of evaluation, which would apprehend more precisely the changes in coagulation. The discrepancy between laboratory and clinical results raises the question, whether the effect of dDAVP upon factor VIII activity is not just a component of its wider intervention into the hemostasis. This assumption is consistent with some recent experimental evidence as well as with the newly demonstrated capacity of the V2 agonist desmopressin to improve hemostasis also in patients with apparently normal factor VIII complex-related activities (see below).

10.4.3 VARIOUS BLEEDING DISORDERS

Also, desmopressin appears to effectively prevent excessive bleeding during minor surgical operations as well as in the treatment of acute hemorrhage accompanying conditions characterized by normal or even high levels of factor VIII. Shortening of bleeding time and of partial thromboplastin time in patients with renal failure and liver cirrhosis, improvement of platelet adhesivity and correction of bleeding time in patients after overdosage of acetylsalicylic acid as well as in those with thrombocytopenia due to storage pool deficiency, after desmopressin might at least partially result from dDAVP-induced increase in VWF:RCo levels. In addition, in a randomized doubble blind clinical trial desmopressin was shown to effectively reduce intra-operative blood losses even in hemostatically normal subjects (Kobrinsky et al. 1984, 1987, Bourroughs et al. 1985, Salzman et al. 1986).

11 VASOPRESSIN AND ANTERIOR PITUITARY FUNCTION

The parvocellular neurosecretory system consists of neurons localized in more or less discrete clusters in the hypothalamus and the basal forebrain, and in their axial projections which end on portal vessels in the external lamina of the median eminence. Via these pathways peptides and amines are delivered to the portal circulation and act to stimulate or inhibit (liberins and statins respectively) the release of anterior pituitary hormones. The view that vasopressin, as another hypothalamic releasing factor, may be involved in the physiological regulation of anterior pituitary function (for review see Hedge and Huffman 1987) has been substantiated by the established projections originating from a distinct subpopulation of parvocellular paraventricular vasopressinergic neurons to the hypophyseal portal circulation (chapter 3.1.2.2).

11.1 VASOPRESSIN AND ADRENOCORTICOTROPIC HORMONE (ACTH) RELEASE

Adrenocorticotropin (ACTH) release has long been recognized as an indicator of a state of stress. Exposure to stressors has been used extensively in studies of the central control mechanisms of ACTH secretion. However, behind the seemingly uniform acute hormonal responses to stress, the trigger may be any of a number of mediators with separate regulatory mechanisms. Since the identification of the corticotropin-releasing factor (CRF) by Vale et al. (1981) it has become evident that, although it is the dominant component in stress-induced release of ACTH, other components may also play important roles (Makara 1985). In a number of studies vasopressin has been reported to potentiate the ACTH secretory potency of CRF, indicating the importance of AVP for the full expression of the anterior pituitary response to stressful stimuli (Tilders et al. 1985, Schwartz and Vale 1988).

An interesting but in physiological terms not fully explored fact is that about half of the CRF producing neurons (i.e. those localized in the median parvocellular subdivision of PVN) release both AVP and CRF into the hypophyseal portal circulation (Whitnall and Gainer 1988). Manipulations of the pituitary-adrenal axis and water balance had differential effects on these neurons, indicating adrenal steroids as primary regulators of both CRF and AVP expression in this system (Sawchenko 1987).

The site of action of AVP in the anterior pituitary is not precisely known. Targets for AVP may be corticotrops or anterior pituitary cells which do not contain ACTH, but act in some paracrine fashion to influence ACTH secretion. Another possibility is that both AVP and CRF act on the same cells. In these cases the primary mechanism by which they operate seems distinct to the point that one can remain operating despite elimination of the other (Schwartz and Vale, 1988). There have been several attempts to categorize anterior pituitary receptors based on the binding of receptor antagonists. Using this approach several investigators suggested that the anterior pituitary vasopressin receptors are neither the V2 nor the "classical" V1 (or V1a) receptors; and that they represent a novel **V3 or V1b**-type receptor (Antoni et al. 1984, Jard et al 1988).

Since blood sampled from individual hypophyseal portal vessels of monkeys showed AVP concentrations 1,000 times higher as compared with the circulating levels of the hormone (Zimmermann et al. 1973) and since AVP secretion from the neurohypophysis and vasopressin release into the portal circulation are under different control mechanisms, it is still doubtful whether plasma AVP concentrations are sufficient to modulate ACTH secretion. Recently an additive effect on ACTH stimulation by human CRF and hypertonic saline infusion have been observed in a large number of normal subjects suggesting physiological importance of this synergism (Milsom et al. 1985, Bahr et al. 1988). On this basis a clinical test including human CRF and AVP injections has been recommended as an alternative to ACTH stimulation by insulin-induced hypoglycemia (Sandler et al. 1986).

In relation to human pathology it appears that if a syndrome of inappropriate hyperactivity of the CRF-AVP system exists, it would be manifested by symptoms similar to those which have already been described in patients with the so-called syndrome of periodic adrenocorticotropin and vasopressin discharge (Sato et al. 1982).

It is believed that stress is associated with elevated plasma AVP concentrations (chapter 5.4.8). On the other hand it has been also supposed that the stress of the underlying illness and/or hospitalization may have led to non-osmotically enhanced AVP secretion in many normovolemic patients (chapter 19.1). For the hypophyseal-portal capillaries that constitute a part of the general circulation it is quite possible that the stress-induced release of AVP (and CRF) from the median eminence might account, at least partly, for the osmotically nonsuppressible plasma AVP levels (vasopressin "leak" in Fig. 20.3) in some of these subjects, although the partial clinical significance of this mechanism has not as yet been specifically tested.

11.2 VASOPRESSIN AND OTHER ANTERIOR PITUITARY HORMONES

More than 20 years ago, vasopressin was characterized as a thyrotropin releasing hormone (TRH). This idea was essentially no further explored after the elucidation of the structure and synthesis of the natural TRH. Recently Lumpkin (1987) reinforced this view suggesting that circulating AVP at physiologic concentrations acts specifically on anterior pituitary cells to enhance the release of TRH. Moreover, AVP was found to be equipotent with TRH, indicating a physiological role of the nonapeptide in promoting thyrotropin (TSH) release. When injected intrahypothalamically, however, AVP specifically inhibited TSH. Thus central and peripheral vasopressin may have differential effects on TSH release.

Interestingly, all of the originally postulated hypothalamic hypophyseotropic hormones that regulate anterior pituitary function have now been isolated and identified except for prolactin releasing factor (PRF). Considerable evidence supports the existence of PRF which is thought to be essential for the large release of prolactin that follows suckling. Several peptides (vasoactive intestinal peptide, oxytocin and TRH) have been nominated to serve such a role based on the ability of their antisera to attenuate suckling-induced prolactin release. Recent experiments have suggested that the 39 amino-acid glycopeptide which is formed from the vasopressin-neurophysin precursor (chapter 2.4.2) is a potent stimulator of prolactin release, without affecting other aspects of anterior pituitary function (Nagy et al. 1988).

12 VASOPRESSIN AND BRAIN FUNCTION

Vasopressin, a peptide of neural origin, which had been transmitting primitive messages in prehistoric brains for millions of years, was selected, on a certain level of evolution, to mediate a new signal for water conservation. This decisive revolutionary change however did not mean the loss of the original neural functions of the nonapeptide; AVP has remained an important member in cell-to-cell communication in the central nervous system. There is now considerable evidence that vasopressinergic nerve fibers originating mainly in the parvocellular subdivisions of the paraventricular nucleus and, to a lesser degree, in other hypothalamic vasopressinergic neurons project to many brain regions other than the neural lobe (chapter 3.1.2.3). Many pertinent neurotransmitter criteria have already been shown to be met by this agent, and increasing evidence for AVP functions within the CNS that are separate from its well known peripheral functions on salt and water balance has accumulated (Barchas et al. 1978, Riphagen and Pittman 1986, VanLeeuven 1987).

12.1 VASOPRESSIN IN CEREBROSPINAL FLUID

Since the brain extracellular fluid communicates freely with the cerebrospinal fluid (CSF) and the blood-brain barrier effectively restricts the movement of the hydrophilic peptide from the systemic circulation into the CSF (Ang and Jenkins 1982) one strategy to better understand the central functions of AVP is to monitor its concentrations in the CSF (chapter 6.2.3). CSF studies have been criticized because of the difficulties in correlating measurements of CSF AVP levels with the hormone concentrations at various brain sites. Nevertheless, despite their limitations CSF studies are convenient and in clinical settings almost the only possible method to study the release of AVP within the brain (Jenkins et al. 1980, Garcia et al. 1981, Sørensen 1986).

12.1.1 THE ROLE OF CSF VASOPRESSIN

The problem whether AVP in the CSF has any physiological function has not been solved as yet. At least some AVP may well be secreted directly into the CSF (Dogterom et al. 1977) which then might have a function of a transport vehicle to distant target areas. If this is true, any physiologic function regulated by changes in the AVP CSF concentrations can be expected to be influenced by administration into the cerebral ventricles of AVP in amounts that only cause changes in the CSF AVP concentration within physiological range. However, the role of CSF as a neurosecretory pathway has not yet been convincingly established. It is more likely that AVP in the CSF may represent peptide released from various sites within the brain and transported via the brain's extracellular fluid to the CSF which would then serve to remove substances from the target sites. The CSF AVP level would then merely indicate the integrated level of activity of the vasopressinergic system projecting inside the CNS, and the concentrations in the CSF would be lower than the local concentrations at any given central target site. In such a case, investigations of any physiologic effect of AVP within the brain would imply intraventricular administration of large doses of exogenous AVP to obtain effective concentrations at the site of action owing to the slow diffusion rate through the cerebral extracellular fluid. The latter possibility is supported by experiments in which vasopressin infusions were most active in behavioral (Kovács et al. 1979, Van Wimersma Greidanus et al. 1986) or other physiological processes (Cooper et al. 1979) when injected directly into brain regions that contain dense AVP innervation.

12.1.2 REGULATION OF VASOPRESSIN SECRETION INTO THE CSF

Separate neurons are responsible for the peptide occurring in the CSF and in blood, and they are regulated by different control mechanisms. Various stimuli that increase blood vasopressin concentration caused either no changes in CSF AVP or, when stimulatory effects were found, vasopressin released into the CSF had a higher threshold than that released in the blood (Sczepánska-Sádowska et al. 1983). Recently Stark et al. (1984) reported that severe hypoxia in sheep led to a pronounced increase in AVP in both CSF and plasma. Again, the increase in CSF vasopressin was delayed in time and was of a less magnitude that the respective increase in plasma. This increase may be due to the peptide leaking from blood in the CSF (which has not yet been studied under extreme conditions that might alter the blood-brain barrier permeability) or, rather, to "spillover" of vasopressin into the cerebral extracellular fluid following synaptic activity in brain regions that normally do not contribute to peptide levels in CSF. In addition, certain factors have been reported to influence AVP levels in the CSF but not in plasma; for example in smaller animals highly organized diurnal rhythms have been observed in the CSF but not in plasma.

12.1.3   CIRCADIAN REGULATION OF CSF VASOPRESSIN

Since its initial discovery in cats the robust endogenously generated daily rhythms of AVP with peak levels during daylight hours have been detected in various mammalian species, including rats, rabbits and sheep; a less prominent rhythm has been found in monkeys, while it is actually absent in humans (Reppert et al. 1987).

The rhythmic nature of vasopressin concentrations in CSF focused attention on the vasopressin containing neurons of the suprachiasmatic nuclei (SCN; see chapter 3.1.1.3) since this region of the hypothalamus may play a critical role as an overall integrator of circadian rhythmicity or as a hierarchical oscillator that imposes phase information on other circadian clocks in mammals (Turek 1985). Earnest and Sladek (1986) demonstrated that SCN explants rhythmically release vasopressin in vitro, and the phase or the rhythm in AVP release from isolated SCN neurons is similar to that observed in the CSF of the donor animal.

12.1.4   VASOPRESSIN IN HUMAN CSF

Elevated levels of CSF AVP can be found in several groups of patients with cerebral disorders associated with increased intracranial pressure (e.g. in those with subarachnoidal hemorrhage, benign intracranial hypertension or meningitis), and the concentrations of AVP in the CSF are directly proportional to the level of the intracranial pressure (Sørensen 1986). These findings are compatible with the proposal that abnormal CSF AVP levels are the result of an increased intracranial pressure (Gauflin et al. 1977). The increased CSF AVP in turn may be involved in the regulation of intracranial pressure and brain water content (Raichle and Grubb 1978, Dóczi et al. 1984). Anorexia nervosa patients were characterized by relatively elevated levels of AVP in the CSF, whereas oxytocin levels were depressed in these subjects. CSF vasopressin levels were also elevated in mania, again with oxytocin shifted in the opposite direction (Gold et al. 1981, 1983a). The reason of these changes is not known, but they might be related to the proposed behavioral effects of AVP and oxytocin.

It might be tempting to regard reduced CSF AVP levels found in aged subjects and in patients with degenerative dementia and Parkinson's disease as supporting the theory which involves AVP in learning and memory processes. However, it must be emphasized that the low CSF AVP in these subjects might be a nonspecific phenomenon accompanying the diffuse loss of cells in the central nervous system (Swaab et al. 1987).

12.2 VASOPRESSIN AND MEMORY

The finding that neurohypophyseal peptides interfere with brain processes related to memory may be regarded as a milestone in neuroendocrinologic research. The pioneering work of deWied and his coworkers stimulated the research in this field and has resulted in the formulation of the neuropeptide concept (DeWied 1984) with the hypothesis that peptides from the brain act directly on the CNS partly after the generation of smaller, more potent and more selectively acting molecules from vasopressin, oxytocin and adreno-corticotrophic hormone.

12.2.1 BEHAVIORAL EFFECTS OF VASOPRESSIN

Peripherally or centrally (intracerebrally or intracerebroventricularly) injected vasopressin has been shown to induce in a rat model marked behavioral effects by affecting the cerebral substrate of learning and memory (for review see Van Wimersma-Greidanus et al. 1986). The peptide improves the performance of normal rats in a variety of behavioral paradigms that measure the acquisition and retention of aversely motivated behavior; in some reports the hormone seemed to affect also positively rewarded behavior. The majority of these relatively complex tasks may be explained by stimulatory influences of the neuropeptide on memory processes involved in information storage and retrieval. In addition, rats characterized by a decrease or lack of endogenous AVP (after neurohypophysectomy; in the Brattleboro rat with hereditary defects in the production of vasopressin or following intracerebroventricular, but not peripheral, administration of vasopressin antiserum) demonstrate impaired performance on learning and memory tasks. In these animals the impaired behavior could be restored by treatment with vasopressin and/or its congeners.

12.2.2 RELATIONSHIP OF AVP TO OTHER BEHAVIORALLY ACTIVE NEUROPEPTIDES (ACTH AND OT)

The behavioral effects of AVP are longer-lasting (days instead of hours) than those of the other hypophyseal hormone (adrenocorticotrophic hormone, ACTH) involved in the memory processes that possess primarily a motivational influence. In this context it is worth mentioning that the N-terminal fragment of ACTH contains the information essential for the behavioral effect of the hormone. ACTH(4—10) was the shortest peptide that was as potent as the parent molecule in restoring avoidance learning in hypophysectomized rats. The fact that ACTH(4—10) was present in ACTH as well as in alpha-MSH

126

and beta-MSH explained why the latter two hormones had the same effects on avoidance behavior as did ACTH (DeWied and Jolles 1982).

In contrast, oxytocin modulates memory function in an opposite manner than does AVP: it has inhibitory effects on information storage and retrieval. Neutralization of endogenous oxytocin by intracerebroventricular administration of oxytocin antiserum induces behavioral effects opposite to those observed following central administration of the neuropeptide. Oxytocin may thus be regarded as a naturally occurring amnesic peptide (Kovács and Telegdy 1982, Fehm-Wolfsdorf et al. 1984).

12.2.3 NATURE OF THE BEHAVIORAL ACTIONS OF VASOPRESSIN

Since the majority of studies reporting positive results after vasopressin administration have employed aversively motivated tasks, one might wonder, whether the behavioral effects of the hormone were due to a central action of the peptide or, alternatively, to its nonspecific activating effects on peripheral V1 receptors. Although there is some dispute on the relative importance of peripheral versus central actions in behavioral effects of the peptide (LeMoal et al. 1984), there are several arguments in support of a direct effect of AVP on CNS.

Animal experiments have suggested that the amount of vasopressin administered intracerebroventricularly (icv) required to elicit behavioral effects is 20—40 times greater than that administered to specific brain nuclei (midbrain limbic structures), and another 100—1,000 times more peptide is needed with peripheral administration (DeWied 1976). The importance of the central AVP system is also supported by experiments, in which antiserum raised against AVP, when administered intracerebroventricularly caused marked alterations in passive avoidance behavior, while intravenous administration of a 100 times as much antiserum was without any behavioral effect (Van Wimersma-Greidanus, 1986). In addition, C-terminal vasopressin fragments devoid of classic (peripheral) endocrine effects (e.g. dGVP) still preserve their behavioral effects (deWied et al. 1972).

The view that AVP metabolites have function in the brain only and are inactive in the periphery makes it tempting to assume that the metabolites are preferentially generated during the activation of the AVP containing neuronal systems in the brain. The identification of such peptides has been approached by studying in vitro conversion of vasopressin by peptidases from rat brain membranes. The major components have been isolated and characterized as [pGlu4,Cyt6] AVP-(4—9) and [pCyt6] AVP-(5—9). In various brain loci that are probably involved in information processing the forms which chromatographically correspond to AVP- (4—9) and -(5—9) fragments account for up to 30 per cent of the AVP content. On icv administration

AVP- (4—9) facilitated passive avoidance behavior already in doses more than 200 times lower than the doses of AVP- (1—9) needed to elicit the same effect (Burbach et al. 1983, 1984b). The recent discovery of separate binding sites for [pGlu4, ^{35}S-Cyt6] AVP-(4—9) in the brain (DeKloet et al. 1985) with a distribution distinct from that of the parent peptide (Brinton et al. 1986) gives further support to the view that AVP metabolites constitute highly potent neuropeptides with selective central effects related to memory processes.

12.2.4 VASOPRESSIN AND HUMAN BEHAVIOR

In the light of the large body of evidence that vasopressin and its fragments may influence memory processes in animals, several clinical trials have been performed to evaluate the ability of the peptide to enhance cognitive functions in both impaired and normal individuals. Unfortunately, there are many differences between these studies with respect to aspect(s) of memory affected, type and severity of the defects, methods used for treatment evaluation as well as to the vasopressin congener administered.

Nevertheless it seems that vasopressin treatment has effects on what is measured as memory in man. This conclusion is based on the fact that most studies result in some effect, be it a clinical impression of improvement, a subjective feeling of patients or subjective test results. Many studies in which the peptide was ineffective were performed on patients with a complex pattern of neuropsychological deficits or other symptoms suggesting profound brain degeneration, while more positive effects have been found in healthy volunteers and in moderately affected subjects. This should not be surprising, because degeneration of the relevant brain structures may well destroy the sites of action of the peptide.

Another important point concerns the nature and amount of the active principle. The amount of vasopressin that can be used in humans is limited due to its peripheral side efects, while high peripheral concentrations are necessary to evoke significant CNS response. dGAVP — [dGlyNH$_2$-9]VP — that lacks the classic peripheral effects of the hormone is favored above vasopressin and desmopressin. Since the blood-brain barrier seems to effectively restrict the access of AVP, LVP or dDAVP from the blood to their central target sites there are certain areas in the CNS devoid of the functional blood-brain barrier, including the area postrema, organum vasculosum of the lamina terminalis (OVLT) and the pineal and pituitary glands, through which circulating hormone may reach the brain to elicit behavioral effects. Finally it may be necessary to treat for a relatively prolonged period of time (for weeks) to allow a relevant treatment effect to develop (Jolles 1986).

It has been suggested that vasopressin may affect human memory through more efficient memory organization and encoding. It may also facilitate memory, improve the speed of motor performace or have an activating effect on rate of working and thinking. A beneficial effect of the peptide has been reported in patients suffering from moderate posttraumatic amnesia or alcoholism, while no beneficial effect was observed in patients with more serious head injuries or after longer periods of alcohol abuse (Laczi et al. 1983a). A similar picture arises from clinical experiments with elderly people or demented patients: subjects at later stages of Alzheimer's disease did not improve after vasopressin treatment, whereas patients with milder forms benefited from this therapy (Jolles 1986). Beneficial effects have been also reported in Lesh-Nyhan syndrome (Anderson et al. 1979), in hereditary central diabetes insipidus (Laczi et al. 1983b) and in depression (Strupp et al. 1984). Positive results with long-term dDAVP treatment have been reported also in minimal brain dysfunction (or in more recent terminology, attention deficit disorder), a common behavioral disorder in childhood affecting approximately 5 per cent of children of elementary school age (Hamburger-Bar et al. 1987).

13   METABOLIC EFFECTS OF VASOPRESSIN

In the light of the stimulating effect of hypoglycemia on AVP secretion (chapter 5.4.3) it might be interesting to consider the significance of the hormone in the control of serum glucose levels, and possibly of other energy-producing substances. The best characterized metabolic actions of AVP are related to the liver, an organ in which the concentration of vasopressin receptors is 5 times greater than in the kidneys (Jard 1983a). Probably glycogenolysis is the most prominent of these hepatic effects, though the peptide also enhances hepatic glyconeogenesis and glycolysis, and reduces hepatic lipogenesis and ketogenesis. Moreover, vasopressin can promote endogenous energy mobilization by stimulating glucagon and ACTH release. Although at present AVP is not regarded as a major counterregulatory hormone, it is possible that it may have a minor role in glucose homeostasis and contribute to the restoration of normoglycemia (Spruce et al. 1985b). In addition to these peripheral effects a potential role of centrally acting vasopressin in the regulation of feeding behavior and in the development of various feeding disorders has been proposed (Gold et al. 1983a, Arawich and Sladek 1986).

14 CLINICAL DISTURBANCES OF VASOPRESSIN SECRETION AND EFFECTS (HYPO- AND HYPERVASOPRESSINISM)

As outlined in chapter 1.4 the dualistic system of regulation of vasopressin secretion and thirst acts in concert to maintain body fluid osmolality by modifying the volume of body water in which solute particles are dispersed (see Fig. 1.4). Anything that interferes with the full expression of either osmoregulatory function (being it an inborn error or acquired defect or, more often, a functional overload of these functions) exposes the patient to hazards of abnormities in the jealously guarded parallelism between body water and sodium content (Robertson et al. 1982).

14.1 HYPOVASOPRESSINISM

There are few pathological conditions which become manifest by dramatic clinical symptoms such as does defect of AVP secretion or its renal action (diabetes insipidus, hypovasopressinism), in which copious amounts of bland, "unsweet" urine are excreted (chapter 17). Probably this is one of the reasons why this syndrome traditionally received more attention than its incidence and seriousness warrant (Czernichow and Robinson 1985, Braden et al. 1985, Vokes and Robertson 1988). But, what has been learned regarding neuroendocrinology and physiology of water metabolism from these studies has been of enormous importance. Moreover, systematic investigations of AVP-dependent and AVP-independent aspects of renal concentrating ability together with the detection of the significance of the thirst mechanism have contributed in a principal manner to the development of modern approaches to fluid replacement therapy (Kerpel-Fronius 1959, Barnett 1966). It may not be exaggerated to state that the introduction of the advanced schedules of fluid therapy — along with the progress in the antibacterial treatment — fundamentally contributed to the impressive decline of general morbidity and mortality in clinical medicine during the last decades.

14.2 HYPERVASOPRESSINISM

Although the neurohypophyseal hypofunction syndrome has been clinically well-defined since long, the existence of a hyperfunction syndrome was denied over long periods assuming that AVP hypersecretion might result in water intoxication in a degree incompatible with life. Paradoxically, it was the widespread use of parenteral fluid therapy (and the associated frequent development of excessive dilution of the internal environment, e.g. hyponatremia) that turned back the attention of clinicians and investigators to problems of secretion and renal action of vasopressin. This time it was hyperproduction rather than deficiency that became the subject of the main interest (Schrier and Bichet 1981, Robertson 1983).

Although it is commonly believed that the function of AVP is to cause excretion of hypertonic urine, its more important function might be better defined as prevention of excretion of diluted urine (Berliner and Davidson 1957). Maximal osmotic suppression of the hormone which permits maximal dilution of urine increases the rate of water excretion in an exponential fashion to a maximum which, if renal function and solute excretion are normal, can offset all but the most pathologically excessive rates of water intake without any disturbances developing in plasma osmolality (see Fig. 8.1). Taking it into account, the occurrence of excessive dilution of body fluids ($P_{osm} <$ < 280 mOsm/kg) in association with only moderately excessive water intake (or water administration) provides evidence that a sustained release of AVP may play an important role in the impairment of the individual's capacity to excrete free water (Robertson 1977, Gross et al. 1986, Kovács et al. 1987b). Accordingly, hypervasopressinism (vasopressin excess) can be defined as a failure to maximally suppress AVP when plasma osmolality falls to the normal threshold level (downward resetting of the osmostat, see Fig. 5.3). When this occurs, the hormone continues to circulate at levels that are excessively high, not always in absolute terms but in relation to the hypoosmolality of body fluids. Hypervasopressinism, in contrast to the opposite disturbance, i.e. hypovasopressinism, is by far no unique phenomenon; rather, it is a frequent concomitant of a number of various pathophysiological conditions (chapter 19).

14.3 ROLE OF WATER INTAKE AND FLUID THERAPY

As far as clinical disturbances of water homeostasis are concerned, there is one important point that warrants comment. Hypovasopressinism (diabetes insipidus) is manifested by excessive losses of solute-free water; nevertheless, clinically significant hypernatremia secondary to dehydration develops only when the water losses are not replaced by adequate amounts of hypotonic fluid (chapter 18). On the other hand, hypervasopressinism per se does not result in any clinically recognizable abnormality unless the intake of solute-free water exceeds the actually limited renal diluting capacity. If this is the case, excess water is trapped resulting in an excessive dilution of body fluid compartments, i.e. hypotonic hyponatremia (chapter 20).

In reality therefore, both hypo- and hypervasopressinism play only a permissive role in the development of clinical disturbances in body fluid compositon; these defects in osmoregulation of AVP usually do not result in clinically evident abnormalities unless water intake also departs from normal. Since primary disturbances in thirst sensation are relatively rare (chapters 17.3 and 17.4), it may not be surprising that the development of severe deviations in plasma osmolality can be expected mainly in those patients who are too young, too old or too sick to seek water (small infants, elderly persons, severely ill individuals or unconscious patients) and who have to be maintained on nondipsogenic water supply (Feig and McCurdy 1977, Friedman and Segar 1979, Goldberg 1981).

14.4   IATROGENIC DISTURBANCES IN BODY WATER HOMEOSTASIS

In view of the still frequently developing hyper- and mainly hyponatremia (Anderson 1986, Kovács et al. 1987c, Snyder et al. 1987) it may not be irrelevant to make an attempt to analyze the most frequent causes underlying the development of these disturbances of body water homeostasis. Generally, it can be stated that the major cause of their development is diagnostic inexactness. The following factors unavoidably must be determined or at least estimated in any patient who is given nondipsogenic fluid therapy:

— qualitative or quantitative volume changes in the individual compartments of the body;
— the basic disease which has resulted in the development of the given disturbance;
— the actual functional capacity of the individual homeostatic control systems;
— the degree of correction reached by the fluid therapy, and further disturbances induced by the therapy.

The above, no doubt extremely demanding, requirements are difficult to meet in routine practice where the clinicians have but a limited number of basic tests available. However, the understanding of pathophysiological mechanisms of the development of most frequently seen "patterns" or "pictures" of disturbances of secretion and renal effects of AVP, and disturbances in water metabolism can supply a very efficient aid. Comparison of clinical and laboratory results obtained for the individual patient with the individual disturbance "patterns" can significantly contribute to the establishment of an exact diagnosis.

Extremely high is the hazard to induce iatrogenic disturbances if the effect and/or expected side effects of the fluid therapy are not checked. Only continuous monitoring allows to establish whether "too much" or "too little" has been administered. It must be also emphasized that the fluids administered and excreted often differ in their composition. Therefore merely comparing intake and output may be insufficient to accurately predict the effects of the therapy. If, for example, urinary sodium and water losses are induced by a diuretic and the fluid losses are replaced by an equal volume of water, the patient will be in water balance, but the loss of unreplaced solute will induce hypoosmolality and hyponatremia.

It arises from what has been said that the diagnosis using a small number of basic tests to comprehensively estimate the actual state of water and salt homeostasis, may often introduce erroneous interpretation in several points. In an aim to prevent the development of iatrogenic disturbances, one possibility might be to make every endeavor to perfect diagnostics. Equally important is to prefer dipsogenic fluid therapy whenever possible by using oral rehydration solutions (Table 14.1) which allow a more appropriate regulation of salt and water balance than does the same solution administered parenterally (chapter 5.1.2) (Sack et al. 1978, Finberg 1980, Boda 1986). However, for the amount

Table 14.1. Oral rehydration solutions (ORS)

	Carboh. (g/100 ml)	Na$^+$ (mmol/l)	K$^+$ (mmol/l)	Cl$^-$ (mmol/l)	HCO$_3$$^-$ (mmol/l)
WHO formula (1)	2	90	20	80	30
Pediatric ORS	4	35	20	37	18
Pediatric ORS for maintenance and preventive purposes	2	49	20	30	29

(1) Anonymus: Treatment and prevention of dehydration in diarrheal disease. Geneva, WHO, 1976.

and the composition of fluid losses are dependent on a myriad of intrinsic and environmental factors and we are still not able to exactly determine the actual maintaining fluid requirements of an individual, fluid therapy is still realized more on the basis of a generalized rather than a really individualized approach. Efforts along this line to more individualized therapy probably would require many years of painstaking trial and error, and even then, would not be assured of success. Therefore, at present, it would seem more rational to favor a careful continuous clinical and laboratory follow-up of patients before, during and after fluid therapy. We may not be wrong to believe that the major cause of severe iatrogenic disturbances of water balance is specifically ignorance of such a continuous follow-up.

15 ONTOGENESIS OF BODY WATER HOMEOSTASIS AND VASOPRESSIN SECRETION

As it has already been mentioned (chapter 14.3), disturbances in water homeostasis most frequently occur in small babies and in elderly subjects. Therefore it seems desirable to review some age-related pecularities in the function of the osmoregulatory system prior to getting down to illustrate the most frequently encountered "types" and "patterns" of disturbed water homeostasis in clinical practice and the role of AVP in their development.

Water as the major single component of living matter has a special position both in physiology and pathophysiology. During ontogenesis mammalian and also human organism undergoes several more or less distinct developmental stages, which may be characterized by more or less pronounced peculiarities in the level of body fluid homeostasis. The responses to changes in external environment are qualitatively identical in every age category but the degree of these responses is different.

The knowledge of the age-related differences at the level of the water homeostasis control has important theoretical as well as clinical implications. From the theoretical point of view each individual stage in the development seems to reflect a prior state and to foreshadow events to follow. Hence a systematic study of longitudinal changes at the level of water homeostasis control might contribute to a better understanding of general principles of ontogenetic development and of the process of aging. On the other hand, the clinical practice suggests an increased hydrolability of persons at the extremes of the age spectrum (newborns, young infants and elderly persons) as reflected in higher frequencies of clinical disturbances in water homeostasis in these age categories. An effective prevention of these disturbances therefore requires approaching each individual period of life (fetal age, immediate perinatal period, neonatal and young infant period as well as old age) as a specific problem and analyzing it as a distinct entity.

15.1 FETAL NEUROHYPOPHYSEAL FUNCTION

Fetal endocrine physiology differs in a number of aspects from endocrinology of postnatal life. The former is characterized by several unique fetal endocrine organs, numerous hormones and metabolites occurring exclusively in the fetal compartment, and by the adaptation of many fetal endocrine systems to specific intrauterine conditions (Fisher 1986). These peculiar characteristics also apply to neurohypophyseal nonapeptides.

15.1.1 ARGININE-VASOTOCIN IN FETUSES

Arginine-vasotocin (AVT), a nonapeptide that differs from AVP by a single amino-acid susbstitution (see Fig. 2.1) and is known as a ubiquitous neuro-hypophyseal principle in nonmammalian vertebrates has been identified in the posterior pituitary, blood and in urine of mammals and humans during the fetal and neonatal period (chapter 2.3). The role of vasotocin during the development is not well understood. Owing to the lack of data concerning the presence of specific vasotocin receptors in the fetus, the hormone (which in standard bioassays shows approximately half the antidiuretic activity of arginine-vasopressin) might act via its binding to vasopressin receptors. It has been suggested that AVT may have a beneficial effect on the maintenance of the fetal homeostatic milieu. During fetal life vasotocin may reduce fetal lung fluid production (Ross et al. 1984), it may inhibit fetomaternal placental water transfer (Leake et al. 1986), may be involved in the regulation of brain maturation (Goldstein 1984) and may play a role in fetal sodium homeostasis (Ervin et al. 1986).

15.1.2 VASOPRESSIN SECRETION IN FETUSES

Arginine-vasopressin has been shown to be present in human posterior pituitary as early as in gestational week 11. There is a progressive increase in neuro-hypophyseal AVP content up to 28 weeks of gestation with relatively little increase thereafter (Schubert et al. 1981). Because ethical considerations justifiably limit the knowledge of the development of human fetuses, most information about the intrauterine neurohypophyseal function has been derived from fetal sheep model (with a length of gestation of 145 days). Leake et al. (1979) demonstrated that neither AVP nor AVT do cross the placenta. Thus the plasma AVP levels measured in the fetus depend on the balance between the rate of secretion and that of removal by the fetal kidney plus the rate of inactivation by placental cystine aminotransferase (oxytocinase).

Both volume and osmoreceptor control of AVP secretion are functional during the last trimester of gestation in the lamb fetus. There is a tendency for progressive increase in responsiveness to hypotensive stimuli from 100 days of gestation onwards (Rose et al. 1981, Ross et al. 1986), whereas there is evidence that the osmoreceptor system is fully functional at 100 days of gestation (Weitzman et al. 1978a). In view of other findings showing that maternal dehydration caused lower plasma AVP levels for a given plasma osmolality in 107—109-day-old fetuses than in those at 126—144 days of development (Bell et al. 1984) however some doubt may exist as to the pattern of development of the osmoreceptor system. In the fetus, as in the adult, AVP also appears to function as a "stress" hormone. Perhaps the major potential stress for the fetus is hypoxia, and the vasopressin response to hypoxia is greatly augmented relative to the maternal response and relative to the fetal AVP responses to osmotic stimuli (Daniel et al. 1984).

15.1.3 EFFECTS OF VASOPRESSIN IN FETUSES

Human kidneys are functional (at least as far as their capacity to produce urine is considered) from gestational week 12—16. Nevertheless, placenta remains the major regulator of the composition of body fluids throughout the intrauterine life. That the fetal renal function is only little more than practice carrying no significant regulatory responsibilities is supported by the fact that renal agenesis and/or hereditary AVP deficiency have no marked influence on the composition of fetal body (Nash and Edelmann 1973, Sokol and Valtin 1982). However, although under basal physiologic conditions the homeostatic effects of AVP seem negligible, the antidiuretic, vasoconstrictor and the ACTH-stimulating capacities of the hormone may become significant under stressful conditions.

Under normal conditions the fetus produces markedly hypotonic urine. Infusion of vasopressin to fetal lamb during the third trimester induces antidiuretic response in the form of the production of slightly hypertonic urine and negative clearance of solute-free water; the fetal renal concentrating ability represents only 20 to 30 per cent of the adult potential. In this regard it has been shown that the fetal nephron is less sensitive to AVP than adult nephron (Table 15.1) and that the ability of the fetal kidney to concentrate

Table 15.1. Factors of reduced responses of fetal and neonatal kidney to vasopressin

Incomplete development of cortico-medullary osmotic gradient
    Lower gomerular filtration rate
    Shortness of the loop of Henle
    Decreased loop solute transport (?)
    Low tubular load of urea (anabolic state)
    High vasa recta blood flow

Increased tubular resistance to vasopressin
    Decreased tubular V2 receptor number
    High renal prostaglandin (mainly PGE_2) production

urine progressively increases with advancing gestation (Robillard and Weitzman 1980, Wintour et al. 1982, Daniel et al. 1982).

Reduced V2 receptor number and/or poor coupling between V2 receptors and the generation of cyclic AMP may contribute to this renal hyporesponsiveness to AVP. It may well be that the late gestational as well as the early neonatal period are critical for the development of renal vasopressin receptors: the administration of desmopressin to pregnant rats as well as the administration of vasopressin to newborn lambs is followed by a significant reduction of maximal renal concentrating capacity in the same animals when reaching adult age (Lichardus et al. 1983, Handelmann and Russell 1983, Ivanova et al. 1987). In addition, high renal production of prostaglandin E in the fetus is thought to attenuate the cellular action of AVP through interference with cAMP production (see Fig. 7.1) (Joppich et al. 1981). Nevertheless, it seems likely that incomplete generation and maintenance of the renal solute gradient (due to the shortness of the loop of Henle, the low tubular load of urea and the relatively high blood flow through the vasa recta) are the most important factors limiting the renal response to AVP (Nash and Edelmann 1973, Robillard and Nakamura 1988, Sulyok 1988).

Despite the limited effect of AVP on the fetal kidney, however, the hormone may contribute, at least to some degree, to water homeostasis during fetal life. This view has been supported by experiments in which infusion of hypertonic saline into the fetus produced a sustained increase in fetal urine osmolality and a decrease in fetal urinary flow rate, and that these changes were completely blocked by an AVP antagonist (Woods et al. 1986). Available evidence suggests that in addition to its renal effects, AVP (similarly as AVT) acts in the fetal environment to conserve water for the fetus by inhibiting flow across the placenta and losses into the amniotic fluid via the lungs (Fisher 1986).

Vasopressin's potent pressor effect may be more important than its antidiuretic action during intrauterine life particularly in response to hemorrhage and possibly to hypoxia (Robillard and Weitzman 1980, Daniel et al. 1982). Intravenous infusion of vasopressin to achieve similar plasma levels as seen in hypoxic fetuses leads to hypertension and bradycardia, and these effects are greater in the fetus as compared to the adult. The hormone also causes redistribution of blood flow in favor of the heart, brain and umbilico-placental circulation, while it reduces perfusion of the gastrointestinal tract and the carcass (Iwamoto et al. 1979). Aside from its cardiovascular effects, administration of vasopressin to the fetus leads to a significant increase in arterial pO_2, probably by promoting placental gas exchange (Rurak and Gruber 1984). As these changes are similar to those that occur during hypoxia in the fetus, they seem to have a definite value for the survival under similar circumstances.

The fetal sheep respond to intrauterine "stress" such as hypoxia, hypoglycemia or hemorrhage, with increased plasma ACTH concentrations. Recent data suggest that AVP released in response to intrauterine "stress" could contribute to stimulation of ACTH release in fetal sheep, but this role seems to be of greater importance in younger fetuses as compared with fetuses of more than 125—130 days of gestational age (Norman and Challis 1987).

15.2 VASOPRESSIN DURING THE LABOR

Neonates delivered vaginally have grossly elevated cord blood AVP (and oxytocin) levels as compared with those delivered by elective Cesarean section. In general, the highest levels have occurred during difficult births in stressed newborns. Values in premature newborns were similar to those found in term babies (DeVane and Porter 1980, Pohjavouri 1983, Pochard and Lutz-Bucher 1986). Increased release together with decreased rates of metabolism by the placenta offer an explanation for these findings.

Several different stimuli may cause hypersecretion of the hormone during vaginal delivery, probably the most important of them are hypoxia/acidosis due to cord occlusion and fetal cerebral compression during the passage of the fetus through the birth channel (Hadeed et al. 1979, Daniel et al. 1984). Physiologic effects of high plasma AVP values during vaginal delivery remain not well understood. They may relate mainly to the vascular and ACTH-stimulating effects of the hormone. Interestingly, the highest concentrations of AVP in cord plasma were found in infants with fetal bradycardia and meconium in the amniotic fluid. AVP is a potent constrictor of the mesenteric vascular bed and a stimulant of the large bowel peristaltics (Iwamoto et al. 1979). It is thus possible that fetal hypersecretion of AVP during asphyxia may be an important mediator of these well known clinical signs of fetal distress (Gaffney and Jenkins 1983).

15.3 REGULATION OF BODY WATER HOMEOSTASIS AND VASOPRESSIN SECRETION IN NEWBORNS AND YOUNG INFANTS

As soon as the baby has been delivered, the kidneys take the function of the major effector of the osmoregulatory system. At the same time, the major role of vasopressin in the organism becomes its involvement in the control of renal excretion and conservation of water.

As compared to adult subjects, the obviously limited functional capacity of the renal osmoregulatory system in newborns and young infants (Fig. 15.1) is frequently still being explained by some "immaturity" of the young organism. In doing so one tends to speak as though the regulations the adult is endowed with are the only adequate ones, superior to those of newborns and infants. Actually, nobody is justified in believing that the adult regulation could sucessfully be imposed upon newborns and small infants. As far as it is known, each stage of development is functionally complete on its own right. So the common assumption has remained because there are no criteria for advantages and disadvantages other than the frequency of survival in natural circumstances.

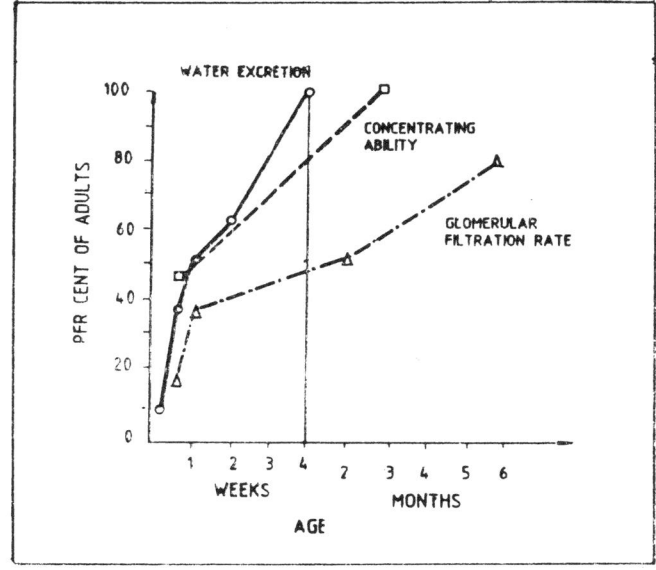

Fig. 15.1. The developmental patterns of renal water excretion, renal concentrating capacity and glomerular filtration rate in healthy term infants (by Kerpel-Fronius, 1959 with permission).

In any case these considerations however do not contradict the observation that under conditions of limited regulatory capacity excess loads may lead to the development of clinical disturbances in water homeostasis more frequently than in any other period of life. This opinion has been expressed already by classics of pediatrics who came to the conclusion that the degree of vulnerability of a young organism depends equally, if not to a greater degree, on the specificities of the level of the control of body water fluid and salt homeostasis and the peculiarities of the immunologic status of the child (Kerpel-Fronius 1959, Barnett 1976).

In trying to characterize the differences in the level of water and salt metabolism in newborns and young infants (to which both central and peripheral mechanisms of the osmoregulatory system are obviously adapted), one must in the first place mention 1. specificities in the volume of body fluids, 2. in the metabolic state of the organism, and also 3. levels of the individual parameters of renal function (Martínek et al. 1964).

15.3.1 DEVELOPMENTAL CHANGES IN BODY FLUID VOLUME AND DISTRIBUTION

One of the major characteristic features of ontogentic development is a gradual isotonic reduction of body water volume from 96% of body weight in 6-weeks-old embryos to 80% of the fat-free weight at term (Fig. 15.2) (Friis-Hansen 1983). The marked postnatal reduction in body fluid volume during the first days of life goes almost exclusively at the expense of extracellular fluid, excess water and sodium being excreted from the body via the kidneys. This postnatal contraction of body fluid volume, with its extent being proportional to the magnitude of the initial decrease in body weight of the newborn, is of adaptational significance for normal transition from fetal into postnatal life (Arant 1987, Kovács et al. 1988a). In fact the possibility exists that preterm infants in whom body fluids have a relatively greater share on their body mass, may not have physiologic stability until their extracellular fluid volume is similar to that of the more mature infant. If this initial decrease in body mass — reaching under normal conditions up to 10 per cent of body mass in term babies, and 20 or more per cent of body mass in preterm babies — does not occur (for example, in excessively hydrated sick preterm infants), the sustained hypervo-

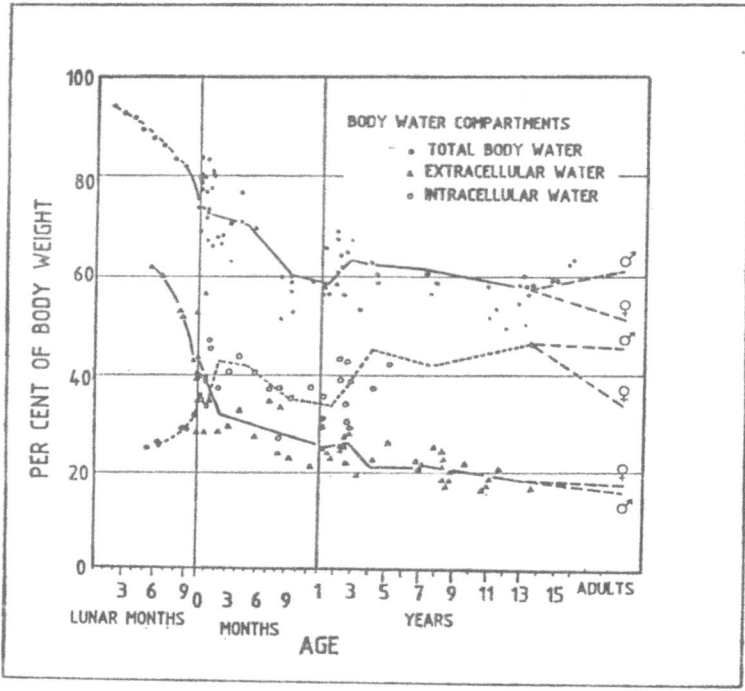

Fig. 15.2. Relative composition of body water compartments during human development from early fetal life to adult life (by Frees—Hansen 1983 with kind permission).

lemia can result in undesirable clinical sequelae, such as bronchopulmonary dysplasia, patent ductus arteriosus and necrotizing enterocolitis (Bell et al. 1979, 1980, Shaffer et al. 1986). The process of water depletion continues throughout the life, though with a decreasing intensity, the most pronounced drop occurring during the first months (see Fig. 15.2). The causes of this tendency remain unknown, although it is obvious that any phenomenon of a general nature, and this is the case with fluid volume contraction, must also have some objective cause.

The above mentioned facts might lead to erroneous conclusion that owing to their larger fluid resources newborns can better tolerate limited fluid supply than do adult subjects. However, when the body fluid volume is compared to functional parameters, other than body weight (such as energy metabolism rates, cardiac output or values of renal clearances), then the young organism is clearly in a water-deficient state in comparison to adults (Kerpel-Fronius 1959). The relatively large body surface area and high rates of energy metabolism result in increased insensible water losses (in particular in newborns maintained under radiant warmers) which tends to further decreasing water resources (Lorenz et al. 1982, Oh 1988). Another critical moment is the ratio of water distribution among the individual compartments. In newborns and young infants rapidly metabolized metabolically unbound extracellular fluid makes up a considerably larger proportion than in adults (see Fig. 15.2). Owing to this, the daily fluid turnover during the first months of life exceeds severalfold values measured in adult individuals. In the organism of normal newborns approximately 50% of the extracellular fluid is exchanged during every 24-hour period, whereas the respective value for an adult is only 10—15%. Inadequate replacement of renal and extrarenal losses of water and salts in younger age may therefore jeopardize the organism by a rapid exhaustion of the internal water reserves and thus by the development of severe volume depletion.

Taking together, the rapidly changing body fluid composition places the pediatrician who provides fluid therapy between the Scylla of volume expansion and the Charybdis of volume contraction. The appropriate calculation of fluid requirements necessitates the understanding of requirements for maintenance, replacement of losses and allowance for growth. In normal situations the estimation of the requirements is generally straightforward since normal values are well known. Furthermore, even if there are variations in individual infants and error is made in the calculations, the compensatory adjustment by a normal kidney normalizes the fluid and electrolyte status. This is not the case in severely ill high-risk newborns and infants since in this group the renal functions are often clinically compromised so that compensatory efforts may not be adequate to correct for the error in calculations (Coulthard and Ney 1985, Oh 1988).

15.3.2 METABOLIC STATE OF NEWBORNS AND YOUNG INFANTS

The volume and composition of the infant feeding can be considered to be the second key factor which determines the different level of water metabolism in newborns and small infants. Mother's milk, which is the only natural source of all nutrients, electrolytes and water, is a markedly hypotonic fluid with considerably lower concentrations of proteins and salts as compared to milks of most mammals. Such a composition is rather advantageous for it assures that the majority of the dietary solutes can be taken up by cells and tissues of rapidly growing organism and thus reducing the renal solute load, i.e. the amount of solutes that must be excreted in the urine. Renal solute load presented by the diet should be a primary consideration in choice of infants with restricted renal concentrating capacity, mainly when volume of food consumed is low and/or extrarenal water losses are high. Therefore cow milk-based infant formulas should be "adapted" to a composition closely resembling that of human milk (Ziegler and Fomon 1971).

A special problem concerns feeding of very low birthweight preterm infants with gestational age of < 34 weeks. Pooled breast milk from term deliveries is used in many hospitals as the primary feeding source for these infants, usually managed in incubators. However, there is now enough incriminating evidence against this practice (Kovács et al. 1985a, Ronnholm et al. 1986). Several investigators found that milk produced during the first weeks after preterm delivery has a higher concentration of sodium (and also some other nutrients) than "mature" milk after term delivery (Fig. 15.3). Preterm infants fed pooled mature human milk grew slower during early postnatal life than infants fed

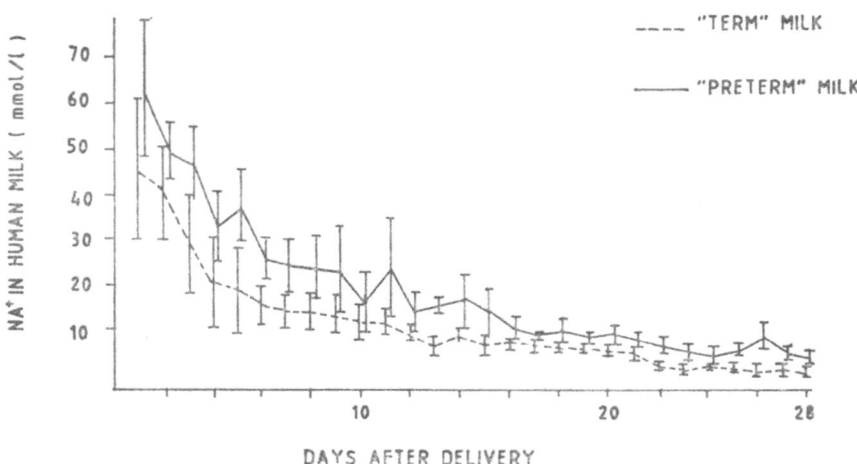

Fig. 15.3. Concentration of sodium in mother's milk of term and preterm infants during the first 28 days following delivery (Kovács et al. 1985a).

their own mother's milk or formulas specially designed for these infants (Atkinson et al. 1983, Chessex et al. 1983). Furthermore it appears that the shortage of sodium in pooled mature human milk may contribute to the development of late hyponatremia often seen in preterm infants during the first 2—3 weeks of life (Kovács and Sulyok 1984) (chapter 20.3.1.8). Therefore, preterm infants should be fed own mother's milk, or, alternatively, formulas specially designed for these infants should be used.

Human and animal studies suggest that the weaning period (i.e. the period between day 14 and 28 in rats and between months 3 and 6 in human newborns) is associated with radical changes in the level of water homeostasis. The organism that has been receiving water and solutes exclusively in the form of breast milk, gradually starts receiving nutrition with substantially less water and higher osmotic load. Therefore weaning constitutes another developmental period critical for the formation of the osmoregulatory system (Dlouhá 1982). It may well be that just the magnitude of the working load imposed upon the kidney is that factor which determines the rate of renal maturation after birth. These changes however occur gradually and smoothly; rapid and excessive pathophysiological loads during the first months, i.e. during the period of adaptation of the regulatory systems, may therefore frequently be associated with disturbances in parameters controlled by them (Nash and Edelmann 1973, Dlouhá 1982).

15.3.3 POSTNATAL DEVELOPMENT OF RENAL HANDLING OF SALT AND WATER

The third factor that determines the different level of water metabolism in neonates and younger infants is the renal functional capacity itself. Parameters that seem to limit renal osmoregulatory capacity in the most significant manner include lower glomerular filtration rate, lower capacity to excrete standard water load, increased distal tubular sodium load and a lower renal concentrating ability in newborns and small infants (see Fig. 15.1), the most profound limitations being observed in preterm newborns delivered before gestational week 34 (Arant 1987, Robillard and Nakamura 1988).

15.3.3.1 Glomerular filtration rate

It has been known for long that glomerular filtration rate, determined as inulin clearance or clearance of endogenous creatinine, does not reach in newborns and infants values measured for adults even after correction for body surface area. In term newborns GFR values corrected for 1.73 m² body surface area and expressed as percentages of the respective values for adults (see Fig. 15.1) do not change during the first month of life; i.e. GFR and body surface area grow proportionally to each other. Between months 1 and 13 of postnatal life however, GFR increases more rapidly than does body surface area, and reaches by the end of this period values comparable with normal values of this parameter for adults subjects (Aperia et al. 1983, Lehotská et al. 1981a).

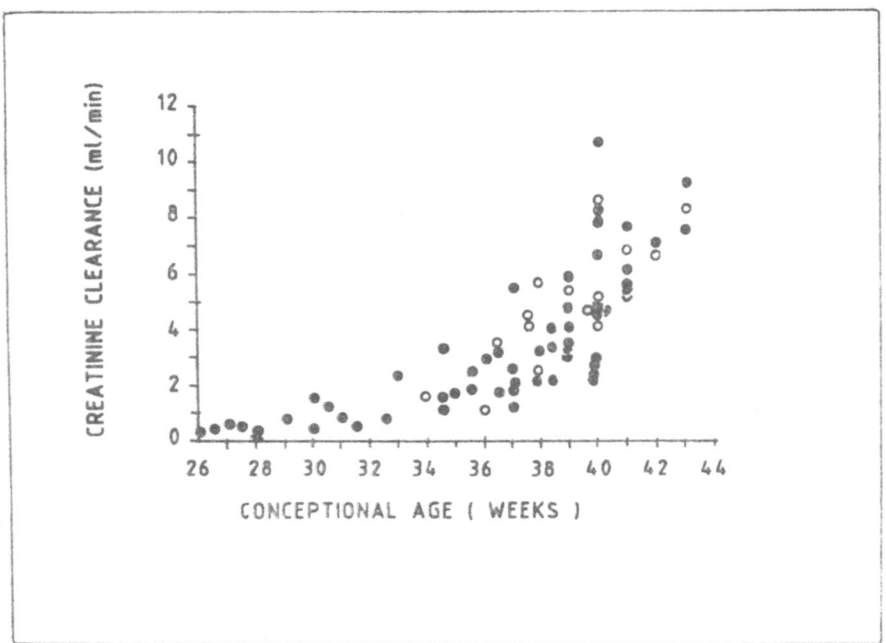

Fig. 15.4. Creatinine clearance as compared with conceptional age of infants at a mean postnatal age of 3.4 days (o) and 7.9 days (●) (by Engle and Arant **1983** with kind permission) (conceptional age = gestational age + postnatal age).

Preterm babies show a different pattern of development of glomerular filtration rate. GFR remains effectively at an unchanged level throughout week 34 of postconception age (i.e. the sum of gestation and postnatal ages) and starts rising only thereafter (Fig. 15.4). Interestingly, this postconceptional age of 34 weeks corresponds to the period when the nephrogenic zone in the developing kidney rapidly disappears. Such a rapid increase in GFR around the period of the completion of nephrogenesis seems to be a consistent phenomenon in mammalian young, and occurs intrauterinely in sheep and postnatally in dogs and rats that are born less "mature" as compared to humans (Guignard et al. 1975, Arant 1978).

146

15.3.3.2 Renal water excretion

Newborns excrete standard water load slowlier than children or adult subjects. A conspicuously delayed excretion of water load is present but for some days after birth, and the excretory capacity reaches adult values as early as by the end of the first month of life (see Fig. 15.1). In interpreting this fact however it should be considered that, based on the fraction of glomerular filtrate appearing in the urine (V/GFR), the kidneys of newborns under normal fluid turnover are in a functionally similar condition as adult kidneys under hyper-hydration of the organism (Aperia et al. 1984). On the other hand, when criteria of diluting capacity are employed, it can be shown that following water load urine osmolality of term babies reaches values of 30—50 mOsm/kg as soon as by day 5 of postnatal life, i.e. values even lower than those measured in adult individuals. The mechanism underlying the "supernormal" diluting capacity in newborns is not entirely clear; a great ability of distal tubules to reabsorb sodium may be a supporting factor (Rodriquez-Soriano et al. 1983). The normal renal diluting mechanism in newborns is thus set to warrant the excretion of highly diluted urine although not in quantities sufficient to readily excrete standard water load (Edelmann and Spitzer 1969). This renders newborns more vulnerable than older subjects to unjudicious admistration of water.

15.3.3.3 Renal sodium handling

A higher fractional urine flow (V/GFR) in preterm and term babies as compared to adults is an unavoidable consequence of a higher fluid turnover at a lower GFR level. At the same time however, the high level of V/GFR is in accordance with the concept concerning the existence of glomerulo-tubular disbalance in newborns, i.e. the concept telling that GFR levels in term and preterm neonates are high owing to the limited capacity of the proximal tubule to reabsorb sodium from the glomerular filtrate (Aperia et al. 1983).

Frequently it has been claimed that increased distal solute load in preterm and term newborns is compensated for by an unlimitedly high distal sodium reabsorption. It has been speculated that the limited renal capacity to excrete sodium load may upon increased sodium supply to the organism result in the development of hypernatremia (Aperia et al. 1983). On the other hand however, clinical data suggest that hyponatremia and salt wasting occur in term and in particular preterm newborns considerably more frequently than does hyper-natremia and salt retention (Sulyok et al. 1980, Al-Dahhan et al. 1983). Nevertheless, both arguments, i.e. inability of the kidneys to excrete sodium load and decreased capacity to retain sodium in the organism have generally been employed to support the view concerning "functional immaturity" of the kidneys. Similar contradictory arguments can only evidence that any of them

Table 15.2. Some parameters characterizing the state of water and salt balance in preterm and term infants (n = 10 each) on the fifth day of life (Lichardus et al. 1986)

Parameter	Preterm infants	Term infants	p <
V (ml/min/1.73 m²)	0.71 ± 0.08	0.58 ± 0.11	n.s.
$U_{Na}V$ (nmol/kg/day)	1.73 ± 0.35	0.20 ± 0.06	0.001
C_{Na} (ml/min/1.73 m²)	0.16 ± 0.03	0.05 ± 0.01	0.05
FE_{Na} (%)	2.02 ± 0.40	0.20 ± 0.05	0.001
FE_{osm} (%)	3.74 ± 0.73	1.25 ± 0.10	0.01
C_{creat} (ml/min/1.73 m²)	8.50 ± 1.40	17.70 ± 2.30	0.01
P_{osm} (mOsm/kg)	284 ± 4.0	288 ± 2.0	n.s.

does not constitute an adequate marker of the process of "maturation" of renal tubules (Aperia et al. 1983, Arant 1987).

Preterm babies appear to have negative sodium balance due to increased fractional renal sodium excretion, (FE_{Na}), during the first two weeks of life (Sulyok et al. 1980, Al-Dahhan et al. 1983) (Table 15.2.). Identical sodium intake makes the sodium balance positive within the subsequent weeks, with EF_{Na} decreasing to low values. Concordantly, the high distal sodium delivery (chapter 8.5.2.2) gradually decreases with the increasing gestational and postnatal age, and by the end of the first year of life reaches values as observed in adults. In this context it could be shown that newborns have increased, though not unlimited, capacity to distally reabsorb sodium. Hence, if distal sodium delivery or V/GFR levels reach values of approximately 15% of the filtered sodium load, larger quantities of sodium can get into the urine and natriuresis develops (Rodriguez-Soriano et al. 1981, 1983). This means that any factor which raises V/GFR (for example, exaggerated physiological postnatal fluid volume contraction in preterm infants (see Fig. 15.2), or volume expansion caused by high rates of fluid administration) can all result in increased natriuresis. The above considerations may have direct clinical application in estimating natriuresis accompanying the syndrome of inappropriate AVP secretion and in the pathogenesis of the late hyponatremia in preterm newborns (chapter 20.3.1.8).

15.3.3.4 Renal water conservation

Following water deprivation or administration of exogenous vasopressin, the urine of newborns and small infants generally fails to concentrate to levels observed in older children and in adults (see Table 8.4). However, little clinical significance can be attached to this single fact since the kidneys of newborns are able to concentrate urine up to 700 mOsm/kg (Poláček et al. 1965, Edelmann and Spitzer 1969), a limitation not considered dangerous to water balance in the adult (see **Fig. 8.1**).

The decreased ability of the newborn and infant to secrete AVP is not a limiting factor in the renal water conservation. Rather, a diminished end-organ responsiveness to AVP is involved in their restricted concentrating performace (see Table 15.1). Towards the end of gestation the kidneys gradually become more and more responsive to the hydroosmotic action of AVP (Robillard et al. 1979), and this tendency continues also postnatally (see Table 8.4). Urinary AVP levels have not been found to correlate linearly with rise in urinary osmolality; rather, urine osmolality rose to a maximum allowed by the age-related renal sensitivity to the hormone and did not rise further despite further increases in urine AVP concentration (Kovács 1985, Wiriyathian et al. 1986).

A major portion of limitation in concentrating capacity in newborns and infants results from the low rates of excretion of urea, owing to the strongly anabolic state that prevails during that period of life (**chapter 15.3.2**). When the infant is fed urea or a high protein diet, a marked increase in concentrating capacity is observed, owing entirely to the additional urea (Edelmann et al. 1960). However, the amount of dietary protein required to induce a similar effect is considered unphysiologic and hence undesirable. Also other studies have pointed to the importance of feeding schedule on the actual concentrating capacity in infants. Following the administration of the V2 agonist dDAVP, maximal urine osmolality has been found to be only slightly higher than the osmolality of plasma in both full term (385 mOsm/kg) and preterm (359 mOsm/kg) newborns. At four to six weeks of age the maximal U_{osm} ranged between 425 and 670 mOsm/kg in both preterm and full term babies (Swenningsen and Aronson 1974). These somewhat lower U_{osm} levels might be related to the lower medullary osmolality in normal infants receiving hypotonic feeding (breast milk) every 3 to 4 hours as opposed to those who were evaluated after fluid restriction (Poláček et al. 1965). On the other hand, the mean urine osmolality of 671 mOsm/kg found by Lehotská et al. (1981b) after dDAVP administration already in 1 month-old infants (see Table 8.4) might be explained by a higher osmolal (i.e. protein) load given to their infants in the form of an insufficiently adapted infant formula.

More recently Rees et al. (1984) have studied the renal response to endogenous AVP in very low birthweight preterm infants with hypernatremic volume depletion and after recovery from hypernatremia. It has been shown that with increasing urinary AVP, urine osmolality rose more steeply and attained a plateau at higher levels in hypernatremic volume depleted infants than in those in a volume repleted state. The importance of volume and composition of body fluid compartments in renal concentrating mechanisms in preterm infants was further substantiated by the observation that in spite of the progressive increase in daily AVP excretion during the course of late hyponatremia of preterm infants (chapter 20.3.1.8) the expected rise in urine osmolality did not occur. What is more, its mean value tended to be the lowest at the end of the second week of life, when plasma sodium concentration approached hyponatremic levels (Fig. 15.5) (Sulyok et al. 1985, Kovács et al. 1986). The exact mechanisms responsible for the impaired renal response to AVP are not apparent. However, on the basis of these observations it appears that 1. disturbances in volume and composition of body fluid compartments have a strong influence on renal concentrating performance: hypernatremic volume depletion enhances and late hyponatremia attenuates the renal action of AVP; 2. the relative contribution of NaCl to the buildup of corticomedullary solute gradient is more important during the early postnatal period than later in life. The limited rate of renal tubular sodium reabsorption and hyponatremia, therefore, is more likely to impair renal concentrating performance in premature infants.

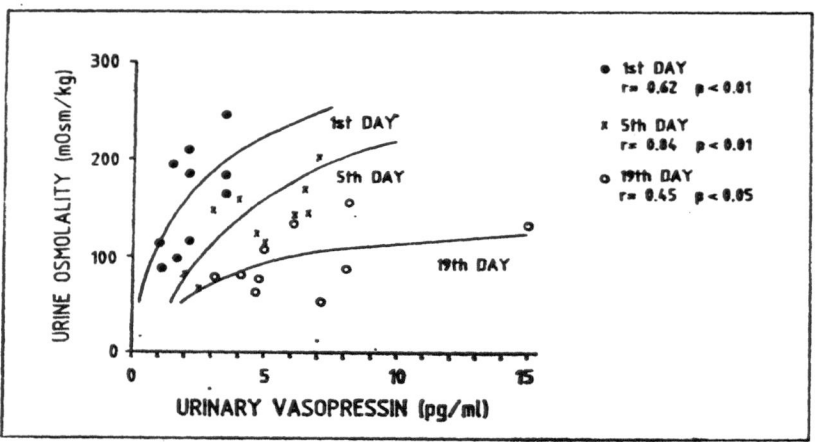

Fig. 15.5. Renal response to AVP in low birthweight preterm infants during development of late hyponatremia (by Kovács et al. 1986).

15.4 ARGININE-VASOPRESSIN DURING THE IMMEDIATE POSTNATAL PERIOD

In normal infants urine and plasma AVP concentrations fall within the first 24 hours following birth to low levels characteristic for this period of life (Table 15.3). The parallel patterns of fall in AVP levels in full term and preterm newborns suggest that the metabolic clearances of AVP are comparable in both groups (Pohjavuori 1983). It has been postulated that this drop could be a result of "pituitary exhaustion" after delivery. However, the decreased ability of the perinate to secrete AVP is not a limiting factor. In contrast,

Table 15.3. Diuresis (V), plasma and urine osmolality (P_{osm} and U_{osm}), endogenous creatinine clearance (C_{creat}) and urinary concentration and excretion of arginine vasopressin (U_{AVP} and $U_{AVP}V$ respectively) in 62 healthy infants and children divided into six age groups (mean ± SEM and range). Asterisks indicate significant differences between groups (* $p < 0.05$, ** $p < 0.01$, *** $p < 0.001$).

Age	n	V ml/min/1.73m²	U_{osm} mOsm/kg	P_{osm} mOsm/kg	U_{AVP} pg/ml	$U_{AVP}V$ ng/day	$U_{AVP}V$ pg/min/1.0m²	C_{creat} ml/min/1.73 m²
2 days	11	0.13±0.01 (0.05—0.18) ***	303±21 (215—440) ***	285±1.1 (282—290)	11.36±2.2 (4.0 —24.0) **	0.21±0.03 (0.04— 0.64) *	0.69±0.1 0.14— 2.24 *	12.3 ±1.1 (8.75—33.3)
5 days	11	0.58±0.11 (0.30—1.38) ***	196±27 (83—320) *	288±1.3 (282—295) *	4.41± 0.9 (1.5 —12.0) *	0.44± 0.13 (0.18— 1.98) **	1.18± 0.16 (0.63— 5.25) **	17.7 ± 2.3 (12.1 —30.2) *
30 days	10	1.48±0.07 (0.58—1.70) ***	120±8 (70—180) ***	283±0.7 (280—285) *	7.2 ± 1.1 (2.5 —20.0) *	1.51± 0.30 (0.24— 5.4) *	5.16± 0.9 (0.80—10.9) *	30.99± 2.3 (18.1 —40.4) *
4 months	10	0.85±0.13 (0.25—1.36)	416±74 (96—896) *	287±1.5 (280—290)	13.3 ± 3.7 (2.5 —33.0) **	3.91± 1.8 (1.05— 9.1) ***	9.06± 4.55 (2.01—17.8) ***	42.46± 2.5 (27.7 —59.6) ***
5—8 years	10	0.95±0.14 (0.40—1.89)	657±63 (311—1036)	288±1.7 (280—295)	32.6 ± 5.3 (9.1 —58.5)	14.32± 2.1 (7.6 —27.5)	11.23± 1.4 (5.68—19.0)	83.69± 4.5 (68.7 —109)
9—13 years	10	0.80±0.13 (0.33—1.50)	664±74 (397—1018)	288±1.8 (280—300)	39.1 ± 9.3 (13.7 —88.0)	19.87± 2.7 (12.4 —43.4)	11.41± 1.5 (6.61—23.9)	91.12± 3.2 (75.7 —108)

recent data suggest that from the first day of life, and from gestational age of 26 weeks in the absence of complicating factors, neonatal AVP secretion occurs appropriately in response to variations in plasma osmolality. Moreover, by using longitudinal sequential measurements of AVP in urine and plasma it has become clear that both preterm and full term infants are capable o-eliciting significant amounts of AVP in response to nonosmotic stimuli accomf panying various perinatal problems. Greatly increased urinary and plasma concentrations of AVP have been reported in infants with hemorrhage, ECF volume contraction, respiratory distress syndrome (hyaline membrane disease), particularly in those who require mechanical positive pressure ventilation; periventricular-intraventricular hemorrhage, meningitis, pneumonia and pneumothorax (Rees et al. 1984, Wiriyathian et al. 1986). How exactly this hormone fits into the intricate pathophysiological responses to perinatal "stress" remains unclear. Nevertheless, it must be considered that in some instances AVP may function as more than a nonspecific "stress" hormone, i.e. it may contribute in a significant manner to the final pathologic state. Moreover, nonosmotically stimulated hypervasopressinism during recent years has been more frequent cause of severe hyponatremia (syndrome of inappropriate secretion of vasopressin, water intoxication) than generally appreciated in severely ill preterm and full term infants on maintenance parenteral fluid and electrolyte therapy (chapter 20.3.1.8).

15.5 DEVELOPMENT OF VASOPRESSIN SECRETION FROM BIRTH TO ADULTHOOD

Little has been known so far about the developmental changes in the osmo-regulatory system under basal physiologic conditions (Godard et al. 1979, 1982, Kovács 1985). Table 15.3 shows AVP urine concentration and excretion values for various age groups of newborns and children in relation to diuresis, urine and plasma osmolality and to glomerular filtration rate. In each individual age-group significant log-linear correlations have been found between urine concentration or excretion of AVP and urine osmolality (Fig. 15.6). After the disappearance of perinatal stress urinary vasopressin dropped on postnatal day 5 to very low values characteristic for the given age category. Importantly, urinary vasopressin started on postnatal day 5 to increase and already in infants reached values similar to those observed in adults. The possibility exists that the lower levels of urinary AVP found in younger age groups might be due to the lower glomerular filtration rate, as urinary AVP correlates with creatinine clearance (Godard et al. 1982). This factor however, may not be entirely responsible, because a similar trend in urine AVP becomes distinguishable after urinary vasopressin levels have been corrected for the corresponding GFR values.

The reasons underlying the lower pituitary secretory activity in healthy neonates and infants are not clear. For although AVP may be present and released in newborns and infants in a similar, but not identical, manner as in the adult, the above developmental phenomenon might reflect age-related peculiarities in the level of water metabolism. The increasing urinary AVP upon identical values of plasma osmolality in individual age categories (see Table 15.3) may be attributed to age-dependently rising sensitivity of the osmoregulatory mechanism of AVP secretion. It is tempting to speculate that the rising sensitivity of the osmoregulatory system of AVP secretion is a general trend from the fetal life (Robillard et al. 1979) through the old age (Os et al. 1985, chapter 16.2). On the other hand, this trend is opposed by a decrease in thirst sensation (an estimation based on the volume of fluid normally ingested) during the human development and aging. As a rule, healthy newborns and small infants daily receive as much as 150 ml per kg body weight and more

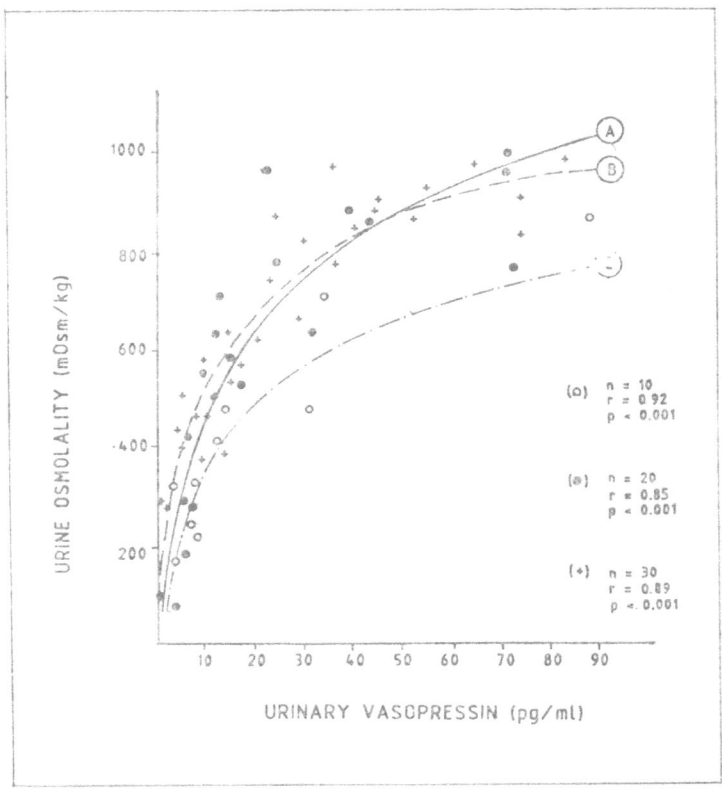

Fig. 15.6. Correlation between urinary AVP and urine osmolality in groups of well-hydrated healthy 4 months-old infants (C, [o] n = 10), children (B, [●] n = 20) and adults (A, [+] n = 30).

fluids, while fluid intake is apparently reduced in aged persons (Ziegler and Fomon 1971, Phillips et al. 1984).

In this respect it may be interesting to recall the proposal that development and aging are the taxes that the organism must pay for general "differentiation" of its structures. According to this it appears that body passes during this "differentiation" from a state in which stability of body fluids depends mainly on fluid intake (as in newborns with a lower sensitivity of the osmoregulatory mechanism of AVP and with high fluid turnover) to a state in which body fluid osmolality depends more on renal water conservation, as it is in aged subjects with higher sensitivity of the osmoregulatory mechanism of AVP and reduced thirst sensation (chapter 16). The question remains open to what degree this trend may relate to developmental changes in body fluid volume (Friis-Hansen 1983, Mann 1987). One may hypothesize based on the above trend that, despite isotonic reduction in extracellular fluid volume (see Fig. 15.2) as a physiologic phenomenon of development and aging, the body tries in the form of an as if biologic paradox maintaining the original extent of the body fluid compartments employing humoral control mechanisms.

15.6 CIRCADIAN VARIATIONS OF VASOPRESSIN SECRETION AND NOCTURNAL ENURESIS IN CHILDREN

Nocturnal enuresis, uncontrolled bedwetting after the age of 4, has been making the life of many individuals and their families unpleasant since prehistorical times when people started clothing and inhabiting closed spaces. Bedwetting among children is a common disorder affecting 30% at age 4, 10% at age 6, 3% at age 12, and 1% at age 20; if untreated, the spontaneous cure rate is about 15% a year (Wille 1986).

The etiopathogenesis of nocturnal enuresis is an enigma to pediatricians and scientists alike. Among other factors a role of a disturbed circadian rhythm of AVP secretion has been proposed (Puri 1980). Recent investigations into the dynamic temporal profiles of vasopressin in cerebrospinal fluid of several mammalian species show that vasopressin really exhibits a highly organized endogenous rhythm with high daytime and low night-time values; however, this rhythm is strictly limited to the liquor and no rhythm is manifested in the plasma (chapter 12.1.3). Although recumbent humans exhibit significant day-night variations in plasma AVP levels (George et al. 1975), an opposite trend with significantly higher daytime urine AVP levels can be generated when healthy subjects are evaluated during their normal daily activities in erect position (Fig. 15.7). Thus it appears that these circadian variations are not a reflection of an endogenously generated rhythm but that they are driven by other bodily functions such as activity and posture which normally influence circulating vasopressin levels by the hemodynamic pathway (chapter 5.4.1).

Owing to the lack of a true endogenous rhythm of AVP in plasma neither bedwetting can be explained by a postulated disturbances in the rhythm. At the same time this does not rule out the possibility that a secondarily (due to

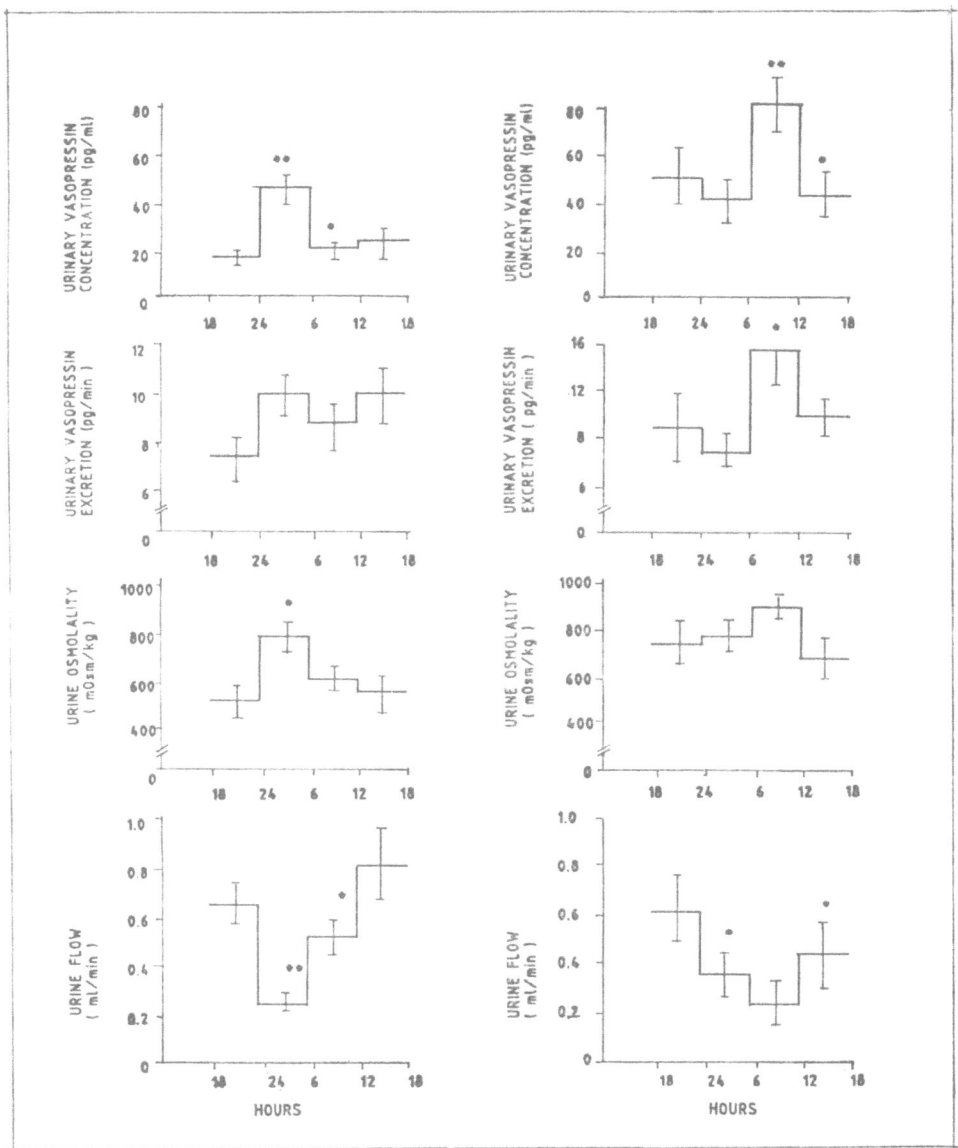

Fig. 15.7. Circadian changes of urinary vasopressin, urine osmolality and urine flow in 10 healthy children (aged 8 to 13 years) during 24 hours of recumbency (left side) and during their normal daily physical activity (right side). Results are shown as mean ± SE.

habitually increased intake of fluids in the evening or to an increased sensitivity of the osmoreceptor control mechanism of thirst) decreased AVP secretion during the night contributes to the development of enuresis. Nevertheless, the estimation of the actual significance of this factor is limited due to the lack of specific and reliable data concerning drinking habits and possible functional characteristics of osmoreceptors that control thirst in enuretics.

15.6.1 DESMOPRESSIN TREATMENT OF ENURESIS IN CHILDREN

In view of the multifactorial etiopathogenesis of the disturbance also the treatment of nocturnal enuresis is "multimodal". It includes in addition to psychotherapy a broad scale of other methods such as pharmacotherapy and electrophysiologic procedures. Pharmacotherapy is aimed mainly at diminishing contractility of the urinary bladder and/or attenuating sleep depth. Currently preferred tricyclic antidepressants have numerous side effects and may do more harm than good (Schmitt 1982). The declared goal of the widely applied electrophysiological technique (in the form of "alarm devices" and pad systems) aimed at establishing a reflex arousal with subsequent development of nocturnal continence is to wake up the patient during micturition (Wille 1986).

A new principle in the treatment of enuresis was recently introduced using the synthetic V2 analog (dDAVP, desmopressin). The theoretical benefit may be that dDAVP might diminish the overnight production of urine and thereby prevent diuresis, since one theory of the pathogenesis of enuresis assumes that bedwetting only occurs when the normal functional bladder capacity is exceeded. This theory is supported by the results of recent sleep investigations in enuretics which showed that enuresis occurred at the individual awake maximum bladder capacity and was independent of depth of sleep (Norgaard et al. 1985). An identical idea has been the basis of the long recommended therapeutic limitation of fluid intake which however is mostly difficult to implement since enuretics frequently violate this recommendation.

Several double blind placebo controlled studies have shown the efficacy of the drug in enuretic but otherwise healthy children (20 µg dDAVP intranasally one hour prior to sleep with subsequently restricted fluid intake). During its short time administration (up to 2 months) the observed success rates (41—86%) were similar, or superior, to those achieved with other forms of treatment (such as tricyclic antidepressants and "enuresis alarm" devices), but often with immediate relapse after the drug withdrawal; the last feature is shared by tricyclic antidepressants (Birkašová et al. 1978, Post et al. 1983, Wille 1986, Dimson 1986). Since the action of dDAVP does not require any conditioning the short time administration of the drug may be useful in exceptional situations such as traveling or camping.

Yet dDAVP also may prove to be another alternative for the long term management of the wetting symptom. Lehotská et al. (1984) evaluated the effect of the prolonged therapy in 87 children who failed to respond to other kinds of treatment (including pharmacotherapy and psychotherapy). Desmopressin was administered for short (3 months) or longer (8 months) intervals (Table 15.4). Prolonged therapy — terminated by gradual withdrawal of the drug or by its replacement by placebo — was applied with the hope that many patients will develop a habit of staying dry. Indeed a permanent disappearence of enuresis after prolonged therapy was observed in 61% of the children, and additional 10% showed a marked reduction in frequency of bedwetting.

Table 15.4. Clinical response to short term (up to 3 months) and prolonged (8 months) desmopressin administration in a group of 87 children with nocturnal enuresis. (A) — full recovery with a frequency of "wet" nights < 1 to 2 per months; (B) — partial recovery with a frequency of "wet" nights < 1 to 2 per week; (C) without effect i.e. with a continued frequency of "wet" nights > 1 to 2 per week; (D) not controlled (p < 0.05) (from Lehotská et al. 1984)

		Effect of desmopressin treatment			
Short term treatment (n = 87)		Prolonged desmopressin administration (n = 72)			
		(A)	(B)	(C)	(D)
(A)	28 (34% ± 13%)	20	—	8	—
(B)	37 (42% ± 12%)	19	7	2	9
(C)	22 (25% ± 12%)	5	—	11	6
		44 (61% ± 14%)	7 (10% ± 11%)	21 (29% ± 13%)	15

Naturally, the question may arise whether therapeutic administration of the synthetic analog of the natural hormone for an essentially benign condition, as enuresis is, is sufficiently justified. However the same question would then be in place concerning desmopressin and partial diabetes insipidus. Also the latter condition does not jeopardize the patient by the development of pathologic shifts in the composition of body fluids, and the drug is being administered exclusively to improve the personal well-being of the subject. In studies using long term desmopressin treatment the drug did not have any significant adverse effects and did not inhibit growth hormone, prolactin or cortisol levels at night (Becker and Foley 1978, Lehotská et al. 1984). Thus the treatment with desmopressin offers many benefits and seems to be a reasonable alternative to other pharmacologic agents, "alarm systems" and hypnosis in the treatment of the child with enuresis.

16 RENAL WATER HANDLING, VASOPRESSIN SECRETION AND THIRST SENSATION IN THE ELDERLY

Another specific problem from the viewpoint of osmoregulation is the period of aging. The normal anatomic and physiologic consequences of aging produce a population that is more susceptible to environmental stress, less adaptable to change, and with impaired recovery from insult or injury. This altered ability to maintain homeostasis may be due to normal functional decline or to superimposed pathologic conditions. Recognition that the geriatric patient may not behave like a younger adult is of paramount importance in medical and surgical management of the aging population.

16.1 AGING AND RENAL FUNCTION

The weight and volume of the kidney decrease 20 to 30% between the ages 30 and 90. This loss is primarily cortical and seems related to intrarenal vascular changes. The number of glomeruli decreases by 30 to 50% with an increasing percentage of sclerotic or abnormal glomeruli. A progressive decline in renal plasma flow is associated with a concomitant decrease in creatinine clearance (Brown et al. 1986).

Renal function in the elderly is thus the function of the residual nephrons. Tubular compensation of the decreased glomerular filtration requires a decrease in the residual nephrons of fractional reabsorption of osmotically active substances. This may relate to the fact that the elderly are unable to respond to sodium deprivation with as effective distal sodium conservation as younger subjects do (Epstein and Hollenberg 1976). Because salt is in ready supply in most circumstances there is not a major problem in maintaining sodium balance. Elderly patients will however respond differently to conditions that involve salt (and water) deprivation, for example, to diuretic therapy which must be given to these patients with caution (chapter 20.3.1.2).

Although renal cortical mass and blood supply decrease in the elderly medullary blood flow is preferentially maintained. This relatively increased medullary blood flow may interfere with the capacity of the countercurrent system to generate hypertonicity and in conjunction with the selective loss of juxtamedullary nephrons and anatomic alterations in renal tubules tends to compromise the urinary concentrating mechanism in elderly patients (see Tables 8.3 and 8.4) (Schück 1984, Brown et al. 1986). Moreover, in rats there is evidence of an age-related fall in water permeability of the collecting duct with a perhaps causative reduction in cAMP response to AVP (Beck and Yu 1982) and the same might pertain to man. In consequence, elderly patients require a larger urine volume to excrete the obligatory daily solute load of approximately 600 mOsm/kg. It is necessary to compensate for the defect with an increased fluid intake. This adaptation however is tedious because there is also impaired thirst perception in these subjects (chapter 16.3).

The interpretation of the decreased diluting capacity present in elderly subjects (U_{osm} min. > 50 mOsm/kg) is difficult. Free water clearance (C_{H_2O}) which under the conditions of maximal water diuresis can be considered an indicator of intensity of the loop solute transport (chapter 8.5.2.2) decreases in an age-dependent manner even when related to glomerular filtration rate ($C_{H_2O}/GFR \times 100$). Thus, renal function in the elderly significantly differs from function of residual nephrons in younger patients with various parenchymatose renal disease, when the value of the $C_{H_2O}/GFR \times 100$ rate does not decrease and the development of osmotic diuresis (with consequent decrease in diluting ability) can be interpreted as being secondary to a decreased reabsorption of solutes in the proximal segment of the nephron. The cause of the increased loop solute rejection in the elderly remains unclear (Schück 1984). Another important fact is that the kindeys of elderly subjects are unable to rapidly excrete a standard water load. The decreased glomerular filtration rate may, in addition to the decreased maximal diluting capacity, be involved in the development of this disturbance.

These physiological alterations undoubtedly represent a normal concomitant of the decremental phase of the life cycle, but at the same time they carry the risk of disturbances in water and salt balance. Impaired thirst sensation (chapter 16.3) and/or the physical disability to obtain adequate fluids is common in the elderly (Snyder et al. 1987). In these circumstances the decreased capacity to conserve water predisposes to hypotonic losses and thus to hypernatremia. On the other hand, the decreased glomerular filtration rate and the consequently decreased distal tubular delivery seen with aging may predispose to hyponatremia, particularly when salt is restricted with free access to water (Ayus 1986). Indeed, in clinical practice it is common for volume depleted elderly patients to respond dramatically to replacement of sodium or fluid deficits.

16.2 AGING AND VASOPRESSIN SECRETION

Recent data support the concept of enhanced secretion of AVP in response to osmotic stimuli in the elderly. Os et al. (1985) reported in 50-year olds basal

AVP levels more than three times higher than in younger men. Halderman et al. (1978) have demonstrated a highly significant age-related increase in osmoreceptor sensitivity, with plasma AVP rising twice as much in older subjects in response to the same osmotic stimulus. An osmoreceptor dysfunction or even resetting with age might be considered a possible explanation for these findings. On the other hand, Rowe et al. (1982) found that failure to release AVP in response to hemodynamic stimuli (orthostasis) is more common in the elderly than in the young (chapter 9.4.5), suggesting a defect distal to the vasomotor center in the afferent limb of the baroreceptor reflex arc.

It is not clear what the relationship between the two alterations in water regulation that occur with aging, i.e. impaired water conservation (see Table 8.4) in the presence of increased vasopressin secretion. It may be speculated that aging leads to the gradual development of an acquired form of partial diabetes insipidus; in this form chronic water losing state might be the initial event causing a secondary increased AVP secretion. Also, the opposite causative relationship of the events is possible: increasing vasopressin secretion may be the primary event occurring as a consequence of age-related changes in osmoreceptor sensitivity which antedate the decline in renal concentrating ability. Now there is some experimental evidence in support for the latter possibility. Assessment of vasopressin release from isolated hypothalamo-neurohypophyseal units by means of an in vitro perfusion system has shown that hormone discharge increased as the animal aged. This was evident by the age of 7 months, whereas impaired water conserving capacity was not present prior to 10 months of age (Miller 1987). Other studies in young and adult rats have shown that exposure of the kidney to increased concentrations of vasopressin produces a state of reduced responsiveness to the hormone, probably resulting in a diminished binding of AVP to its receptors on renal medullary cells (Handelmann et al. 1983). Thus it appears that the two events are somehow linked so that the increase in circulating AVP with advancing age may contribute to the secondary reduction in water conserving capacity of the kidney.

16.3 AGING AND THIRST

Not only sick but also healthy old people lack appropriate thirst when dehydrated and drink adequately well when encouraged by nursing staff (Phillips et al. 1984). The reasons for deficient thirst but enhanced AVP secretion in elderly subjects are not evident. Decreased sensitivity or selective loss of osmoreceptors that control thirst is possible since thirst and vasopressin pathways seem to be separate (Hammond et al. 1986).

17 CLINICAL SYNDROMES ASSOCIATED WITH HYPOVASOPRESSINISM

Clinical syndromes associated with absolute or relative hyposecretion of vasopressin and/or with diminished renal responsiveness to the antidiuretic effect of the hormone (hypovasopressinism) are usually classified in four main classes depending on the nature of the primary defect (Table 17.1). Each of the four syndromes is the end result of several pathogenetic mechanisms and can have diverse etiologies. In the first two of them — central diabetes insipidus (CDI) and nephrogenic diabetes insipidus (NDI) — the underlying disturbance is a diminished response of the AVP secretion mechanism to physiological stimuli, or a diminished renal response to hydroosmotic action of AVP respectively; this is manifested by solute-free polyuria and secondary polydipsia. In the other two — polydipsic diabetes insipidus (PDI) and essential hypernatremia (EH) — the clinical picture is determined by the primary disturbance of thirst osmoregulation, but hypovasopressinism is also involved, at least secondarily, in the abnormalities associated with these syndromes.

Table 17.1. Clinical syndromes associated with hypovasopressinism

Diagnosis	Vasopressin secretion	Vasopressin action	Thirst	Clinical presentation
Central diabetes insipidus (CDI)	decreased	normal	normal	polyuria and polydipsia
Nephrogenic diabetes insipidus (NDI)	normal	decreased	normal	polyuria and polydipsia
Polydipsic diabetes insipidus (PDI)	normal	normal	increased	polyuria and polydipsia
Essential hyper-natremia (EH)	decreased or normal	normal	decreased or absent	hypodipsia and hypernatremia

17.1 DISTURBED VASOPRESSIN SECRETION (CENTRAL DIABETES INSIPIDUS, CDI)

Central diabetes insipidus may result from any condition which impairs synthesis, transport and release of neurohypophyseal AVP. This rare condition affects both sexes equally, and its onset is at any age (most frequent onsets however are observed between 10 and 20 years of age). There may be no evidence of ill health or physiologic disturbance associated with the condition other than the annoyance of polyuria and (secondary) thirst, unless the patient suffers from the underlying disease which destroyed the hypothalamo-neurohypophyseal system. Nocturia is usually present and results in chronic tiredness, poor school or work performance and malaise. In children the presenting symptom may be enuresis. Patients who due to additional reasons are unable to sufficiently empty the urinary bladder, may develop enlarged atonic bladder and hydronephrosis, although more typically, these features are seen in individuals with hereditary nephrogenic diabetes insipidus (Coggins and Leaf 1967, Czernichow et al. 1985).

In complete forms of central diabetes insipidus the daily diuresis may reach as many as 8—12 l, occasionally even more; the maximal urinary osmolality does not exceed the isotonicity level (U_{osm} max < 290 mOsm/kg) even if the patient is deprived of water. Water deprivation for even a short period of time results in rapid dehydration which is associated with compulsive thirst: it wakens the subject up even during the night. As a rule, these patients prefer ice water, and if they cannot replenish their water losses from normal sources, they not infrequently drink water from flower vases, from air humidifiers, or even their own urine.

However, central diabetes insipidus not always is an all-or-none disease. Partial forms of the syndrome, characterized by only moderately excessive diuresis and urine osmolality reaching, upon dehydration, values between isotonicity and the lower limit of normal range for the respective age category (see Tables 8.3 and 8.4), are much more frequent than complete forms of the disorder. The daily urine volume however, only weakly correlates with the actual extent of the damage to the hypothalamo-neurohypophyseal tract, and it may depend on a number of other factors, in particular on the actual setting of the thirst threshold in the individual (see Fig. 5.7) and on the amounts of dietary solutes ingested (chapter 8.4.2.1).

The frequently encountered assumption that patients with diabetes insipidus suffer from severe dehydration is not supported by measurements of plasma sodium or total solute concentrations. As long as the thirst center remains intact and the individual is able to seek water, the osmotic concentration of body fluids usually oscillates around values only slightly exceeding 290 mOsm/kg, although at the expense of polydipsia and large fluid turnover characteristic of this condition. The slightly higher values of plasma osmolality in these patients may relate to relatively high osmotic threshold in humans (see Fig. 5.5). Owing to this, individuals with central diabetes insipidus begin replenishing their water deficit with a certain latency, i.e. after their plasma osmolality has exceeded the thirst threshold. Following a period of water restriction, of course, the increment of plasma osmolality may become more pronounced and have greater diagnostic value (Moses 1985, Kovács et al. 1985).

17.1.1 ETIOLOGY OF CENTRAL DIABETES INSIPIDUS

Roughly, almost one third of cases of central diabetes insipidus are usually claimed to result from tumors localized in the hypothalamo-neurohypophyseal region, either primary or metastatic. A second third of patients include those with idiopatic forms of the syndrome with currently no obvious etiology. Finally, the remaining third of cases of central diabetes insipidus can be ascribed to various other mechanisms, including rare hereditary forms of the syndrome (Table 17.2).

Table 17. 2. Causes of central diabetes insipidus

A. Trauma (accidental, surgical)
B. Neoplasms (hypothalamic, pituitary, metastatic, lymphoma, leukemia)
C. Granulomatous diseases (histiocytosis, sarcoidosis)
D. Infectious processes (encephalitis, meningitis, syphilis, Guillain—Barré)
E. Vascular diseases (Sheehan's syndrome, aneurysms, brain arrest, hypoxic brain damage)
F. Congenital intracranial defects
G. Autoimmune processes
H. Idiopathic
I. Congenital
   — isolated, familial
   — sporadic
   — DIDMOAD syndrome

Although these conditions still account for a significant number of cases of central diabetes insipidus, the increasing incidence of traffic injuries, but mainly surgical pituitary stalk sections and other neurosurgical procedures in the region of the hypothalamo-neurohypophyseal system, have affected the relative frequencies. Currently the latter conditions constitute the major causes of central diabetes insipidus, accounting in developed countries for more than 40 per cent of cases. At the same time, the partial proportions of the idiopathic forms of the syndrome drop, especially thanks to the development of modern clinical methods of investigation which have enabled to separate a number of new etiological forms from this heterogenous group (inborn defects of the septal-optic brain area, and also autoimmune variants of CDI) (Moses 1985, Greger et al. 1986, Scherbaum et al. 1986).

17.1.1.1 Postoperative and posttraumatic central diabetes insipidus

The clinical course of these etiological forms of CDI depends largely on the anatomical localization of the primary insult to the hypothalamo-neuro-hypophyseal tract (Verbalis et al. 1985). More proximally sited lesions, localized more closely to cell bodies, are associated with the death of larger numbers of neurons of the hypothalamo-neurohypophyseal tract. In these cases, accounting for about 30—40% of all posttraumatic and postoperative diabetes insipidus, the primary insult is accompanied by an abrupt onset of grave polyuria. During subsequent weeks and months, the urine volume remains definitely, or at least sustainedly, copious (permanent or prolonged CDI; Fig. 17.1 (B)). On the other hand, with low sitting lesions (below the median eminence, 50—60% of cases), only a small proportion of magnocellular neurons degenerates, and intact preserved cell bodies are able, within a certain period of time, to produce new axonal terminals, the neurohemal organs, at the level of the portal vessels of the median eminence, thereby resolving CDI. Clinically, this

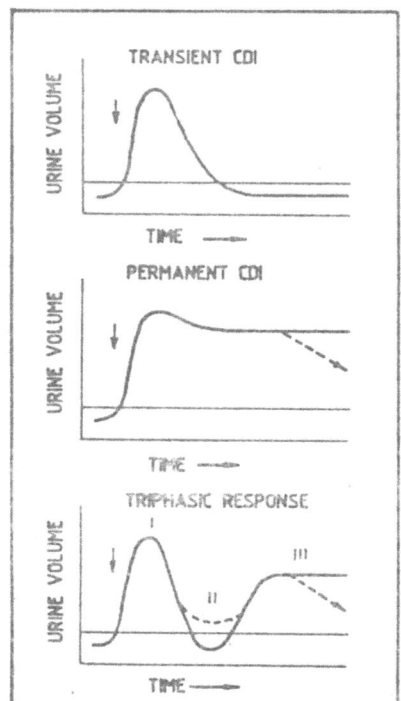

Fig. 17.1. Diagrammatic summary of the major patterns of postoperative and post-traumatic central diabetes insipidus (CDI). The abscissa represents time following the initial injury (arrow) and the ordinate urinary volume relative to a hypothetical "normal" urine output of 2 to 3 l/day (solid line) (the variability of real time periods is described in the text) (by Verbalis et al. 1985 with kind permission).

pattern is manifested by abrupt onset of pronounced polyuria during the first 24 h, and by a gradual improvement, or even total disappearance, of clinical symptoms within the subsequent days or weeks (transient CDI; Fig. 17.1 (A)). Finally, the rarest (10—20% of cases) but potentially the gravest pattern is that in which abrupt onset of polyuria is followed in several hours or days by an "antidiuretic interphase" lasting as a rule only 2—14 days before the persistent CDI is established (Fig. 17.1 (C)). This triphasic response can be expected to occur following neurosurgical or traumatic injury to the pituitary stalk, when the entire neurohypophysis (or at least a significant part of it) has been left in situ.

Although the development of the triphasic response can be supposed based on the nature of the neurosurgical intervention, this pattern may remain a source of serious diagnostic and therapeutical problems in individuals with head traumatism. Perfunctory investigation of these patients may lead to the erroneous conclusion that the "antidiuretic interphase" reflects regeneration and normalization of the neurohypophyseal function. One may oversee that it is, in fact, an inappropriate antidiuresis resulting from neurohypophysis degenerating in situ in the sella, which underlies the condition and which may result, if fluid intake is not limited, in excessive retention of water in the body with resulting brain edema (Ikkos et al. 1955, Hollinshead 1964). Owing to this, each patient with recent severe head traumatism should be considered to potentially have the neurohypophysis injured, even if the actual values of plasma and urinary osmolality are normal. The finding of hyponatremia and plasma hypoosmolality in a patient with cerebral traumatism, and the excretion of inadequately concentrated urine should prompt the assumption of "antidiuretic interphase" in the development of central diabetes insipidus, requiring limitation of fluid intake; a third phase should then be anticipated.

Diagnostic problems may also be due to concurrent anterior pituitary failure, specifically hypocortisolemia. The inability of patients with hypocortisolemia to excrete maximally diluted urine is generally known, and amelioration of central diabetes insipidus following the anterior pituitary failure has been described (Jamison 1983, chapter 20.3.1.7). As a rule, this is rarely a problem after surgical interventions, since patients after sellar or suprasellar interventions are usually given high hydrocortisone doses. Nevertheless, individuals with extensive cerebral traumatism not always receive the hormone, and hypophyseal injury may remain ignored. Hence, this possibility should be considered in patients after cerebral traumatism.

17.1.1.2 Idiopathic central diabetes insipidus

It is not unusual that the primary cause of CDI is established only after repeated investigations of the subject. For example, histiocytosis cannot always be ruled out with certainty, and a delay of several years between the onset of vasopressin sensitive polyuria and the establishment of the primary disease is not infrequent (Sims 1977). Despite all efforts spent, in many patients the exact nature of the primary disease may remain obscure. Various, so far insufficiently defined pathological processes may be involved in the development of these idiopathic cases of CDI.

The few autopsic studies have reported atrophic neurohypophysis as well as supraoptic and paraventricular nuclei in idiopathic CDI (Green et al. 1967). The presence of circulating antibodies against AVP-secreting hypothalamic neurons in one third of patients with idiopatic forms of CDI favors the hypothesis concerning the existence of an autoimmune variant of the syndrome. This opinion is supported also by the relatively frequent association of CDI with various other autoimmune endocrinopathies, mainly with thyroidal autoimmune processes. In addition AVP-cell antibodies have been also demonstrated in many patients with CDI secondary to histiocytosis suggesting a role of autoimmune mechanisms in the genesis of this clinical syndrome (Scherbaum et al. 1986).

17.1.1.3 Hereditary variants of central diabetes insipidus

In addition to the above mentioned secondary forms, also primary, hereditary variants of the syndrome are known, making up not more than 1—2 % of all cases of CDI.

The classic variant, inherited by an autosomal dominant trait, is usually manifested clinically already in infancy, although cases of delayed manifestation have also been reported (Brugnier et al. 1981). The few autopsy findings reported have consistently shown neuronal degeneration and gliosis of variable numbers of supraoptic and paravetricular nuclei, usually accompanied by a small neurohypophysis (Braverman et al. 1965). Although similar findings have been reported in idiopathic CDI, the relationship between these observations remains unclear. Nevertheless, these data suggesting a pathological process of a still not defined nature affecting individual AVP-**produc**ing cells, may explain the considerable differences in the age at the syndrome onset as well as the conspicuous differences in its clinical significance, even between members of the same family. Some members of families affected by the syndrome can have subclinical deficiencies of vasopressin secretion that become evident upon a careful examination only. Though not studied systematically, the other posterior pituitary hormone, oxytocin, appears to be secreted normally in patients with hereditary CDI. It is important to note that this human disorder is in several aspects different from hereditary CDI in Brattleboro rats (chapter 4.4) (Table 17.3).

Less known is another variant of CDI which is inherited by an autosomal recessive trait (Page et al. 1976, Zerbe 1985, Chu et al. 1986). In this form, deficient AVP secretion is manifested concomitantly with diabetes mellitus,

Table 17.3. Genetic variants of central diabetes insipidus

	Isolated familial CDI	DIDMOAD syndrome	Brattleboro rat
Inheritance	autosomal dominant	autosomal recessive	autosomal recessive
AVP secretory defect	complete/partial	partial	partial
Associated abnormalities	none	diabetes mellitus, optic atrophy, neural deafness, other	growth retardation
Etiology	neurosecretory defect, degeneration	neurosecretory defect, degeneration	synthetic defect

optic atrophy and neural deafness. This variant, referred to as **DIDMOAD** syndrome or Wolfram's syndrome (see Table 17.3), is characterized by clinically significant polyuria with an onset before the age of 10. However, the recognition of diabetes insipidus may be delayed if polyuria is explained as resulting from osmotic diuresis due to uncontrolled diabetes mellitus. Neural deafness and other associated abnormalities (e. g. neurogenic bladder and hydronephrosis) develop as a rule but at later age. The above combination of typical manifestations cannot be explained by a single abnormality; most likely, the syndrome is secondary to some so far unidentified metabolic disorder resulting in cell degeneration of specific neural structures and pancreatic beta-cells.

17.1.2 CENTRAL DIABETES INSIPIDUS IN INFANCY AND CHILDHOOD

As a rule, neither acquired nor hereditary vasopressin deficiency are manifested in newborns; significant polyuria usually develops in infancy. Mechanisms protecting newborns from excessive renal water losses in the absence of vasopressin remain unknown. However, there is an interesting analogy to rats of the Brattleboro strain; also these animals start increasing diuresis as late as 3—4 weeks after the birth, i.e. during the weaning period, when requirements of the body for water conservation significantly increase (Dlouhá et al. 1982).

Due to their inability to seek water, small infants usually present with chronic dehydration, unexplained fevers, obstipation and failure to thrive.

167

Chronic water deficiency can cause serious neurologic disturbances and may, under unfavourable conditions, result in long-term neurological consequences (Vest et al. 1963, Czernichow et al. 1985). Because of the increased hydrolability of the young organism, the management of CDI in infants is mostly difficult. Plasma osmolality should be frequently monitored as episodes of plasma hyper- and hypoosmolality can frequently occur despite careful adjustment of water. When early diagnosed and adequately treated, infants affected by this syndrome may mentally and physically develop in parallel with their normal counterparts (Némethová et al. 1979, Waggoner et al. 1978).

The major symptom of central diabetes insipidus in childhood is dramatic polyuria. However, its gravity mostly does not closely correlate with the actual seriousness of AVP deficiency. Most patients develop maximal diuresis between the age of 15 and 25, with the polyuria tending to diminish thereafter. This diminution of diuresis however is not necessarily parallelled by an increase in urinary osmolality as measured by the dehydration test; hence, factors other than a possible return of the neurohypophyseal capacity to secrete AVP into the circulation may be assumed to underlie this improvement.

17.1.3 CENTRAL DIABETES INSIPIDUS IN PREGNANCY

The coexistence of central diabetes insipidus and pregnancy is rare, probably because the former is uncommon (Hime and Richardson 1978). It is unlikely that neurohypophyseal deficiency without concomitant loss of adenohypophyseal hormones would alter fertility, cause spontaneous abortions, or interfere with normal labor and delivery. Even women with posterior pituitary failure of any etiology usually have normal lactation.

Pregnancy itself may modify the development of CDI in various ways. Aggravation of polyuria observed in some pregnant women with CDI might result from the presence in the plasma of pregnant women of placentary cystine aminopeptidase, an enzyme which inactivates oxytocin and vasopressin (Rosenbloom et al. 1975, Amico 1985, Durr et al. 1987). In other cases polyuria of unchanged intensity may be present throughout the pregnancy, or it sometimes may partially subside from reasons that remain unknown (Oravec and Lichardus 1972, Baylis et al. 1986, Durr et al. 1987). Most likely, these changes are independent of physiological parallel downward resetting of the thresholds of the osmoregulatory systems of thirst and vasopressin secretion, that accompanies pregnancy (see Fig. 5.6). This physiological alteration stabilizes plasma osmolality at levels lower than in nonpregnant women, while not inducing either polyuria or secondary polydipsia.

Diabetes insipidus developing during pregnancy and remaining post partum most likely suggests tumor etiology of the syndrome, requiring thorough examination of the patient.

Transient vasopressin deficiency during the post partum period may develop in Sheehan's syndrome. Association of vasopressin deficiency with Sheehan's syndrome is however extremely rare, most likely owing to different blood supply to the anterior and the posterior pituitary. If this association occurs, significant polyuria may ensue, but only after supplementation of glucocorticoid hormones.

17.1.4 THERAPY OF CENTRAL DIABETES INSIPIDUS

Water is emphasized as therapy for diabetes insipidus, because water alone taken in sufficient quantity will correct any metabolic abnormality secondary to excessive dilute urine. Since the patient with uncomplicated diabetes insipidus who has an intact thirst mechanism and an ample supply of water suffers no known harm but only inconvenience from lack of vasopressin, the indications for replacement therapy may not be pressing. However, the marked polydipsia and polyuria may be disturbing and distract during the day and prevent sleep at night, and for reasons of convenience replacement therapy or some other therapeutic modalities are usually justified.

Owing to their antidiuretic activities all of these therapeutic modalities can cause excessive water retention and hyponatremia. This is particularly true for patients with polydipsic diabetes insipidus. Therefore, one must be certain to exlude polydipsic DI (chapter 17.4) as the cause of polyuria before starting therapy for CDI (or nephrogenic diabetes insipidus). Moreover, since the neurologic symptoms of hyponatremia can mimic those of hypernatremia, but the therapy is diametrally opposite (water restriction versus water loading) it is important to establish the correct diagnosis rather than assume the presence of hypernatremia because of the history of central diabetes insipidus.

Finally, it should be emphasized, that the description of CDI as a benign condition is based upon the assumption that the patient has normal thirst and is able to drink sufficient water to maintain normal water balance. Any factor that interferes with the normal expression of thirst function (e.g. loss of consciousness after trauma) unavoidably converts this in fact benign condition into a dangerous one: sustained excessive water losses may within several hours after the therapeutical agent reaches the end of its normal duration of action lead to life-threatening dehydration, plasma hypertonicity and cardiovascular collapse. To avoid this, patients should carry with themselves medical cards indicating the presence of the syndrome (Verbalis and Robinson 1985).

17.1.4.1 Conventional substitutional therapy

The earliest commercially available preparation of vasopressin was a crude acetone dried extract from bovine or porcine posterior pituitary given by nasal insufflation ("pituitary snuff"). However its antidiuretic potential and thus the interval of activity, varied. Further problems concerned local irritation of nasal mucosa resulting in chronic rhinitis and loss of efficacy, in part due to antibodies which developed against multiple antigens present in crude preparations (Pepys et al. 1965).

A subsequently developed application form of antidiuretic hormone, pitressin tannate in oil, was a substantially more purified preparation that provided relief of symptoms for 24 to 72 hours. Its major disadvantage, particularly in the pediatric age category, was the discomfort associated with the necessity of repeated intramuscular injections once in 2—4 days, associated with the possibility of the development of sterile abscesses at the site of administration. The prolongation of the effect of the preparation was paralleled with the hazard of water intoxication, in particular in patients with CDI accompanied by concomitant abnormalities of the thirst mechanism.

Synthetic arginine-vasopressin or lysine-vasopressin has almost no place in the treatment of uncomplicated CDI. When administered parenterally by injection there is a brief and variable period of antidiuretic activity because of prompt absorption into the bloodstream and subsequent rapid inactivation (Moses 1964). Moreover, with an adequate dose vomiting, flushing, dizziness, increased small bowel motility or syncope may occur due to the V1 receptor related effects of the hormone.

17.1.4.2 Oral therapeutic agents

Disadvantages of the above mentioned hormone preparations along with efforts aimed at oral treatment of CDI prompted in the 60ies the introduction of a number of drugs originally used for other purposes.

The antidiuretic effect of chlorpropamide, an oral hypoglycemic sulfanylurea preparation, was disclosed by chance in relation with a patient who had treated himself for presumed diabetes mellitus (Arduino et al. 1966). Chlorpropamide decreases the clearance of solute-free water but only in the presence of a residual secretory capacity of the neurohypophysis (partial central diabetes insipidus). Usual doses of the agent (100—500 mg orally daily) induce maximal antidiuresis since day 4 of the drug administration. However, the clinical employment of the antidiuretic activity is substantially limited by the risk of hypoglycemia, particularly in children and patients with concomitant failure of the anterior pituitary. Antidiuresis observed following chlorpropamide is likely due to raising the sensitivity of the collecting duct epithelia to low concentrations of circulating vasopressin (Moses et al. 1973) (chapter 17.2.2.5).

Carbamazepine, an anticonvulsant, potentiates in doses of 200—600 mg/day antidiuresis in patients with partial central diabetes insipidus. The mechanism of its antidiuretic action is complex. The drug reduces the sensitivity of the osmoregulatory system of AVP secretion and simultaneously raises the sensitivity of the collecting duct to the hydroosmotic action of the hormone (Gold et al. 1983b).

Clofibrate, a lipid lowering agent, enhances in doses of 2 g/day antidiuresis in patients with partial central diabetes insipidus, most likely by stimulating residual endogenous AVP production (Bonnicci 1973). However, in view of increased incidence of cholecystopathies and of cancer of the gall bladder, the drug has not been recommended for routine use.

Finally, the paradoxical antidiuretic effect of thiazide diuretics has its firm place in the treatment of central diabetes insipidus (Crawford et al. 1960), though these drugs are more commonly used in the therapy of nephrogenic DI (chapter 17.2.3.1).

17.1.4.3 Desmopressin treatment

Since the first report concerning the clinical use of desmopressin (1-deamino-8D-arginine vasopressin, dDAVP) by Vávra et al. (1968), this agent has received enthusiastic support from patients who previously preferred drinking liters of water every day to taking other forms of therapy. Really, desmopressin is currently the safest therapeutic agent to be the drug of choice for therapy of CDI (Némethová et al. 1979, Richardson and Robinson 1985).

Desmopressin can be given parenterally and orally; the most frequent route of administration however is intranasal (chapter 7.3.1). With the intranasal route the patient must acquire some skill to use the "rhinyl" catheter so that the solution does not flow out of the nose and does not get deep into the pharynx where its resorption is considerably worse. The patient should understand the therapy so that individual judgement can be used for flexibility of therapy depending upon daily activities. He should be aware that the aim of the therapy is not to reach the smallest urine volume possible. Diuresis should be reduced to a degree only allowing the patient normal life and working activities.

Despite marked individual variations in dDAVP halflife (chapter 7.3.1) the duration of the effect of the synthetic peptide in an individual is well reproduci ble (Pliška 1985). Hence, desmopressin dose and scheduling should be adjusted individually. This can be done by titrating the duration and effectivity of different desmopressin doses (5 µg, 10 µg, and 20 µg) under controlled clinical conditions, if possible, allowing to longitudinally follow up changes in diuresis and urinary osmolality (or specific gravity). Any other previous treatment should be discontinued, and the first titration dose of desmopressin (5 µg = = 50 µl) is administered after the effects of the previous therapy have completely disappeared. As a rule, the first desmopressin dose reduces urine volume within 1—2 hours, and the antidiuretic effect may last as long as 6—24 hours. Subsequent testing doses (10 and 20 μg) are administered but after the effect of the preceding dose dissipates and baseline diuresis has returned to at least 4 ml/min.

The titration of desmopressin effect allows then to flexibly schedule the dosage according to the actual needs of the patient. Generally, it is recommended to administer repeated lower doses rather than one large dose. The administration of the drug in the early morning hours is usually sufficient to prevent mid-morning polyuria. The second and third dose can then be given around the noon or late in the afternoon to allow undisturbed afternoon activities and sleep (Richardson and Robinson 1985).

To prevent the development of volume expansion, natriuresis and hyponatremia (i.e. a condition resembling the syndrome of inappropriate secretion of ADH) after desmopressin, it is recommendable to delay, once or twice a week, the drug administration until marked polyuria accompanied with thirst occurs. This may be particularly important for long-term follow up of posttraumatic and postsurgical CDI where endogenous AVP production may recover even after longer intervals (even after several years) after the initial insult If hyponatremia occurs, which cannot be explained by too large doses of des

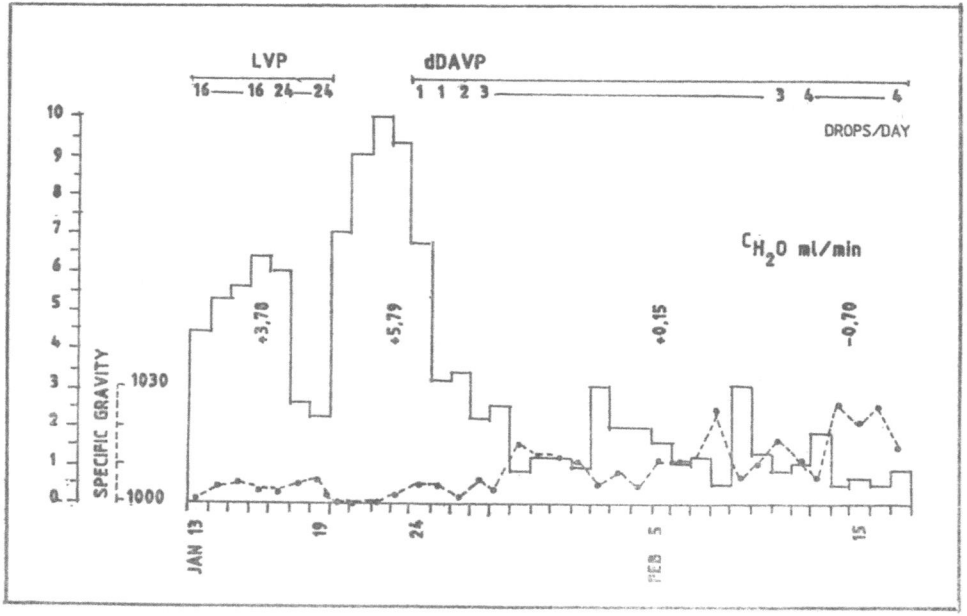

Fig. 17.2. Effects of desmopressin treatment in a child with central diabetes insipidus (by Némethová et al. 1979).

172

mopressin, abnormalities of the thirst mechanism (polydipsic diabetes insipidus) should be considered and the diagnosis of CDI should be reevaluated.

In children with CDI, doses required to obtain sufficient antidiuresis are generally lower as compared to those needed by adult patients (Fig. 17.2). However, the doses do not correlate with the size of infants and children. Dosage should be carefully set individually, and it is advisable to start with lower doses (1.25 and 2.5 µg). In patients requiring very small doses which cannot be exactly dosed with the tube accompanying the drug, adequate dosage can be obtained by diluting the drug solution with normal saline. Infants and children may occasionally require but one daily dose of desmopressin. However, to prevent undesirable oscillations in plasma osmolality, it is more adequate to administer smaller doses 2 to 3 times daily. Frequent infections of the upper airways may alter absorption of desmopressin from the nasal mucosa. In similar cases the drug can be administered orally, naturally in adequately larger doses (chapter 7.3.1) (Némethová and Lichardus 1974, Fjellestad and Czernichow 1986).

Desmopressin, which contrary to lysine-vasopressine, does not induce myometral contractions, is an ideal drug to treat central diabetes insipidus in pregnant women (Oravec and Lichardus 1972). A weaker response to desmopressin during pregnancy would not be expected as the cystine aminopeptidase of human pregnancy does not degrade desmopressin. Even lactation does not represent a contraindication of its administration. It is highly unlikely that minimal doses of desmopressin which get into the milk can induce hyponatremia in newborns and infants (Burrow et al. 1981).

In patients with altered consciousness who are not able to report thirst desmopressin administration must be extremely cautious. Owing to possible development of symptomatic hyponatremia, fluid balance by intravenous administration of hypotonic solutions is often preferred in patients during the acute phase of posttraumatic or postsurgical CDI. However, this approach has no advantages over desmopressin therapy: both procedures require measurements of plasma and urinary osmolality several times a day. If however, desmopressin is started during the first days after the insult, one dose of the agent should be omitted daily to ascertain whether or not a triphasic pattern of CDI develops (see Fig. 17.1).

17.2 NEPHROGENIC DIABETES INSIPIDUS (NDI)

A major hallmark of nephrogenic diabetes insipidus is the inability of the kidneys to produce maximally concentrated urine in the presence of sufficient amounts of vasopressin in conditions when the renal concentrating mechanism has been maximally stimulated by prolonged water deprivation. In patients with complete nephrogenic diabetes urinary osmolality remains consistently

Table 17.4. Causes of nephrogenic diabetes insipidus (NDI)

A. Congenital nephrogenic DI

B. Acquired nephrogenic DI

    Potassium depletion

    Hypercalcemia

    Drugs
    — lithium salts
    — demeclocycline
    — sulfanpureas
    — amphotericin B
    — gentamycin
    — cis-dichlorodiamine (II) platinum
    — colchicine
    — vinca alcaloids

    Renal and systemic diseases (see Table 8.2)

    Dietary abnormalities
    — excessive water intake
    — decreased sodium chloride intake
    — decreased protein intake

    Osmotic diuresis (see Table 17.5)

less than plasma osmolality (U_{osm} max < 290 mOsm/kg) in cases of complete NDI, but considerably higher levels can be met (ranging between isotonicity and the respective age-related normal levels) in subjects with partial forms of the syndrome.

The many causes of nephrogenic diabetes insipidus can be divided in two categories: familial and acquired (Table 17.4). The complex pathogenesis of the various forms of NDI is characterized by one of the three ways (and, most frequently, by their various combinations): 1. disturbed generation and/or maintenance of the cortico-medullary osmotic gradient serving as the driving force for the osmotic water flow from collecting ducts into the interstitial tissue; 2. disturbance of osmotic equilibration between the tubular contents and the medullay interstitium due to a defect of the proximal component of the AVP-cAMP system (i.e. those processes which determine the intracellular concentration of cAMP, the mediator of AVP effect) and/or of the distal component of this system (i.e. processes whereby cAMP induces the hydro-osmotic response of epithelial cells); and/or 3. osmotic diuresis producing rapid flow of the tubular fluid and thus preventing its complete osmotic equilibration with the medullary interstitium. The situation is further complicated by the fact that certain acquired forms of NDI are associated with concomitant alterations of central elements of the osmoregulatory mechanism:

174

with primary polydipsia (e.g. in hypercalcemia, potassium depletion and during the administration of lithium salts), or with a defect in vasopressin secretion (e.g. during the administration of the "diuretic" sulfanylureas).

17.2.1 FAMILIAL NEPHROGENIC DIABETES INSIPIDUS

The first modern descriptions of vasopressin-resistant diabetes insipidus concerned the rare hereditary form of the syndrome. The disorder is usually transmitted in a sex-linked fashion, either as an X-linked recessive trait or as an X-linked dominant trait with variable penetrance in females. Thus complete or partial nephrogenic diabetes insipidus can occur in both males and females, but the complete disorder is much more common in males, and the partial forms usually occur in females (Bode and Crawford 1969).

The leading symptoms include polyuria, polydipsia, constipation and recurrent febrile episodes which usually become manifest during early infancy. The occurrence of febrile episodes correlates with the hydration status of the individual; following adequate rehydration body temperature also normalizes. However, since detection of polyuria and polydipsia in infants may often present difficulties, not infrequently the diagnosis of NDI is established relatively late, with a delay of several months or even years. Nocturia, enuresis, megaureter and hydronephrosis are all frequent complications of the syndrome occurring during the later childhood (Schoen 1960, Dicker and Eggleton 1963, Némethová et al. 1984). Unfortunately, growth retardation and also mental disturbances of varying degree (from slight memory disturbances up to imbecility) still remain a frequent finding in children with familial nephrogenic diabetes insipidus. It is the more regrettable since these defects seem not genetically determined but rather they are consequences of inadequate caloric intake (growth retardation) and of repeated episodes of hypertonic dehydration during the infancy (mental dullness). Both the mental and physical development of patients who were receiving "generous water supply" since their first months of life parallel that of their healthy counterparts (Reuss and Rosental 1963, Uttley et al. 1972).

Despite extensive evaluation of renal morphology and function, the only abnormality that is consistently found in patients with hereditary NDI is the inability to respond to vasopressin by producing maximally concentrated urine. The absence of enhanced excretion of cAMP in urine in response to vasopressin or desmopressin administration observed in many cases of hereditary NDI suggests that the primary defect likely is in the proximal component of the AVP-receptor-cAMP system. However, other patients with this disorder have been reported who responded with increased urine cAMP excretion to exogenous AVP. These contradictory data prompted the proposal of at least two different types of familial nephrogenic diabetes insipidus: type 1 not responding by enhanced urinary cAMP excretion to AVP administration (proximal type), and type 2 which though being capable of cAMP response to AVP, does not respond to AVP by increasing urinary osmolality due to the defect in the distal component of the AVP-cAMP system (distal type) (see Figs 7.1 and 8.5) (Fichman and Brooker 1972, Zimmermann and Green 1975, Ohzeki et al. 1984).

It cannot be ruled out that, at least in certain cases, the disturbance may concern a more general defect of utilisation of the vasopressin effect; then, the defect is not limited to the kidneys but may become manifest also in other tissues, e.g. the vascular epithelium and hepatic sinusoids, i.e. at sites of the supposed production of factor VIII. If reports concerning the lack of increased FVIII: Ag following administration of dDAVP to patients with NDI, and a 50% reduction of the response in carriers of the genetic defects will prove true (Kobrinsky et al. 1985), the test might be useful as an additional information in genealogic investigation of families with hereditary NDI.

17.2.2 ACQUIRED NEPHROGENIC DIABETES INSIPIDUS

During the last decade it has been widely appreciated that in addition to several well-known causes of acquired NDI (hypercalcemia and potassium depletion as well as various renal and systemic diseases) administration of several widely used pharmacological agents may also be associated with the development of an AVP-resistant renal concentrating defect (see Table 17.4). Indeed, drugs, in particular lithium salts, are responsible for most cases of NDI seen in general clinical practice (Singer and Forest 1976, Braden et al. 1985). Acquired forms of NDI are much more frequent, but rarely are as severe as is the familial variant of the syndrome. The former forms are usually accompanied by a partial defect in concentrating ability and moderate polyuria, usually not exceeding 4—5 l per day.

17.2.2.1 Potassium depletion

A clinically significant potassium deficiency always means potassium depletion from the intracellular fluid; this may, but needs not, become manifest as hypokalemia. Thus, normokalemia does not rule out deficiency of body potassium; on the contrary, hypokalemia cannot be taken as evidence for this condition, though it does suggest it. Potassium depletion due to reduced dietary intake of the cation and/or more frequently, due to increased losses (e.g. due to gastroenteritis, hypermineralocorticism, renal tubular defects or metabolic acidosis) is usually associated with the development of polyuria, polydipsia and renal concentrating defect resistant to vasopressin.

Experimental potassium depletion in animals has suggested a very complex nature of the associated disturbance in water homeostasis (Berl et al. 1977). By the end of the first week of potassium depletion animals developed polyuria which was solely due to increased fluid intake (i.e. due to primary polydipsia); however, after two weeks of potassium depletion a vasopressin resistant concentrating defect was also present. Although the role of primary polydipsia in human potassium depletion has not been completely delineated, this primary dipsogenic effect may explain the known clinical observations suggesting that in patient with potassium depletion polyuria usually is more significant than might be expected from the actual degree of the concentrating defect present in the patient (Jespersen et al. 1987).

Two major mechanisms have been proposed to explain the renal concentrating defect in potassium depletion. The first of them is related to an alteration of the generation and maintenance of the medullary osmotic gradient, while the other one concerns the resistance of the collecting ducts to hydroosmotic effect of AVP. With regard to gradient generation and maintenance, direct measurements of medullary and papillary solute content in potassium depleted animals revealed decreased interstitial concentration of sodium (Kim et al. 1984, Gutsche et al. 1984). In addition, in humans with severe potassium depletion decreased clearance of solute-free water (C_{H_2O}), decreased tubular reabsorption of solute-free water ($T^c_{H_2O}$) and increased values of minimal urine osmolality (U_{osm} min) were reported (Rubini 1961). This combination of disturbances indicates a decreased reabsorption of NaCl (i.e. disturbed gradient generation) in the thick segment of the ascendent limb of the Henle's loop (chapter 8.4.2.2).

With regard to the second mechanism proposed, experimental data have shown that tubular fluid fails to achieve osmotic equilibrium with the interstitium, implying that the response of the collecting duct to vasopressin is also impaired in potassium depletion. The biochemical defect responsible for this disturbance most likely is localized within the proximal component of the AVP-cAMP system; however, a simultaneous presence of a post-cyclicAMP defect in this electrolyte disturbance cannot be ruled out (Raymond et al. 1985). Although prostaglandins have been implicated in the development of the tubular resistance to AVP, other studies with inhibitors of prostaglandin synthesis have not confirmed this attractive hypothesis (Stoff et al. 1979, Berl et al. 1980).

17.2.2.2 Hypercalcemia

The syndrome of combined polyuria and polydipsia has been referred in association with hyperparathyroidism and later on also with other clinical conditions characterized by hypercalcemia (idiopathic hypercalcemia, vitamin D intoxication, hypercalcemia accompanying prolonged immobilization of patients, etc.). Chronic hypercalcemia may result in renal interstitial calcification and fibrosis with secondary anatomic disruption of the renal concentrating mechanism. Anatomic damage may represent a significant factor under certain circumstances. However, renal concentrating capacity in many patients improves within several days following the correction of chronic hypercalcemia; this would favor the role of the functional component in the genesis of the syndrome (Goldfarb and Agus 1984).

Hypercalcemia can modify water turnover by influencing central mechanisms of the osmoregulatory system. The cation may in fact be an important mediator of the central release of the hormone, and it may well raise the sensitivity of the osmoregulatory mechanism (Robinson et al. 1983). However, the osmotic threshold for thirst is simultaneously decreased. At an unchanged threshold level for AVP secretion, this becomes manifest as a slight, though significant, narrowing of the gap between the osmotic thresholds (see Fig. 5.6, panels 5, 7 and 9). In theory, the narrowing of the threshold gap itself is sufficient to induce increased water turnover independently of any other concomitant alteration of AVP secretion or activity. This is in agreement with the observations suggesting that hypercalcemia in experimental animals as well as in humans may be a primary dipsogenic stimulus (Levi et al. 1983, Aycinena and Robertson 1983).

However, polyuria in hypercalcemia is not entirely due to polydipsia; it is also a consequence of defective renal water conservation. As in potassium depletion, both a decrease in renal interstitial hypertonicity and a cellular defect in the response to vasopressin may be involved in hypercalcemia - associated polyuria. Direct measurements of tissue tonicity have shown that medullary solutes are decreased in hypercalcemia, but the mechanism(s) underlying this phenomenon has not been fully defined. A decreased glomerular filtration rate may result in less solute delivery to the loop of Henle, an impairment in NaCl reabsorption may cause a decreased solute accumulation in the medulla, and an increased inner medullary plasma flow may contribute to the dissipation of the existing medullary osmotic gradient (Galla et al. 1986).

The observation that some hypercalcemic subjects excrete urine that is hypotonic to plasma even in the presence of vasopressin (Gill and Bartter 1961) strongly suggests a concomitant defect in water permeability of the collecting duct. Calcium has multiple potential sites of action within the AVP responsive cell including the adenylate cyclase complex, cAMP phosphodiesterase and microtubule metabolism in addition to a number of other sites (Levine and Schlondorff 1984). However, it is important to appreciate that it is intracellular calcium that is the critical determinant of the influences of this ion on cellular transport processes, and a mechanism must thus exist which transforms changes in extracellular calcium concentration into changes in intracellular content of the ion. The majority of studies have pointed to a defect at the level of the adenylate cyclase complex, whereas there have been some data suggesting an additional post-cyclic AMP defect which could relate to defective assembly of cytosolic microtubules (Berl 1987).

Prostaglandins may play a contributory role in the development of concentrating defect in hypercalcemia, and indomethacin has been reported to reduce polyuria and to partially restore the tubular response to AVP. Nevertheless, the antidiuretic action of prostaglandins may not be entirely dependent on their effect at the level of the collecting duct epithelial cells; these agents may well reduce the renal concentrating ability also by their actions at other sites of the renal concentrating mechanism (Serros and Kirchenbaum 1981, Levi et al. 1983).

17.2.2.3 Lithium salts

Symptoms of disturbed water balance frequently occur with lithium therapy. Polydipsia and polyuria accompany the initiation of treatment in as many as 60% of patients and persists in about 20 to 25%, even with plasma lithium levels within the "therapeutic range" (Baylis and Heath 1978). The number of patients who complain of polyuria and/or polydipsia may be considerable, as more than 1 in 1,000 people in developed countries are receiving long-term lithium therapy for prophylaxis of affective disorders (Battle et al. 1985). As a result of the widespread use of lithium salts, lithium administration is now the most common cause of nephrogenic diabetes insipidus.

Most humans with lithium induced polyuria are unresponsive to exogenous AVP. Their plasma and urinary levels of AVP are generally elevated or normal during chronic lithium administration (Gold et al. 1983c). Thus lithium seems to induce the same reciprocal changes in the secretion and activity of vasopressin as seen in hypercalcemia: it diminishes the sensitivity of the antidiuretic response to vasopressin, and on the other hand, it increases the sensitivity of the vasopressin secretory response to osmotic stimulation. Although lithium may directly stimulate thirst in animals, there is no evidence that lithium induced polydipsia plays an important role in humans.

Lithium-induced polyuria is generally characterized by normal solute-free water generation (C_{H_2O}) and by impaired solute-free water reabsorption ($T^c_{H_2O}$) (Martinez-Maldonaldo et al. 1975). Since lithium may also produce polyuria by affecting processes that are AVP independent (e. g. a decreased fluid reabsorption in the proximal tubule can increase solute-free water generation and thereby increase the delivery of water to the collecting duct), these findings strongly suggest that lithium has a major effect on the AVP-dependent aspects of water homeostasis (chapter 8.4.2.2). At the cellular level, lithium likely has a significant effect on the proximal component of the AVP-cAMP second messenger system, most probably by inhibiting the hormone-stimulated activity of adenylate cyclase. However, there is also evidence for other sites of action, including cAMP-dependent protein kinase, microtubules, cellular calcium, and prostaglandin metabolism (Cogan and Abramow 1986).

The lithium-induced diabetes insipidus is generally believed to be an easily reversible condition which rapidly subsides following lithium withdrawal. However, recent reports have repeatedly stressed that the concentrating defect may be present for several months (and perhaps indefinitely) after the drug discontinuation. The persistence of the renal concentrating defect even after the drug withdrawal may, at least in certain patients, result in long-term renal injury and in the development of chronic interstitial nephritis and renal failure (Simon et al. 1977, Salata and Klein 1987).

Because of its ability to induce nephrogenic diabetes insipidus, lithium has been proposed for the treatment of the chronic syndrome of inappropriate secretion of vasopressin (chapter 20.4.2). However, in testing this possibility demeclocycline proved to be a more effective therapy, and because of its several side effect, lithium is rarely being used for this purpose (Forrest et al. 1978).

17.2.2.4 Demeclocycline

Demeclocycline, an antibiotic of the tetracycline series, when given in doses commonly used by the dermatologists to treat acne (900—1,200 mg/day) induces prominent polyuria and polydipsia. The administration of lower doses (600 mg/day) is not associated with this side effect in every patient, or only a slight partial concentrating defect occurs. Resistance to hydroosmotic action of AVP usually develops gradually, and no clinically evident polyuria may occur within the first days or week of drug administration. Similarly, complete restoration of the renal concentrating capacity requires several weeks after the drug withdrawal (Forrest et al. 1973, 1978).

In healthy volunteers demeclocycline induces polyuria which is characterized by selectively reduced reabsorption of solute-free water ($T^c_{H_2O}$) and is essentially unresponsive to the administration of exogenous vasopressin (Singer and Forrest 1976). A different picture is seen in subjects with renal failure, liver cirrhosis or congestive heart failure in whom demeclocycline administration is frequently accompanied by marked renal salt wasting, and decreased glomerular filtration rate. Demeclocycline (as an "aqueretic" agent or antibiotic) is therefore better avoided in similar conditions until the pathogenesis of demeclocycline-induced natriuresis and renal failure has been understood (Geheb and Cox 1980).

The demeclocycline-induced inhibition of osmotic water flow in renal epithelia has been suggested to involve the binding of the drug to a cellular protein (or proteins) that may play a major role in the proximal component of the AVP-cAMP second messenger system. The antagonism against the hydroosmotic effect of AVP provided the rationale for the successive use of demeclocycline in the treatment of hyponatremia associated with the chronic syndrome of inappropriate AVP secretion (chapter 20.4.2). This therapy permits unrestricted water intake in most patients with this syndrome, while the side effects in these subjects with otherwise normal renal function are minimal (Forrest et al. 1978).

17.2.2.5 Sulfanylureas

Sulfanylureas are widely used in the therapy of diabetes mellitus. Initially, it was postulated that polyuria occurring after the administration of glyburide, tolazamide, or acetohexamide is due to inhibition of the hydroosmotic effect of AVP (Radó and Borbély 1975). In contrast, two other sulfanylureas, chlorpropamide and tolbutamide, have antidiuretic effects. Indeed, chlorpropamide has been successfully used to treat partial central diabetes insipidus (Moses et al. 1973). Moreover, the development of hyponatremia, closely resembling the syndrome of inappropriate vasopressin secretion, has been reported in patients with diabetes mellitus treated by chlorpropamide (Garcia et al. 1971). The observation that drugs of the same category may have conspicuously different effects on renal water excretion, has been sufficiently surprising to prompt numerous studies into the interactions of these agents with the mechanisms of renal water excretion.

It seems that the effect of "diuretic" sulfanylureas on collecting ducts may be qualitatively (and not necessarily also quantitatively) similar to that of "antidiuretic" sulfanylurea (chlorpropamide) in that all these compounds increase the hydroosmotic effect of submaximal AVP concentrations. Nevertheless, it remains obsure how these agents can increase diuresis despite increasing the sensitivity of collecting ducts to AVP. Their diuretic action might rest in the inhibition of AVP secretion and in the production of more solute-free water. "Diuretic" sulfanylureas resembling chlorpropamide may also decrease vasopressin secretion by decreasing the sensitivity of the osmoregulatory system of the hormone secretion. Then, "diuretic" sulfanylureas may sensitize human collecting ducts to hydroosmotic effect of AVP considerably less strongly than does chlorpropamide (i.e., these agents in fact induce the development of partial central rather than renal diabetes insipidus) (Braden et al. 1985).

17.2.2.6 Miscellaneous drugs

Numerous other drugs can induce the development of nephrogenic diabetes insipidus, while a number of still other drugs have been shown to be able to inhibit AVP mediated water transport in experimental animals and/or in vitro model systems (such as the toad urinary bladder), but they have not been reported to produce nephrogenic diabetes insipidus in humans (Singer and Forrest 1976).

Amphotericin B is the currently most effective agent available for the therapy of fungal infections. The main limitation of its use is set by its nephrotoxicity. Renal dysfunction of varying extent accompanies its administration to every patient (Butler et al. 1964, Barbour et al. 1979). A decrement in glomerular filtration rate itself does not seem to be sufficient to fully explain the drug-induced concentrating defect. Rather, the latter is due to disturbances in the generation and maintenance of the medullary osmotic gradient, and perhaps also to irreversible damage caused by the drug to cell membranes.

Many patients with gentamycine induced acute renal failure are nonoliguric; indeed urine volume may increase prior to the appearance of renal insufficiency. No studies to determine the etiology of polyuria in such patients have been reported so far. However, experimental data seem to support the view that the defect in cellular response to AVP may play a significant role in the genesis of polyuria (Bennett 1981).

Cis-dichlorodiamine (II) platinum, cis-platin, which has found wide applications in the therapy of solid tumors, presents a variety of side effects. The main limiting factor of the use of this compound is its considerable nephrotoxicity. In experimental animals, cis-platin decreases renal concentrating ability, most likely by inducing some abnormalites in the generation of the medullary gradient (Blachley and Hill 1981, Safirstein et al. 1981). In humans, a defect in renal concentration may be masked by the common practice of volume expansion prior to the administration of cis-platin.

Colchicine and vinca alcaloids inhibit the hydroosmotic effect of vasopressin in experimental animals and also in toad urinary bladder; their site of action is distal from the site of cAMP production. Since these agents are potent inhibitors of microtubule assembly, it has generally been assumed that they inhibit the action of the second messenger by disrupting microtubule function (Dousa and Barness, 1974). Despite the obvious potential for the development of AVP unresponsiveness in humans treated with these agents no cases of nephrogenic diabetes insipidus have been reported.

V2 receptor antagonists, "aquaretic" agents (chapter 7.3.4), produce in experimental animals hyposthenuria and polyuria by competitive inhibition of the hydroosmotic effect of the natural hormone. As yet, these analogs have not been tested in humans. If free of significant side effects, such specific antagonists of the antidiuretic hormone will prove invaluable in the evaluation and treatment of hyponatremic states secondary to hypervasopressinism (e.g. the syndrome of inappropriate secretion of AVP).

17.2.2.7 Renal disease

A large variety of renal diseases unrelated in terms of etiology, anatomy and abnormalities, are characterized by a urinary concentrating defect. Several factors contribute to this problem, including osmotic diuresis induced by the necessity to increase solute excretion in the remaining functioning nephrons, decreased tubular responsiveness to AVP, and interference with the counter-current mechanism (see Table 8.2). Diseases which primarily affect the papillary and the medullary zone of the kidney (such as medullary cystic disease, amyloidosis, chronic interstitial nephritis, obstructive uropathy, etc.). tend to have earliest and most severe defect (Schück 1984).

A defect in the renal concentrating capacity is a uniform feature of most forms of advanced chronic renal failure. The degree of impairment in renal concentrating capacity correlates most closely with the level of renal impairment, and is mostly pronounced when the serum creatinine levels exceed 600 μmol/l. In these cases hypotonic urine is excreted even after maximal doses of vasopressin. However, because of the profound decrease in GFR, the excretion of hypotonic urine is not associated with massive polyuria. The recognition of the concentrating defect is of primary significance for an adequate therapy. For example, an individual with a maximal concentrating capacity as low as 300 mOsm/kg must produce 2 l of urine to be able to excrete normal daily solute load (approximately 600 mOsm/kg). Consequently, his daily water intake must be at least 2,500 ml to compensate for insensible losses and to maintain water balance. If due to any causes the subject is not able to ingest this quantity of water, he may develop serious dehydration within several days just because of his kidneys being unable to preserve water by concentrating urine.

17.2.2.8 Sickle cell anemia

Diminished concentrating ability is an early and consistent finding in sickle cell anemia. The disease is characterized by painful hemolytic crises and multiplex thromboses in various organs. Low partial oxygen tension, low pH and high osmolality of the renal medulla favour sickling in the vasa recta also in intervals between crises (as suggested by the frequency of asymptomatic hematuria in this disease), thereby causing anatomical damage to the medulla. This results in an insufficient trapping of solute in the inner medulla, and an impairment of the countercurrent function.

In a homozygote child the net effect is that by the age of 10 to 15 years, U_{osm} max is only about half the normal value; the concentrating defect is reversible after multiple transfusions with normal blood, which presumably restore the flow in vasa recta. However, such a beneficial effect is lost by the age of 15 as no improvement in maximum urine osmolality has been observed after red blood cell transfusions to patients above this age. Heterozygotic patients show a gradual decrease in their concentrating capacity with age, and subjects over 50 to 60 years are no more able to raise their urine osmolality above 450 mOsm/kg (deJong and Statius van Eps 1985).

While sickling may be enhanced by increasing plasma sodium concentration, it decreases in a hypotonic medium. Although oral and intravenous hydration have long been a standby in the treatment of sickle cell crisis, even rapid intravenous hydration with fluids low in sodium is generally ineffective in reducing serum sodium very much below normal because of the unimpaired renal diluting ability in these patients. Preliminary studies have suggested that the production of controlled hyponatremia ranging between 120 and 125 mmol/l (by asking the patients to drink 3,500 to 4,000 ml water daily and ensuring that their kidneys are constantly under the influence of vasopressin by administering desmopressin intranasally) shortened the duration and reduced the frequency of hemolytic crises (Rosa et al. 1980, Epstein et al. 1984). However, the practical difficulties in adjusting serum sodium during long-term treatment, and the potential hazards of water intoxication emphasize that induced hyponatremia should not be applied indiscriminately; this approach should be reserved only for severely affected patients treated in properly controlled conditions.

17.2.2.9 Dietary abnormalities

Large water ingestion during several days has been reported to washout the medullary osmotic gardient, and to decrease maximal concentrating capacity of the kidneys in healthy volunteers (DeWardener and Herxheimer 1957). A similar mechanism is obviously operative in primary polydipsic diabetes insipidus (chapter 17.5.2.2). The severity of the concentrating defect changes directly proportional to the degree of solute-free polyuria, while being independent of its origin. The decreased maximal concentrating ability is transient and the renal concentration capacity is restored after the fluid intake has been reduced.

Also, starvation and/or continuous massive protein losses may generate AVP-resistant polyuria by altering the available urea which accounts for 50 per cent of osmols in the inner medulla (Epstein et al. 1957).

17.2.2.10 Osmotic diuresis

Increased delivery of solutes to the distal nephron sites produces osmotic diuresis characterized by a vasopressin-resistant concentrating defect. At high rates of solute excretion the level of urinary osmolality asymptotically approaches isotonicity, even under the administration of supraphysiological doses of vasopressin (see Fig. 8.7.). Both an increase in collecting tubule fluid flow and an impairment in countercurrent function may contribute to this blunted response (Table 17.5) (Gennari and Kassirer 1974, Singer 1981).

Nonelectrolyte osmotic diuresis can almost always be attributed to glucose or urea; occasionally other solutes (e.g. mannitol, fructose or amino-acids) are involved, particularly if given by rapid intravenous infusion. Poorly controlled diabetes mellitus with glucosuria is the most common cause of osmotic diuresis.

Table 17.5. Causes of osmotic polyuria

A. Electrolytes
   Sodium chloride
   — increased tubular load (dietary habit, iatrogenic NaCl intoxication)
   — decreased tubular reabsorption (renal salt wasting, diuretic administration, mineralocorticoid deficiency)
   Sodium bicarbonate
   — increased tubular load (dietary habit, iatrogenic $NaHCO_3$ intoxication)
   — decreased tubular reabsorption (proximal renal tubular acidosis, carbonic-anhydrase inhibition)
B. Non-electrolytes
   Urea
   — increased tubular load (postobstructive diuresis, chronic renal failure, protein hypercatabolism, urea administration)
   Glucose
   — increased tubular load (diabetes mellitus, iatrogenic osmotic diuresis)
   Other (mannitol, sorbitol)

Polyuria in these patients occurs despite the fact that insulin deficiency per se increases vasopressin by some as yet unrecognized mechanism (see Fig. 5.4) (Vokes et al. 1987). Although nonelectrolyte osmotic diuresis may be caused by therapeutic administration of urea or by high protein tube feeding, urea diuresis more often is due to accumulation of endogenous urea. The most common clinical settings associated with endogenous urea diuresis are probably chronic renal failure and postobstructive diuresis (Kramer 1985).

Electrolyte osmotic diuresis is almost always due to a sodium salt, either chloride or bicarbonate. Sodium diuresis may be due to excessive sodium delivery to the kidney (overflow osmotic diuresis), or to excessive rejection of sodium salts by renal tubules (tubular osmotic diuresis) (Singer 1981).

Although excessive sodium might be ingested for different reasons, the most common causes of sodium chloride diuresis are iatrogenic (e. g. hyperalimentation, intravenous solutions). Overflow osmotic diuresis of sodium bicarbonate may be associated with self-treatment (e.g. in chronic gastric disease with soda); more commonly however it is the result of medical treatment of acidosis. Some patients may have solute diuresis in excess of 10 liters per day because of an initial infusion of 1 to 2 l of saline followed by orders to replace urine output by equivalent volumes of saline. As a result, urine output gradually increases since the patient remains volume expanded.

If salt is lost at the renal level, the defect may reside in the kidney (e.g. in chronic renal failure) or may be due to extrarenal hormonal deficiency (e.g. in Addison's disease or in isolated hyperaldosteronism). The administration of diuretics may be viewed as a iatrogenic renal defect, and is probably the single most common cause of primary excessive renal loss of sodium chloride.

Primary tubular disorders can sustain bicarbonate osmotic diuresis in proximal renal tubular acidosis and in Fanconi syndrome. The administration of carbonic anhydrase inhibitors (sulfonamide diuretics) can cause renal sodium bicarbonate wasting which is limited only by the fall in the filtered load of bicarbonate.

17.2.3 THERAPY OF NEPHROGENIC DIABETES INSIPIDUS

Chronic treatment of nephrogenic diabetes insipidus is required by patients with symptomatic polyuria in whom the renal concentrating defect cannot be readily corrected. This mainly concerns subjects with hereditary NDI and those on lithium salts. No specific treatment is required when the concentrating defect is reversible (hypokalemia, hypercalcemia, drugs, dietary abnormalities, osmotic diuresis) or when polyuria is not a problem (renal diseases, sickle cell anemia).

By definition, nephrogenic diabetes insipidus does not respond to vasopressin, and the administration of desmopressin or of drugs that potentiate AVP secretion (such as chlorpropamide or carbamazepine) is thus ineffective. Obviously, employment of the thirst mechanism and free access to water are very important to prevent dehydration. Newborns and infants with hereditary NDI should receive water continuously with gastric tube during the first months of life and during the nights thereafter (Némethová et al. 1985, Niaudet et al. 1985).

17.2.3.1 Diuretic treatment

The major form of therapy of NDI are diuretics (hydrochlorothiazide 25 mg once or twice daily) and a low-sodium low-protein diet. Although it seems paradoxical to treat polyuria with a diuretic, as little as $1.0\%-1.5\%$ weight loss due to diuretic therapy can reduce urine output to apparently normal or only slightly elevated values (from 10 l to below 3.5 l per day) (Shirley et al. 1982). It seems likely that the decrease in urine flow is secondary to sodium loss and extracellular fluid volume contraction (Fig. 17.3). ECF volume depletion in turn decreases GFR and increases proximal tubular sodium and water reabsorption. As a result less water is delivered to the collecting tubules and less water is therefore excreted. At the same time, renal losses of potassium during thiazide therapy should be substituted as potassium depletion alone may be the cause of polydipsia and AVP-resistant polyuria. The ECF volume contraction can be maintained with a low sodium intake after discontinuation of the diuretic, and the therapy remains effective. In addition, a moderate protein restriction which reduces renal solute load has also potential therapeutic importance in the control of polyuria (Blalock et al. 1977). When U_{osm} is relatively fixed as in both NDI and CDI, the rate of solute excretion becomes the primary determinant of urine volume. If, for example, urine can be concentrated to 75 mOsm/kg, the daily urine volume will be 8 liters with 600 mOsm solute load excreted, but only 4 liters with 300 mOsm excreted.

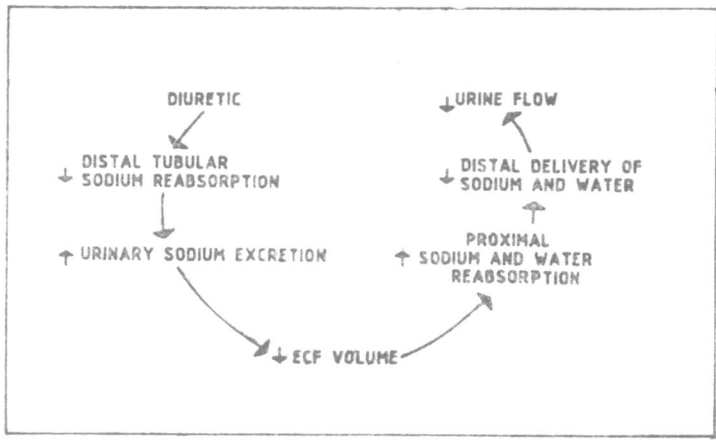

Fig. 17.3. Mechanism of antidiuretic effect of diuretics in nephrogenic diabetes insipidus.

17.2.3.2 Treatment of lithium-induced nephrogenic diabetes insipidus

In patients receiving lithium the symptoms of NDI can be bothersome. If polyuria persists it places the patient at an increased risk of dehydration which in turn leads to a lowered renal clearance of lithium, elevated serum lithium levels and lithium intoxication. The ensuing volume depletion is also the reason why thiazide diuretic therapy may be of some risk in patients on continuous lithium therapy. However, the considerable morbidity and mortality of manic-depressive psychosis and the recognized effectiveness of lithium in the treatment of this disorder often makes it difficult to discontinue lithium maintenance therapy simply because of the development of NDI. Recently, amiloride, a new potassium sparing diuretic, has been shown to ameliorate polyuria in patients receiving maintenance therapy with lithium. The effect of this diuretic seems to be specifically related to partial restoration of the sensitivity of the collecting duct to AVP. It has been suggested to start diuretic treatment of patients with lithium-induced polyuria with 10 mg/day amiloride; the dose can be increased to 20 mg if polyuria is not substantially reduced within 7 to 10 days (Battle et al. 1985). Others have suggested that blood levels lower than those typically reported (i.e. below 0.7 mmol/l) may be effective in most patients with bipolar affective disorders, and the reduction of lithium dose may reduce polyuria without the need of diuretic administration (Goodnick and Fieve 1985).

17.2.3.3 Inhibitors of prostaglandin synthesis

Another therapeutic strategy that has been effective in some patients with hereditary NDI or lithium toxicity is the administration of indomethacin which inhibits renal prostaglandin synthesis (2 mg/kg per day in three divided doses alone or in combination with thiazides) (Usberti et al. 1985, Libber et al. 1986).

Renal prostaglandin (mainly PGE_2) synthesis is often increased in patients with NDI. Prostaglandins have a variety of effects leading to impairment of concentrating ability: they reduce proximal tubular sodium reabsorption, lower the medullary osmolality by increasing the medullary blood flow, and inhibit vasopressin-induced cAMP production. However, since indomethacin reduces water excretion also in Brattleboro rats known to lack vasopressin, as well as in humans with central diabetes insipidus, the presence of vasopressin seems not a prerequisite for the antidiuretic action of the drug. Consequently, the antidiuretic action of indomethacin cannot be explained simply by the restoration of a state of relative sensitivity of the collecting duct to vasopressin (Ponec and Lichardus 1980). Other effects of indomethacin (such as direct rise in permeability of the collecting duct to water, enhanced proximal sodium reabsorption, and increased corticomedullary osmotic gradient) may be responsible for the drug induced reduction of urine output in NDI. A good correlation found between the reduction of diuresis and the reduction of distal sodium delivery (chapter 8.5.2.2) seems to indirectly support this view (Turi et al. 1981, Niaudet et al. 1985).

17.3 DISTURBED OSMOREGULATION OF THIRST AND VASOPRESSIN SECRETION (HYPOVASOPRESSINISM WITHOUT POLYURIA; ESSENTIAL HYPERNATREMIA)

This syndrome is characterized by chronic or recurrent episodes of severe hypernatremia associated with moderate volume depletion — as reflected by high basal levels of plasma renin activity — and lack of thirst. Hypodipsia or adipsia is the definitive abnormality of this condition, and is both necessary and sufficient to account for all fluid and electrolyte abnormalities observed with this syndrome. In addition, usually, though not without exception (Hammond et al. 1986), hypodipsia or adipsia has been associated with some defect in vasopressin secretion (Robertson et al. 1982, Baylis and Thompson 1988).

This constellation of deficits suggests that the syndrome is due to hypoplasia or destruction of the hypothalamic osmoreceptors that regulate thirst and AVP release (chapter 5.2). Lesions noted to cause this disorder in infants and adults typically involve the anterior hypothalamus (most notably aneurysms of the anterior communicating artery, neoplastic lesions in the anterior hypothalamus and the third ventricular region, and granulomatous processes infiltrating the hypothalamus), often giving rise to various other signs and symptoms of hypothalamic disease (polyphagia, poikilothermia, anterior pituitary deficiency of hypothalamic origin, etc.) in addition to polydipsia. In animal studies discrete lesions in the AV3V region, specifically in the circumventricular organ, the organum vasculosum of the lamina terminalis (OVLT) (see Fig. 3.4), produces disorders that closely resemble essential hypernatremia in humans (Brody and Johnson 1980) (Table 17.6).

Table 17.6. Characteristic features found in patients with essential hypernatremia and in AV3V-lesioned animals

	Essential hypernatremia	AV3V-lesioned animals
Hypothalamic damage	+	+
Chronic hypernatremia	+	+
Persistently reduced thirst	+	+
Disturbed osmoregulation of AVP	+	+
Reduced blood volume	+	+
Increased plasma renin activity	+	+

Chronic hypernatremia may be well tolerated and many reported cases are asymptomatic although neurologic and muscular problems may arise (chapter 18.1). Thirst deficiency is most dramatically apparent when insensible extrarenal fluid loss is likely to be increased (fever, increased ambient temperature, etc.). This abnormality can be diagnosed at the bedside simply by observing that the subject does not drink spontaneously or even shows marked aversion to fluids offered to him, at plasma sodium concentrations and effective osmolality above 150 mmol/l and 310 mOsm/kg respectively. The therapy of patients with "essential hypernatremia" is alleviation of the degree of hypernatremia and plasma hyperosmolality by increased nondipsogenic water intake. Trying to prevent the extremes of hypernatremia and hyponatremia these patients cannot be managed by prescribing a fixed rate of water intake.

17.3.1 CLINICAL PATTERNS OF VASOPRESSIN SECRETION AND THIRST

Hypodipsia or adipsia due to loss of osmoreceptor function might not be as rare as previously supposed. Because of the absence of polydipsia and polyuria, the defect in AVP secretion remains often inapparent and can be demonstrated only by direct assay of the hormonal response to osmotic stimulation and suppression. At least four different patterns of defective osmoregulation of vasopressin have been observed in patients with essential hypernatremia which probably depend on the nature and extension of the primary hypothalamic disorder (De Rubertis et al. 1974, Halter et al. 1977, Robertson et al. 1982, Dunger et al. 1985, Villadsen and Pedersen 1987, Baylis and Thompson 1988).

The most serius type of the syndrome is the so-called adipsic hypernatremia, which is thought to be due to complete destruction of the osmoreceptors. These patients completely lack thirst sensation irrespective of plasma sodium concentrations and are never motivated to drink spontaneously. Interestingly, vasopressin is released persistently in small quantities (Fig. 17.4. (C)), a finding which well fits the theoretical concept concerning the "bimodal" nature of the osmoregulatory system (chapter 5.1.3.1). Although vasopressin secretion appears to be totally refractory to osmotic influences, it responds normally to hemodynamic and other nonosmotioc stimuli. In principle this is an opposite condition as compared to that present in patients with autonomous insufficiency (Shy-Drager syndrome, chapter 9.4.5) who have intact AVP osmoregulation, whereas their ascendent projections from autonomous centers in the brainstem to magnocellular hypothalamic neurons are affected.

This goes to show that these individuals are devoid of active protection against both underhydration and overhydration. If not forced to take water they become progressively hypernatremic and eventually manifest the numerous neurological features of severe hypernatremia. Equally important

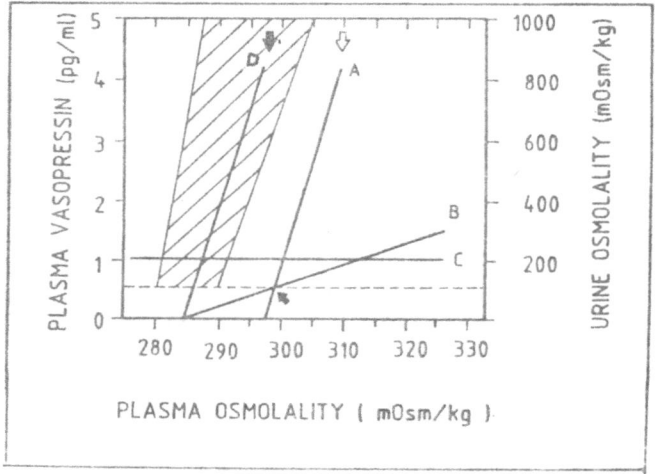

Fig. 17.4. Schematic representation of abnormalities in AVP osmoregulation observed or postulated in patients with essential hypernatremia. The vertical arrows at the end of lines A and D indicate the osmotic threshold for thirst in the respective conditions. The solid lines depict the relationship of plasma AVP to plasma and urinary osmolality. For details see text. (By Robertson et al. 1982 with kind permission.)

is to appreciate that these subjects should be unable to develop maximal water diuresis because vasopressin secretion continues, albeit at a low rate (Robertson 1980). Therefore, if given fluids injudiciously, they may go from severe hypertonic dehydration to a condition clinically indistinguishable from the syndrome of inappropriate secretion of antidiuretic hormone. Trying to prevent the extremes of hypernatremia and plasma hypoosmolality, these patients cannot be managed by prescribing a fixed rate of water intake. The fluid therapy is best accomplished by adopting a regimen of water intake based on defined objective measures (plasma sodium concentration or body weight). In an ambulatory setting, the follow-up of deviations from an age-related "ideal" weight provide the only practical guide; in the presence of increased extrarenal fluid losses the daily fluid intake must be increased proportionately.

The second type (see Fig. 17.4. (B)) represents a decrease in the sensitivity or slope of osmoregulatory lines for thirst and vasopressin release with no change in osmotic thresholds, probably due to partial destruction of the osmostat. The range in plasma osmolality in these patients is wide but they are protected from both over- and underhydration because they are able to experience thirst, and at high plasma osmolalities will secrete sufficient amounts of vasopressin to maximally concentrate urine. Patients with partial central diabetes insipidus are differentiated from these hypernatremic patients by their normal thirst sensation which leads to polyuria and polydipsia (see Fig. 5.7). In addition, patients with partial destruction of the osmostat usually have normal vasopressin responses to nonosmotic secretory stimuli whereas those with partial central diabetes insipidus tend to have subnormal responses.

In addition, some hypernatremic syndromes have been attributed to an upward resetting of the osmostats for both thirst and vasopressin release (see Fig. 17.4. (A)). Since vasopressin secretion remains under osmotic control, water balance can be maintained as the kidneys are still able to concentrate and dilute urine maximally. Furthermore, these patients are protected from extreme hypernatremia because they still experience thirst which will motivate them to drink. The only abnormality of water balance is that the whole osmoregulatory system operates around a higher setpoint (see Fig. 5.6., panel 3). Therefore management of this form of hypernatremia is not difficult; these patients should be encouraged to drink normally, about 2 l per day.

Finally, Hammond et al. (1986) described a fourth type of defect in hypernatremia with absent osmoregulated thirst in association with apparently normally osmoregulated vasopressin release (see Fig. 17.4. (D)). On theoretical ground, this observation suggests that there are two distinct populations of osmoreceptor cells, one serving the vasopressin release and the other thirst sensation. Patients with a similar abnormality should be managed by ensuring fluid intake of about 2 l per day.

17.4 INCREASED THIRST WITH SECONDARY HYPOVASOPRESSINISM -POLYDIPSIC DIABETES INSIPIDUS, PDI

Increased thirst is classified as either symptomatic or pathologic. Symptomatic thirst results from body fluid depletion; consequently, thirst represents here a normal physiologic response to a true water deficit (Fitzsimmons 1985). In contrast, pathological thirst represents an inappropriate activation of drinking: the patient remains thirsty despite his body being well hydrated or even over-hydrated and the plasma osmolality being reduced below the level ($P_{osm} >$ > 280 mOsm/kg) which is normally necessary to stimulate AVP release (Barlow and deWardener 1959, Cronin 1987). In these cases the secondarily decreased AVP secretion is an appropriate response to the ingestion of excessive quantities of water. Nevertheless, this condition is usually discussed in the context of other forms of hypovasopressinism, in particular owing to problems in differentiating this disorder from other forms of free water polyuria (chapter 17.5.2).

Isolated (independent of AVP secretory function) activation of thirst has been clearly demonstrated by experimental studies indicating that destructive lesions in certain parts of the brain can increase water intake. Moreover, hereditary polydipsia occurring in certain species of experimental ani-mals (with certainty in the STR/N strain of mice and possibly in Penn State chicken) is another significant argument in favor of the idea that the analogic condition observed in humans needs not necessarily be of "psycho-genic" origin. Although this hypothesis has been generally accepted, the use of terms such as "compulsive water drinking" or "psychogenic polydipsia" to refer to the syndrome still tends to conserve the idea that this disorder in humans is an emotional or character disorder. Examples of pathologic thirst in humans include polydipsia caused by continued irritation of osmoreceptors for thirst (e.g. by tumors, granulomatous disorders, trauma, or by inflamma-

Table 17.7. Causes of polydipsic diabetes insipidus (PDI)

A. Organic damage of hypothalamus
   — tumors
   — granulomatous disorders
   — trauma
   — inflammation
B. Electrolyte disorders
   — potassium depletion
   — hypercalcemia
   — lithium administration
C. Psychiatric diseases (primary polydipsia)
D. Idiopathic disorders ("reset osmostat"?)

tion); rare idiopathic defects; direct stimulation of thirst centers by electrolyte abnormalities (such as hypokalemia or hypercalcemia); and the so-called primary polydipsia (Table 17.7) (Valtin et al. 1985, Cronin 1987, Robertson 1988).

Most patients with primary polydipsia have serious psychiatric disturbances, and the majority are women. The clinical features of primary polydipsia include hysteria, delusions and depression. Usually, the presenting complaint is polyuria due to the ingestion of large quantities of water. Bizarre reasons are offered for such behavior, e.g. that the water will flush out worms, poisons or cancer; an attempt to rid the body of hiccups or to prevent formation of renal stones. Up to one third of chronically psychotic patients become polydipsic in 5 to 15 years from the onset of their illness; typically, these patients reside in mental hospitals and are readily identified by the staff as consuming fluid almost constantly throughout the day. Since many antipsychotic drugs are anticholinergic, mouth dryness could be a factor that stimulates thirst. However, primary polydipsia clearly occurs in schizophrenic patients who are not on antipsychotic medication (Vieweg 1987, Cronin 1987). Early data indicated few harmful consequences from this excessive drinking behavior. Recent studies however have documented episodic water intoxication, characterized by profound hyponatremia and diverse neurologic signs ranging from ataxia to irreversible coma, as a frequent source of morbidity and mortality in patients with primary polydipsia (see chapter 20.3.1.6).

17.5 DIFFERENTIAL DIAGNOSIS OF POLYURIC SYNDROMES

Polyuria is a relatively common clinical complaint; it should be suspected when the daily urine volume is more than 3 to 4 liters in adults, or when the age-related maintenance rate of urine excretion is increased by a factor exceeding 2.5 in infants and small children. Hypovasopressinism almost always causes polyuria, unless the thirst sensation is defective or fully absent (as in patients with essential hypernatremia). Differential diagnosis of polyuric states begins with the establishment whether diuresis is primarily solute-free or whether excess solutes excreted in the urine are responsible for polyuria (osmotic, solute diuresis).

17.5.1 OSMOTIC POLYURIA

The simplest way to determine whether a polyuric patient has a solute or water diuresis is to measure the urine osmolality. In general, a very low osmolality in random urine samples (less than 200 mOsm/kg) suggests a free-water diuresis, whereas values close to isotonicity suggest a solute diuresis or a combined solute and water diuresis (Table 17.8). If solute diuresis is suspected, the next step is to disclose the solute responsible for diuresis. As a rule, detailed analysis of case history and preceding therapy records provides sufficient information about the solute which most likely plays a role in the condition, and suggests which confirmatory tests can provide a useful tool to exactly determine the nature of osmotic diuresis (Gennari and Kassirer 1974, Singer 1981, Schück 1984).

Table 17.8. Differential diagnosis of polyuric states

Parameter	Free water diuresis	Osmotic diuresis	Combined diuresis
Uosm	$< P_{osm}$	$\geq P_{osm}$	$< P_{osm}$
FE_{H_2O}	increased	increased	increased
FE_{osm}	normal	increased	increased
$(C_{H_2O}/GFR) \times 100$	> 0	< 0	> 0

A solute diuresis caused by a nonelectrolyte can almost always be attributed to glucose or to urea (chapter 17.2.2.10). Hyperglycemia causes glycosuria and glucose osmotic diuresis; negative (or but slightly positive) results of semi-quantitative urine test effectively unequivocally reject glucose as the cause of polyuria. Uremia and high protein feeding also result in osmotic diuresis; low levels of blood urea nitrogen (BUN) prove against the involvement of this nonelectrolyte solute in polyuria. Occasionally other sugars or sugar alcohols are involved (e.g. mannitol and glycerol employed in the management of cerebral edema); even more rarely, other solutes (e.g. amino-acids) can produce a nonelectrolyte diuresis, particularly if administered in rapid intravenous infusions.

For electrolyte-induced solute diuresis are almost always responsible sodium salts (chapter 17.2.2.10). The estimation of the degree of fractional excretion of osmotically active agents (FE_{osm}) and of the excretory fraction of sodium (FE_{Na}) is practically always suggestive of the definitive cause of the solute osmotic diuresis. If sodium plays a major role in osmotic diuresis, the FE_{Na}/FE_{osm} ratio is expected to be increased. Acid urine reaction (pH below 7.0) excludes bicarbonate diuresis, leaving sodium chloride as the responsible solute. Examples of sodium chloride diuresis may be the administration of diuretics or intravenous administration of excessive NaCl solutions. Although true salt wasting can occur also with renal failure, polyuria is unusual complaint in this disorder since for the low GFR the obligatory urine output is usually less than 2 liters per day.

17.5.2 SOLUTE-FREE WATER POLYURIA

Once osmotic diuresis has been excluded, there are several anamnestic and laboratory data that may aid in establishing the correct type of diabetes insipidus present. Diabetes insipidus — central, nephrogenic or polydipsic in nature — is a generic term applied to a large number of disorders presenting with similar clinical features (free water polyuria and polydipsia). Sudden onset of polyuria, nocturia, and also an interesting preference for very cold, iced water are all signs more characteristic of complete central diabetes insipidus. Familiar occurrence, patient's age at the onset, symptoms suggesting renal or systemic disorders and/or electrolyte disorders, as well as records of previous pharmacotherapy (e.g. lithium therapy) also reveal important clues to the diagnosis. Severe polyuria with an urine output exceeding 4 to 5 liters per day is seen only with severe concentrating defects, primarily with complete central DI or congenital nephrogenic DI, or with polydipsic DI.

There is no single definitive diagnostic standard for the differential diagnosis of the 3 major solute-free polyurias, but the diagnosis can be established on the basis of some relatively simple clinical tests (Table 19.7) by the use of a combination of factors.

Table 17.9. Diagnostic tests for differentiation of solute-free water polyurias (for details see text)

Hypertonic saline infusion
The two-part concentrating test
Parallel determination of plasma and urine osmolality
Radioimmunoassay of vasopressin in plasma or urine
Short-term therapeutic trial with desmopressin

17.5.2.1 Hypertonic saline infusion

The Hickey-Hare test, which consists of checking changes in diuresis and urine osmolality during the infusion of hypertonic NaCl solution (most commonly 2.5% saline at the rate of 0.05 ml/kg/hour for no more than 2 hours) to patients previously hyperhydrated by oral water load (Vallotton et al. 1986a), in fact repeats the classic experiments employed by Verney (1947) to define the osmoregulatory system of AVP secretion. Currently this test is rarely used in clinical setting except where there is a problem to define the basic functional characteristics of the osmoregulatory system (i.e. its threshold and sensitivity) by employing direct measurements of plasma or urine vasopressin (chapter 17.5.2.4). It may be of interest that hypertonic saline may produce in patients with essential hypernatremia a paradoxical fall in urine osmolality, since in this disorder urine osmolality is governed primarily by volume rather than osmolality (chapter 17.3).

17.5.2.2   The two-part concentrating test

Although hypertonic saline infusion may be somewhat cumbersome, the two part concentrating test is more suitable for routine clinical requirements.

The first part of this test, the classic dehydration test (chapter 8.4.1.2), involves induction of plasma hyperosmolality by complete water restriction, thereby stimulating endogenous AVP secretion. To allow a correct interpretation of this part of the test, it is necessary to 1. eliminate with certainty any access to water throughout the test and 2. obtain plasma osmolality levels as high as 295 mOsm/kg, a level at which normally endogenous AVP is expected to have maximum effect on the kidneys. If neither urine, nor plasma osmolality increases during this part of the test and the body weight does not decrease by an amount consistent with urine output, surreptitious drinking should be suspected. In that event, either the dehydration test should be repeated with closer supervison or hypertonic saline should be infused instead (chapter 17.5.2.1).

The other part of the two-part standard concentrating test involves the

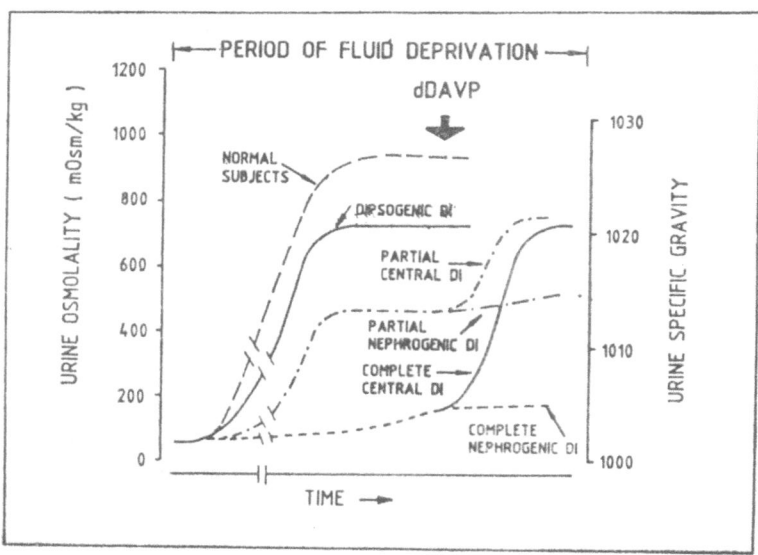

Fig. 17.5. The two-part concentrating test for differentiating the major types of free-water polyuria. In normal subjects as the P_{osm} reaches 295 mOsm/kg during fluid deprivation, there will be maximum AVP effect on the kidney and exogenous vasopressin (or desmopressin, dDAVP) will be without effect (for details see text).

196

administration of exogenous vasopressin (5 units subcutaneously or 10 µg dDAVP by nasal insufflation) immediately after the completion of the thirst test, and monitoring of changes in urinary osmolality during a subsequent 4-hour interval (chapter 8.4.1.3).

Although the determination of the response to the two-part concentrating test has been the standard approach to patients with polyuria, this test is still indirect since Uosm is used as an index of AVP secretion or effect. Fig. 17.5 summarizes the different patterns of the response. In normal subjects water restriction raises urine osmolality above the lower limit for the respective age category, i.e. above 800 mOsm/kg in young adults and older children, and exogenous vasopressin does not cause any further rising in Uosm. In complete CDI the value of U_{osm} reached before the exogenous vasopressin administration remains below isotonicity ($U_{osm} < 290$ mOsm/kg), and vasopressin induces a rise in U_{osm} of $> 50\%$; while in patients with partial CDI Uosm rises above P_{osm} during dehydration, and further increases (by 9—50%) after vasopressin. Subjects with complete NDI have a plateau in U_{osm} below P_{osm}, followed by a 0—45% rise in U_{osm} after exogenous vasopressin. In partial NDI a rise in U_{osm} above the level of P_{osm} during dehydration is followed by an additional, exogenous vasopressin-induced rise in U_{osm} by about 100 mOsm/kg. In subjects with polydipsic (dipsogenic) diabetes insipidus the dehydration-induced increase in U_{osm} is diminished in relation to normal subjects, and urine osmolality rises by $< 9\%$ in response to exogenous vasopressin administration (Table 17.10) (Miller et al. 1970).

Table 17.10. Responses to the two-part concentrating test (data from Miller et al. 1970)

	Number of cases	Mean U_{osm} with dehydration	U_{osm} after vasopressin	% change in U_{osm}
Normal subjects	9	$1,067 \pm 68.7$	978 ± 79.4	-8.9 ± 3.0
Complete CDI	18	168 ± 13.0	445 ± 52.0	180 ± 41.4
Partial CDI	12	437 ± 33.6	548 ± 28.2	28.5 ± 4.7
Polydipsic diabetes insipidus	7	738 ± 52.9	779 ± 73.1	5.0 ± 2.2

This simple, generally available and safe two-part concentrating test is of principal value in differentiating patients without abnormality in vasopressin function from those with complete central or nephrogenic diabetes insipidus. However, if dehydration increases urine osmolality above that of plasma (i.e. the patient has either polydipsic DI or a partial defect in vasopressin secretion or action) these indirect criteria do not differentiate reliably between these three possibilities. In fact, the incidence of both false-positive and false-negative results approximates 30 to 40 per cent (Zerbe and Robertson 1981). Several factors may be responsible for this ambiguity (Robertson, 1985a). First, as shown in Fig. 17.5, U_{osm} max achieved in PDI and CDI (after vasopressin) is appreciably less than in normal subjects. This is because a chronic polyuria of any etiology interferes with the maintenance of medullary osmotic gradient ("washout effect"), and the maximum urine osmolality cannot exceed the osmolality of the medullary interstitium, even in the presence of saturating AVP concentrations. Thus, both polyuric conditions represent reversible forms of acquired NDI which is readily correctable by the control of water intake or by chronic administration of desmopressin to these patients (see below). Another factor which may cause diagnostic confusion in distinguishing between the partial forms of CDI and NDI, is illustrated in Fig. 5.7. The plasma vasopressin rises in direct proportion to plasma osmolality. The sensitivity of the system depends on the severity of the underlying impairment of the secretory capacity, as depicted by a series of regression lines in Fig. 5.7, the greater the degree of the disturbance, the larger increment of plasma osmolality is needed to induce the same vasopressin response and the same increment of urine osmolality. Thus depending on the level of plasma osmolality achieved during the dehydration test, the urine osmolality may or may not reach the maximum permitted by washout of the medullary concentration gradient. Consequently, subsequent administration of exogenous vasopressin (or dDAVP) may or may not induce a further elevation of urine osmolality. The problem is further complicated by the fact that many patients with central diabetes insipidus respond in a supersensitive manner to even low levels of circulating vasopressin (Block et al. 1981). It follows that relatively slight increases in plasma osmolality and plasma vasopressin during water deprivation may, even in the presence of markedly reduced secretory capacity, be sufficient to raise urine osmolality to maximum permitted by washout of the medullary concentration gradient.

17.5.2.3 Parallel determination of plasma and urine osmolalities (P_{osm} versus U_{osm})

The two-part concentrating test as described above has provided much important information about the status of the vasopressin function in many polyuric patients. Nevertheless, it eventually became obvious that U_{osm} has to be carefully related to plasma osmolality (Richman et al. 1981, Moses 1985, Kovács et al. 1985b). Accurate measurement of P_{osm} is an essential component of the test. For its correct interpretation appropriate corrections have to be introduced for substances such as urea and ethanol which have actually no effects on osmotic water movement across the cell membrane. An alternative, and possibly a better approach, might be to relate urine osmolality values to effective plasma osmolality calculated as $2 \times P_{Na}$ (equation 1.2).

For diagnostic purposes the normal P_{osm}/U_{osm} relationships have been determined during ad libitum water intake and during water loading in healthy subjects, and the distribution of normal values has been described (Fig. 17.6, the larger and the smaller ellipse respectively) (Kovács et al. 1985). The evaluation of P_{osm}/U_{osm} values obtained for polyuric patients, according to this nomogram usually allows to distinguish polydipsic diabetes insipidus from complete forms of CDI and/or NDI, based on the initial investigation. For equivocal cases the diagnosis can be established by short-term water restriction. The concentrating test can be discontinued as soon as a clear-cut dynamic pattern of P_{osm}/U_{osm} changes has been obtained, even before urine osmolality reaches its plateau; at the same time, this avoids the potential hazards of long-term water deprivation. In addition, serial determination of the P_{osm}/U_{osm} ratio is of special value in bedside follow-up of the individual

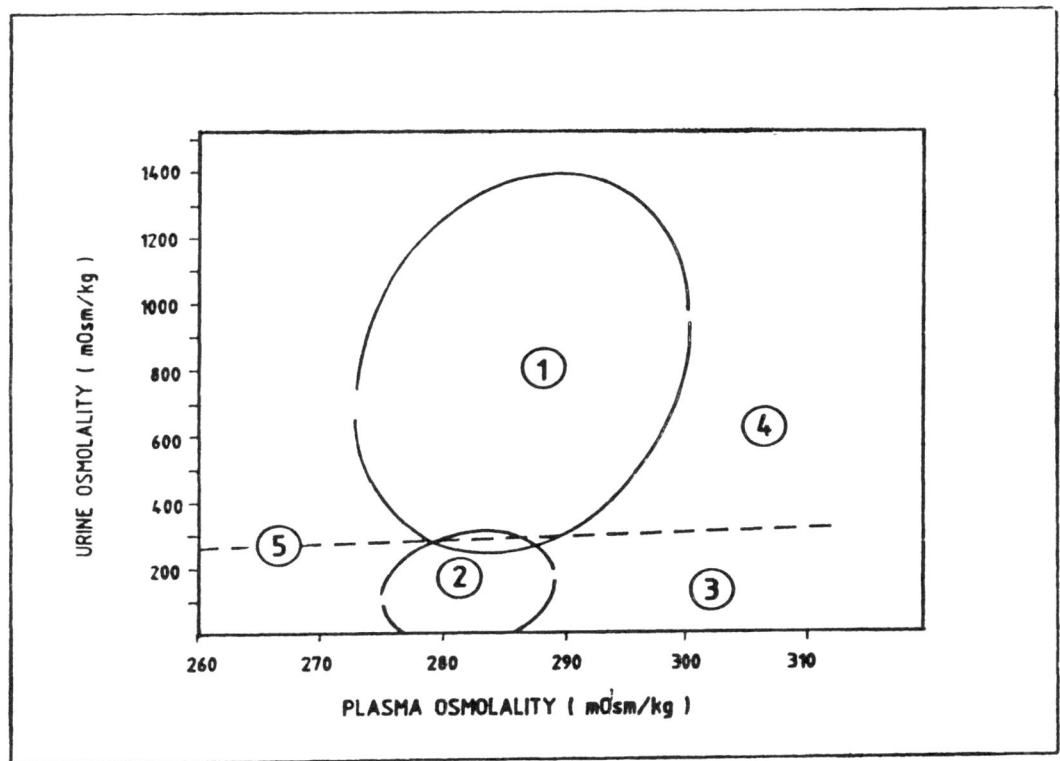

Fig. 17.6. Urine and plasma osmolality relationships in normal subjects during unrestricted access to fluids (greater ellipse 1) and after a standard water load (smaller ellipse 2) indicating the 95 per cent confidence region for normal renal concentrating and diluting performace respectively. The U_{osm}/P_{osm} relationships in patients with disturbed osmoregulation or effect of vasopressin are indicated by numbers (for details see text).

patterns of the development of postoperative and posttraumatic central diabetes insipidus (see Fig. 17.1).

If the point representing the P_{osm}/U_{osm} ratio for a polyuric patient with unrestricted fluid intake is within the area delineated by the larger ellipse (Fig. 17.6 (1)) any marked disturbance in the osmoregulatory system as well as the presence of significant diabetes insipidus can be excluded with a high probability even without any further testing. Points lying in the area to the right from the smaller ellipse (with sustained urine hypotonicity) suggest the presence of complete central or nephrogenic diabetes insipidus; these two forms can then be distinguished from each other by the administration of desmopressin. With complete nephrogenic diabetes insipidus the point remains in the same area after the administration of the synthetic AVP analog, whereas it is shifted into the area delineated by the larger ellipse in patients with complete central diabetes insipidus, i.e. the P_{osm}/U_{osm} ratio shifts to normal range.

If the point characterizing the P_{osm}/U_{osm} ratio in the initial test lies in the area delineated by the smaller ellipse (Fig. 17.6 (2)), further differentiation of the solute-free polyuria is required by monitoring the dynamics of changes in the point location during a short-term (4 to 6 hrs) concentrating test with restricted oral and intravenous intake of fluids. If with water restriction the point shifts to the larger ellipse, the patient was hyperhydrated and his disturbance most likely is polydipsic diabetes insipidus. On the contrary, if with sustained urine hypotonicity the point is shifted into the area on the right to the smaller ellipse (Fig. 17.6 (3)), the disturbance is complete central or nephrogenic diabetes insipidus. If a short-time water restriction is accompanied by the production of hypertonic urine, however only at the expense of an abnormal increase in plasma osmolality (i.e. the point shifts to the right from the larger ellipse, Fig. 17.6 (4)), the disturbance underlying the solute-free polyuria in the given patient most likely is partial central or nephrogenic diabetes insipidus; further differentiation requires monitoring of changes in the location of the P_{osm}/U_{osm} point following desmopressin administration.

With the point representing the P_{osm}/U_{osm} ratio obtained during the initial testing without any water restriction, lying to the right from the larger ellipse (i.e. plasma hyperosmolality and the production of hypertonic urine, Fig. 17.6 (4)) suggests a primary disturbance of the thirst mechanism; in conscious patients this is a finding consistent with the diagnosis of essential hypernatremia (chapter 17.3).

Finally, the location of the point for the P_{osm}/U_{osm} ratio obtained during the initial testing in the area to the left from both ellipses (Fig. 17.6 (5)) suggests the presence of some form of inadequate antidiuresis (hypervasopressinism) (chapter 20.3).

17.5.2.4 Radioimmunoassay of vasopressin in plasma and urine

The accuracy of indirect tests has recently been evaluated by concomitant direct measurements of plasma and urinary vasopressin. In the category of polyuric patients who were able to concentrate their urine to varying degrees when water deprived, the error rate of the indirect tests approximated 30 to 40%, the most common mistakes occurring in the distinction between partial CDI and polydipsic DI as well as between partial forms of CDI and NDI. Therefore, in patients who concentrate their urine to any extent during fluid deprivation plasma or urinary vasopressin should be measured at the end of the dehydration test and related to the concurrent plasma and urinary osmolalities. In doing so, considerable care should be taken to avoid interferences by nonosmotic stimuli (hypotension and nausea). In patients with renal disease, plasma instead of urinary AVP measurements have to be done.

This approach differentiates unambiguously between the three basic types of free-water polyuria in over 90 per cent of patients and is of direct clinical value, when simpler means of differentiation between the type of diabetes insipidus gave uncertain results (Zerbe and Robertson 1981). Some authors have recommended measuring urine rather than plasma vasopressin when evaluating a patient with polyuria. The advantage of this approach is that the amount of vasopressin is higher in urine and can therefore be measured more accurately by less sensitive radioimmunoassays (Miller and Moses 1972, Moses 1985). The urine output of AVP represents the secretion rate of this hormone in a defined period of time ("integrated secretion rate"). A simple water deprivation test, utilising measurements of urinary AVP concentration has been recenly described in order to avoid the need for accurately timed urine samples which are often difficult to obtain or incomplete in children (Dunger et al. 1988).

17.5.2.5 Short-term therapeutic trial with desmopressin

An adequate alternative to the currently still limitedly available direct determination of plasma and urinary vasopressin for the diagnosis of partial forms of diabetes insipidus is to institute a closely monitored therapeutic trial with desmopressin. If a 2 to 6-day administration of standard desmopressin doses (25 μg intranasally twice daily) significantly reduces diuresis and increases urine osmolality, the presence of nephrogenic diabetes insipidus can be effectively excluded, and the problem is reduced to differentiation between the remaining two types of solute-free polyuria: they can then be distinguished from each other by monitoring water balance during the desmopressin trial. If both polyuria and polydipsia subside and plasma osmolality does not drop to abnormally low values, the basic disturbance most likely is partial central diabetes insipidus. On the contrary, if desmopressin administration is followed by a reduced diuresis with no or a lesser reduction of water intake, and the body fluid volume excessively expands as evidenced by weight gain and by the development of plasma hypoosmolality, the patient most likely suffers from polydipsic diabetes insipidus (Zerbe and Robertson 1981).

The trial should in any case be undertaken in a hospital setting under closely monitored conditions because the administration of dDAVP to a patient with polydipsic DI can lead to overt water retention as manifested by severe symptomatic hyponatremia. Moreover, there is a slight possibility of false diagnosis, because about 5 per cent of the patients with central DI drink excessively during dDAVP administration either because of an associated abnormality in thirst or for some other reasons, probably habit (Vokes and Robertson 1988).

18   HYPERTONIC SYNDROMES

By definition hypertonicity reflects an increased concentration of nonpermeable solutes in plasma ($P_{osm} > 300 \, mOsm/kg$) which create an osmotic concentration gradient across the cell membrane and result in water moving out of cells. The number of solutes capable of causing hypertonicity is rather limited. Hypernatremia always represents hypertonicity, but all the other ions present in the extracellular fluid (potassium, magnesium, calcium) would cause specific lethal effects even before reaching concentrations sufficient to produce hypertonicity. From nonelectrolytes, only glucose and certain exogenous substances (as mannitol, sorbitol and glycerol when administered in sufficient amounts) can cause hypertonicity.

18.1   HYPERTONICITY AND THE CENTRAL NERVOUS SYSTEM

Independently of their cause, the common denominator to all hypertonic syndromes is cellular dehydration. Acute cell shrinking may be well responsible for the symptoms of hypertonicity that are primarily of neurologic nature: lethargy, weakness and irritability are the earliest findings which then culminate in seizures, coma and death (Arieff 1984, Mattle 1985). The severity of the neurologic symptoms of hypertonicity is related to both the degree and, more importantly, the rate of rise in effective plasma osmolality, i.e. to the speed of water flow out of brain cells down the osmotic gradient. A clinically significant water shift in animals and humans appears to require an acute change in P_{osm} of approximately 30—35 mOsm/kg, which represents a 15 mmol/l change in plasma sodium concentration (Arieff and Guisado 1976). Abrupt onset of severe hypertonicity causes the shrunken brain to tear away from its vascular attachment to the rigid calvarium, capillary and venous congestion, rupture of the cerebral veins: focal intracranial and subarachnoidal bleeding may occur. The mortality of acute hypernatremia is very high: reported mortality rates range from 40 to greater than 70%. Unfortunately, in survivors irreversible damage of the CNS is common and encountered in as many as in two thirds of these patients (Matulay and Watson 1967, Finberg 1973, Himmelstein et al. 1983).

When hypertonicity persists for hours or days the brain possesses a unique mechanism to respond to the osmotic stress by gaining osmotically active solutes within the tissue (chapter 1.4.2, Fig. 18.1). This results in an increase in brain cell osmolality, water osmotically moves back to the brain, and brain volume is restored to normal. Up to one half of the solute gained in this way seems to originate from the plasma and the cerebrospinal fluid (sodium chloride and, in the case of hyperglycemia, glucose), while the other half is made up by newly generated intracellular osmoles (amino acids and mostly other, so far unidentified solutes called idiogenic osmoles). The time course of this homeostatic adaptive response seems to depend on the nature of the osmotic stimulus: in hypernatremia this process begins early and restores brain cell volume to normal by one week, while in experimental hyperglycemia it takes only four hours for the brain volume to return to normal (Arieff et al. 1976). The resulting intracellular salt gain has at least two important clinical consequences. First, patients with more gradually developing or chronic hyperosmolality (e.g. subjects with essential hypernatremia) may be relatively asymptomatic despite plasma osmolalities as high as 350—370 mOsm/kg for days or months. As a consequence, also mortality of chronic hypertonicity is much lower than

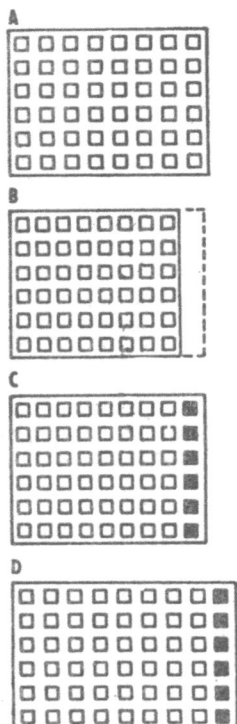

Fig. 18.1. Schematic representation of hyperosmolality induced alterations in volume and osmolality of brain cells. The normal state is depicted on panel (A). In this and subsequent panels, open squares represent the normally present impermeant solutes in ICF; newly generated "idiogenic" osmoles are shown by solid squares. The density of the symbols reflects solute concentration and their number total intracellular solute content. Brain cells respond to acute hyperosmolality mainly by osmotic water loss (panel B). During sustained ECF hypertonicity the cells partially reverse osmotic water loss to ECF by gaining additional intracellular solutes (panel C). In that situation rapid correction of ECF osmolality to normal values would unavoidably produce cell swelling with resulting brain edema (panel D).

in acute cases, the ultimate outcome primarily depending on the basic disease process (Snyder et al. 1987). Second, the removal or inactivation of the newly gained solutes is, as their generation, also a process that takes certain time. Therefore, overly rapid correction of extracellular hyperosmolality before the complete disappearance of these solutes, would unavoidably result in cell hyperhydration and appearance of neurologic signs of cerebral edema, a phenomenon that might be termed "the syndrome of isotonic water intoxication" (see Fig. 18.1) (Feig 1981).

18.2 HYPERNATREMIA

The normal defense against the development of hypernatremia ($P_{Na} > > 150$ mmol/l) is the stimulation of both AVP secretion and thirst by the hypothalamic osmoreceptors. Although AVP release occurs earlier it is thirst that provides ultimate protection against hypernatremia. Thus, hypernatremia is almost always due to deficiency of water intake; increased output via the skin, lungs, gastrointestinal tract or kidneys may contribute to its generation, but is rarely if ever a sufficient cause if thirst is normal and access to water is unlimited. The same can be said about excessive intake of salt. Although hypernatremia has been reported after accidental overdoses of sodium, the disturbance is only transient unless the patient is unable to compensate by increasing water intake.

Since primary hypodipsia (chapter 17.3) is relatively rare, hypernatremia occurs much more commonly in infants, elderly or comatose patients who have an intact thirst mechanism but are unable to ask for water or lack the necessary motor responses to seek and ingest water. More than 1 per cent of hospitalized patients older than 60 years may have hypernatremia which is usually iatrogenic, and its presence often suggests clinical neglect (Himmelstein et al. 1983, Snyder et al. 1987). High plasma sodium level is a known and justifiedly feared complication of many diseases of newborns and small infants (Matulay and Watson 1967, Finberg 1973). In recent years, the incidence of hypernatremic dehydration following gastroenteritis has fallen in infants, primarily because of the use of low solute feedings as well as pediatric oral rehydration solutions (see Table 14.1), which supply more free water to replace the insensible losses (Samadi et al. 1983).

Hypernatremia is not a uniform syndrome. Rather, it is a biochemical sign that reflects a state of relative deficit of body water in relation to body sodium, but is not indicative as to the absolute level of total body sodium (see Fig. 1.2). Total body sodium is a bedside judgement based on signs of adequacy of intravascular volume and, as shown in Fig. 18.2, hypernatremia can develop with either low, normal, or more rarely, high total body sodium. Thus in addition to the neurologic changes, hypernatremic patients

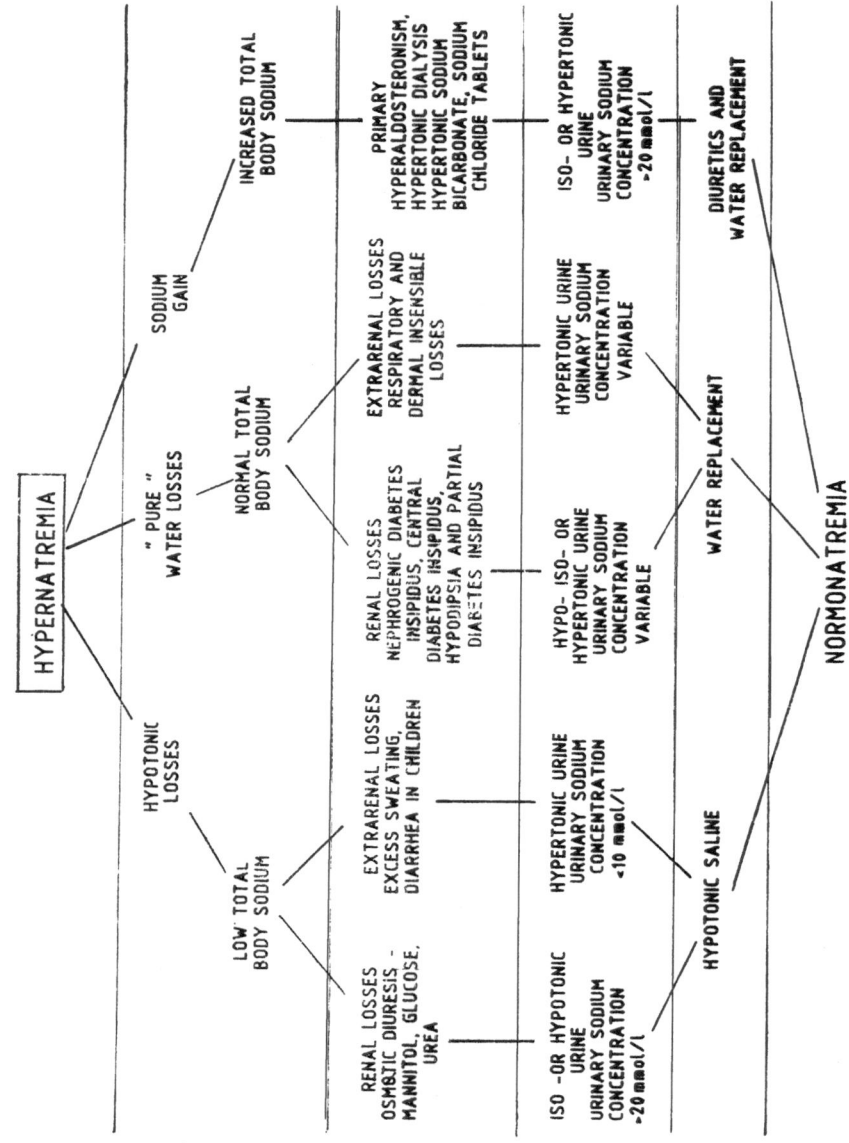

Fig. 18.2. Diagnostic approach to hypernatremia.

may show on clinical investigation signs of volume depletion (flat neck veins, decreased turgor and postural hypotension) or volume expansion (manifested as peripheral and/or pulmonary edema).

18.2.1 HYPERNATREMIA DUE TO "PURE" WATER LOSS (HYPERNATREMIA WITH NORMAL TOTAL BODY SODIUM)

Hypernatremia, although rarely, can be generated by loss of water alone (see Fig. 18.2). In patients with "pure" (solute-free) water losses only 1/3 of the water will originate from the extracellular compartment. Moreover, plasma volume which comprises only about one fourth of the ECF volume will share only one twelfth ($1/3 \times 1/4$) of the total volume loss. Thus, in this setting the signs of extracellular volume depletion are usually absent, unless marked water losses (10 to 15 per cent of body weight) have occurred that raised the plasma sodium level usually greater than 165—170 mmol/l. Consequently, these patients are likely to exhibit the neurologic symptoms of hypernatremia before those of ECF volume depletion. With marked dehydration moderate azotemia is common. Urine osmolality is at least twofold higher than the plasma osmolality, unless the source of "pure" water loss was renal. Urinary sodium excretion will vary according to the patient's sodium intake.

18.2.1.1 Extrarenal losses

Insensible loss of water occurs continuously via the skin and lungs in an average amount of 500 ml/day in adults; appropriate replacement of these obligatory losses by supplying the same amount of electrolyte-free water to patients is mandatory for preservation of the isotonicity of body fluids. This problem is amplified in many conditions associated with increased insensible losses: increased rate and/or depth of breathing, in preterm infants treated under radiant warmers and/or phototherapy (because of thin skin and relatively large body surface area), in patients with fever, thyrotoxicosis or burns, and also in subjects maintained in too hot and dry environment (Engle et al. 1981, Mahowald and Himmelstein 1981). Inappropriate replacement of daily water losses with normal saline is the most commonly encountered in-hospital cause of hypernatremia associated with normal total body sodium content (Snyder 1987).

18.2.1.2 Renal losses

The other major potential route of excess water loss is renal either due to a defect in the production or release of vasopressin, or due to a defect in the renal response to the hormone (chapters 17.1 and 17.2 respectively).

18.2.2 HYPERNATREMIA DUE TO HYPOTONIC LOSS (HYPERNATREMIA WITH LOW TOTAL BODY SODIUM)

Hypernatremia most commonly occurs in patients with sustained losses of hypotonic fluid. In terms of the free-water concept hypotonic losses can be viewed as a mixture of two fractions. One fraction is "pure" water which originates homogenously from total body water, raises body fluid tonicity and has relatively minor effect on extracellular fluid volume; the other, isotonic fraction, which contains mostly sodium salts, originates from the ECF compartment, causes ECF volume depletion but obviously has no effect on body fluid tonicity.

As a consequence, for any given volume lost the extracellular volume contraction is more severe while the increment in tonicity is less marked (P_{Na} only rarely exceeds 160—165 mmol/l) than if losses were "pure" water alone. An important fact to remember is that the ECF volume contraction caused by sodium loss is usually far more life threatening than hypertonicity per se. Since vascular volume contraction reduces GFR and, together with hypertonicity, stimulates AVP secretion, these patients typically excrete scant amounts of highly concentrated urine, except if persistent osmotic diuresis is the cause of the syndrome. When marked hypernatremia is present, urine sodium concentration usually does not drop to values as low as are typical of hypovolemic states ($U_{Na} < 20$ mmol/l) (see Fig. 18.2).

18.2.2.1 Extrarenal losses

The most common mechanism is the loss of hypotonic fluids from the gastrointestinal tract in the form of diarrhea, particularly in children (Bruck et al. 1968, Samadi et al. 1983). Such losses are often aggravated by vomiting or, most importantly, by the simultaneous administration of relatively hypertonic diets and/or solutions.

Enteral tube feeding can cause hypernatremia on the basis of either osmotic diarrhea, hyperglycemia with glucosuria and/or osmotic diuresis from high protein supplements (Cataldi-Betcher et al. 1983).

During the early 1970ies there was a high incidence of hypernatremia complicating acute gastroenteritis in infants. As subsequently recognized, this was the result of feeding infants dangerously high solute foods (overconcentrated dried milk) which supervened the limited ability of the infant's kidneys to maintain osmolal homeostasis in the face of hypotonic losses associated with gastroenteritis. The introduction of low-solute infant formulas have led to a considerable decline in the incidence of infantile diarrhea and hypernatremia (Davies et al. 1979).

The past few years have seen the widespread application of the World Health Organization oral rehydration solutions to treat infantile gastroenteritis.

208

Their improper preparation and/or application of formulas designated to adults instead of those developed for children (see Tab. 14.1) resulted in hypernatremia because of the net ingestion of a high solute load (Walker 1981). In this case the resolution seems to involve the use of specific infant rehydration solutions along with a clear instruction on the package how to prepare them (Finberg 1980, Boda 1985).

Hypertonic peritoneal or hemodialysis can also lead to hypernatremia by removing extra "pure" water as well as isotonic fluid. In addition, since sweat in humans is hypotonic (normally up to 60 mmol/l), heavy hypotonic losses from the skin may occur in subjects in extremely hot and humid environment (Quinton 1987).

18.2.2.2 Renal losses

Another major cause of hypotonic fluid loss is that which occurs during an osmotic diuresis (from high protein tube feeding, due to prolonged glucosuria in diabetes mellitus or during the therapeutic use of osmotic agents such as mannitol). In such patients the urine is usually isoosmotic or hyperosmotic to plasma (see Table 17.8). However, since the osmotic agent itself constitutes a substantial fraction of the urinary osmoles, the net result is loss of hypotonic body fluids with sodium concentration below that of the plasma (Gennari and Kassirer 1974).

18.2.3 HYPERNATREMIA DUE TO SALT GAIN (HYPERNATREMIA WITH INCREASED TOTAL BODY SODIUM)

Hypernatremia due to an acute or chronic salt gain is the least common type of the syndrome. The immediate consequences of the sudden hypertonicity involve water flow out of the cells down the osmotic gradient with consequent acute cell dehydration and ECF volume expansion. Accordingly, the severe sodium overload is often manifested by pulmonary and/or peripheral edema in addition to the neurologic signs of hypernatremia. ECF expansion leads to brisk natriuresis and, when renal function is normal, the sodium load may be excreted rapidly in the urine.

In clinical settings most cases of acute salt intoxication are accidental or iatrogenic resulting from ingestion or infusion of hypertonic Na^+ solutions (Finberg et al. 1963, Mattar et al. 1973). This problem can occur in infants given sodium bicarbonate for correction of metabolic acidosis or during cardiopulmonary resuscitation (Simmons et al. 1974). The inadvertent administration of only one tablespoon NaCl to a newborn can raise the plasma sodium concentration by as many as 70 mmol/l (Saunders et al. 1976). Patients with primary hyperaldosteronism and Cushing syndrome have slight and clinically unimportant chronic hypernatremia. There are also occasional reports of excessive oral intake of sodium chloride in the form of salt tablets or chicken soup which have resulted in hypernatremia (Addleman et al. 1985, Fujiwara et al. 1985).

18.3 TREATMENT OF HYPERNATREMIA

In treating patients with hypernatremia, it is important to realize that usually disturbed water balance is only one of many concomitant electrolyte and acid-base disorders found in these patients. In order to determine the realistic priority of hypernatremia the nature of the primary disturbance or disease which has resulted in the pathologic alteration should be established, and symptoms attributable to either of them should be differentiated.

Less severe chronic hypernatremia (P_{Na} < 160—165 mmol/l) usually subsides upon adequate therapy of the basic disease (e.g. the administration of desmopressin to treat central diabetes insipidus). Acute symptomatic hypernatremia is a medical emergency requiring more specific measures aimed at restoring plasma sodium concentration to normal levels. In patients with water (and sodium) depletion reduction of P_{Na} may be attempted by administering hypotonic solutions, while excess sodium may be removed by administering loop diuretics such as furosemide. Since diuretics remove more water than sodium, it is necessary to simultaneously administer sufficient amounts of hypotonic solutions to prevent worsening of the hypertonicity. Peritoneal dialysis using 4.25 per cent glucose solutions, or hemodialysis also have been successfully used to acutely lower P_{Na}.

The rate at which the serum sodium can safely be lowered depends on the duration of hypernatremia. Therapy using minimal concentrations of sodium or, occasionally, 5 per cent dextrose alone, can safely be initiated if it can be unequivocally documented that the duration of hypernatremia has been less than a few hours. In most clinical settings however, the duration of hypernatremia is much longer, additional intracellular osmoles (see Fig. 18.1) may have formed, and P_{Na} should be lowered slowly. Since it still remains unknown how rapidly these "volume-protecting" additional intracellular osmoles can be removed or inactivated, the ideal rate of correction of the plasma sodium abnormality remains a matter of debate. At present most investigators agree that P_{Na} should be lowered by no more than 15 mmol/l in any 8-hour period, i.e. a maximum reduction by 2 mmol/l per hour (Gruskin et al. 1982, Snyder et al. 1987). If, after initial improvement, at any time during water replacement, deterioration of sensorium and signs of cerebral edema occur, they must be considered as signs of "isotonic water intoxication", and treated as one would treat cerebral edema in the face of hyponatremia (Feig 1981).

The following imprecise formula can be helpful in estimating the amount of water which is theoretically required to lower the serum concentration to normal (i.e. to 140 mmol/l):

$$\text{Water deficit (liters)} = 0.6 \times \text{lean body weight (kg)} \times \left[1 - \frac{P_{Na}}{140}\right] \quad \text{(equation 18.3)}$$

This calculated value is only approximate, and does not include the ongoing losses which must also be replaced. Another disadvantage of the calculation is that it only estimates the actual "pure" water deficit, but ignores any isoosmotic fluid deficit which is usually also present. Thus it may be relatively accurate for a patient with diabetes insipidus who loses only water, but it underestimates the deficit in hypernatremic patients with diarrhea who lose both Na and water.

If a patient is avid with intact thirst the best choice is giving replacement fluid therapy orally. The initial oral fluids should contain electrolytes as well as dextrose (e.g. the WHO oral rehydration solution; see Table 14.1) so that P_{Na} will fall slowly. This approach, probably through oropharyngeal or other gastrointestinal receptors (chapter 5.1.2) allows to self-regulate the volume of the ingested fluids according to the actual needs of the body, and appears to reduce the frequency of potentially dangerous complications from this therapy. The intravenous route of fluid therapy should be reserved for those patients who do not drink spontaneously when offered fluids (as unconscious or severely ill subjects), for those who have nausea or vomit, or for cases when appreciable volume depletion and hypotension is also present (Boda 1985).

The therapeutic approach to volume depleted subjects consists of two parts. If volume depletion is severe (more than 10 to 15 per cent of body weight lost) a rapid infusion of physiologic saline (15 to 40 min) should be given in an attempt to restore adequate tissue perfusion as rapidly as possible. Since physiologic saline solution (0.9 per cent) in these states is hypotonic to the patient's body fluid, it will also at the same time tend to decrease the degree of hypernatremia. Plasma albumin solutions or, in the presence of blood loss or severe anemia, whole blood may be used when required to treat hypovolemic shock. Only after the reversal of signs of intravascular collapse should hypotonic replacement (e.g. 5 per cent dextrose in half or quarter physiologic saline or, when possible, appropriate oral rehydration solutions) be initiated; potassium should be added only after urine formation is assured. The total quantity and rate of administration of water should be carefully controlled until the serum sodium has been in the normal range for 8 to 12 hours (Gruskin et al. 1982).

19 HYPERVASOPRESSINISM

According to its definition (chapter 14.2), the diagnosis of hypervasopressinism rests ultimately on the demonstration that vasopressin is present in plasma and urine in the face of hyponatremia and hypotonicity of body fluids. Consequently if a patient does not have hyponatremia it is impossible to either diagnose or exclude hypervasopressinism. If a patient, in whom excessive AVP secretion is suspected, is given "water loads" and these loads are retained in body fluid compartments producing hyponatremia instead of being normally lost via urine hypervasopressinism is likely. The definitive proof depends on the demonstration that plasma or urinary vasopressin remains inappropriately high for the degree of hypotonicity produced. This approach is adequate to investigate the causes of hypervasopressinism in experimental work as well as in closely controlled clinical investigations. It is obvious however that a similar approach is undesirable in routine clinical practice because of the risk of severe induced hyponatremia. On the other hand, the knowledge derived from animal studies and clinical investigations may have direct therapeutic implications. It increases the ability of the clinician to anticipate vasopressin-mediated water retention and by judicious administration of free-water and monitoring of serum sodium concentration to prevent the development of severe plasma hypotonicity.

19.1 CAUSES OF HYPERVASOPRESSINISM

The many diverse causes of hypervasopressinism and inappropriate antidiuresis in relation to body fluid osmolality may be divided into three categories.

The most important category of causes of vasopressin excess are nonosmotic stimuli that act by lowering the threshold of the osmoregulatory mechanism (see Table 5.1). Specifically, recent data indicate a major importance of a decreased "effective circulating blood volume" (ECBV) and/or blood pressure which result in baroreceptor-mediated nonosmotic release of AVP in hypovolemic and edematous patients. In view of the demonstrated relationship of plasma norepinephrine (NE) and, to a lesser degree, plasma renin activity (PRA) to sympathetic vasomotor outflow and baroreceptor activation (Grossman et al.

1982, Levine et al. 1982a, b) the role of decreased "effective arterial blood volume" has been exemplified, albeit indirectly, by observations that documented abnormally elevated concentrations of NE and PRA in association with stimulated vasopressin in edematous states and a reversal of these humoral changes after maneouvres that are believed to improve ECBV (e.g. head-out water immersion, non hypotensive afterload reduction in cardiac failure, and plasma volume expansion with albumin in nephrotic syndrome (Tulassay et al. 1987, Kovács et al. 1987e, Gross et al. 1987)).

It is important to emphasize that blood redistribution within the vascular bed resulting in "regional hypovolemia" within the capacitance vessels of the chest including the left atrium (i.e. within the structures in which the principal volume receptors are localized) is also a frequent cause of vasopressin excess, particularly in patients with asthma, pneumonia, during positive end-exspiratory pressure (PEEP) ventilation and in pure right-sided heart failure (Friedman and Segar 1979, Kovács et al. 1984b). "Regional hypovolemia" may account, at least partly, for hypervasopressinism that occurs in severely ill subjects; motionless lying in bed permits blood to pool in the dependent portions of the vascular compartment with a subsequent decrease in left atrial filling (Segar and Moore 1968).

In addition to alterations in generalized or "regional" hemodynamics, other recognized nonosmotic stimuli may also cause hypervasopressinism (see Table 5.1). Emetic stimuli eliminate the capacity to osmotically suppress AVP release. Since nausea is of common occurrence during the course of various disease states, emetic stimuli may be a more important mechanism than is usually appreciated, contributing to the development of vasopressin excess, althought documentation is still lacking. Also hypoxemia as well as hypercapnic acidosis can stimulate AVP release by decreasing the set point of the secretory mechanism. Head trauma, intracranial infections and conditions associated with increased intracranial pressure are common causes of hypervasopressinism, probably secondary to their direct central effect on the secretory mechanism. In this respect also stress of hospitalization and/or the underlying disease appears to be an important stimulus for excessive vasopressin release (Felsl et al. 1978). Indeed, a recent study reported increased plasma NE levels in normovolemic patients with vasopressin excess, suggesting increased sympathetic efferent neural traffic (Anderson et al. 1985). In addition, pain afferents may directly stimulate the hypothalamus and lead to excessive AVP secretion (e.g. during postoperative period).

The second category of causes includes ectopic AVP production by humorally active malignant tissues (chapter 20.3.1.9), while the third category consists of administration of exogenous AVP, dDAVP or oxytocin or various other drugs that stimulate AVP secretion or potentiate its hydroosmotic effect (chapter 20.3.1.10).

19.2 HYPERVASOPRESSINISM — IS IT ALWAYS INAPPROPRIATE?

Sustained AVP release which continues even at abnormally low values of plasma osmolality (hypervasopressinism) is often entitled as "inappropriate" AVP secretion. The latter term implies that the mechanisms regulating AVP release are not functioning normally. However, it needs not be true. Instead, in most instances well-known physiologic and pathophysiologic nonosmotic secretory stimuli are responsible for the elevated circulating levels of the hormone (chapter 19.1). From an evolutionary viewpoint, this nonosmotic release of AVP might be considered an integral part of autonomic neural response of the organism to a variety of stressors (Schrier and Berl 1975). In earlier sea living species in which water conservation was less critical, perhaps the pressor effect rather than the antidiuretic action of the hormone was more important. In the context of this hypothesis perhaps all nonosmotic release of vasopressin from the posterior pituitary constitutes an integral component of an appropriate response of the autonomic nervous system to stress reactions. In other words, although nonosmotically elevated AVP secretion might be inappropriate from the narrow viewpoint of body fluid tonicity, in most clinical settings (for example in hypovolemic states) it is quite appropriate from the broader perspective of the patient's survival. Perhaps then only the uncontrolled, ectopic release of AVP-like activity from tumors should be classified as "inappropriate".

These different points of view can only lead to confusion in clinical situations and mislead the physician who ideally is expected to determine why a patient has excessive plasma AVP levels and initiate appropriate treatment of the underlying condition in an aim to improve renal water excretion. Nevertheless the term "syndrome of inappropriate secretion of antidiuretic hormone" has become established to describe hyponatremia in apparently normovolemic subjects (chapter 20.3.1) so that it is almost impossible to exclude it from clinical terminology. The requirement not to use terms "appropriate" and "inappropriate" independently is more acceptable in this respect; these terms should always be further specified by characterizing the volume status of the organism (Berl et al. 1976, Kovács et al. 1984c, Gross et al. 1986).

20 THE HYPOTONIC SYNDROME

Hypotonicity ($P_{osm} < 280$ mOsm/kg) reflects a relative increase in body water in relation to the body solute content, i.e. it is in a simplistic sense always dilutional. Sodium is the only plasma solute the concentration of which can decrease sufficiently, upon plasma dilution, to induce hypotonicity. Hypotonicity therefore always means also hyponatremia. However, it should be remembered that the opposite needs not be always true. Hence if low plasma concentration of sodium has been found in a patient ($P_{Na} < 130$ mmol/l) it should be decided first whether the condition represents "true" hypotonic hyponatremia or whether some of the non-hypotonic forms of hyponatremia is present (Fig. 20.1).

20.1 NON-HYPOTONIC HYPONATREMIAS

Non-hypotonic hyponatremias do not reflect excess water in body spaces. Therefore, nothing needs be done specifically about them, except to suspect and confirm this problem (see Fig. 20.1). Treatment of non-hypotonic hyponatremia should be directed to the elimination of the underlying condition which will result in the restoration of plasma sodium concentration to normal.

20.1.1 PSEUDOHYPONATREMIA

Solids (proteins and lipids) normally occupy only 7 per cent of total plasma volume. Electrolytes are virtually restricted to the remaining plasma water fraction. Replacement of salt containing plasma water with salt-poor lipid or protein reduces the content of sodium in each newly reconstituted liter without changing the concentration of cations in the remaining water. Thus sodium concentration per unit of volume of total plasma is decreased (as reflected by low P_{Na} as measured by flame photometry) without changing the concentration of cations in the remaining water. This is shown by analytical procedures which measure the solute concentration in the aquous phase, i.e. by directly determining plasma osmolality (Faye and Payne 1986). Various forms of

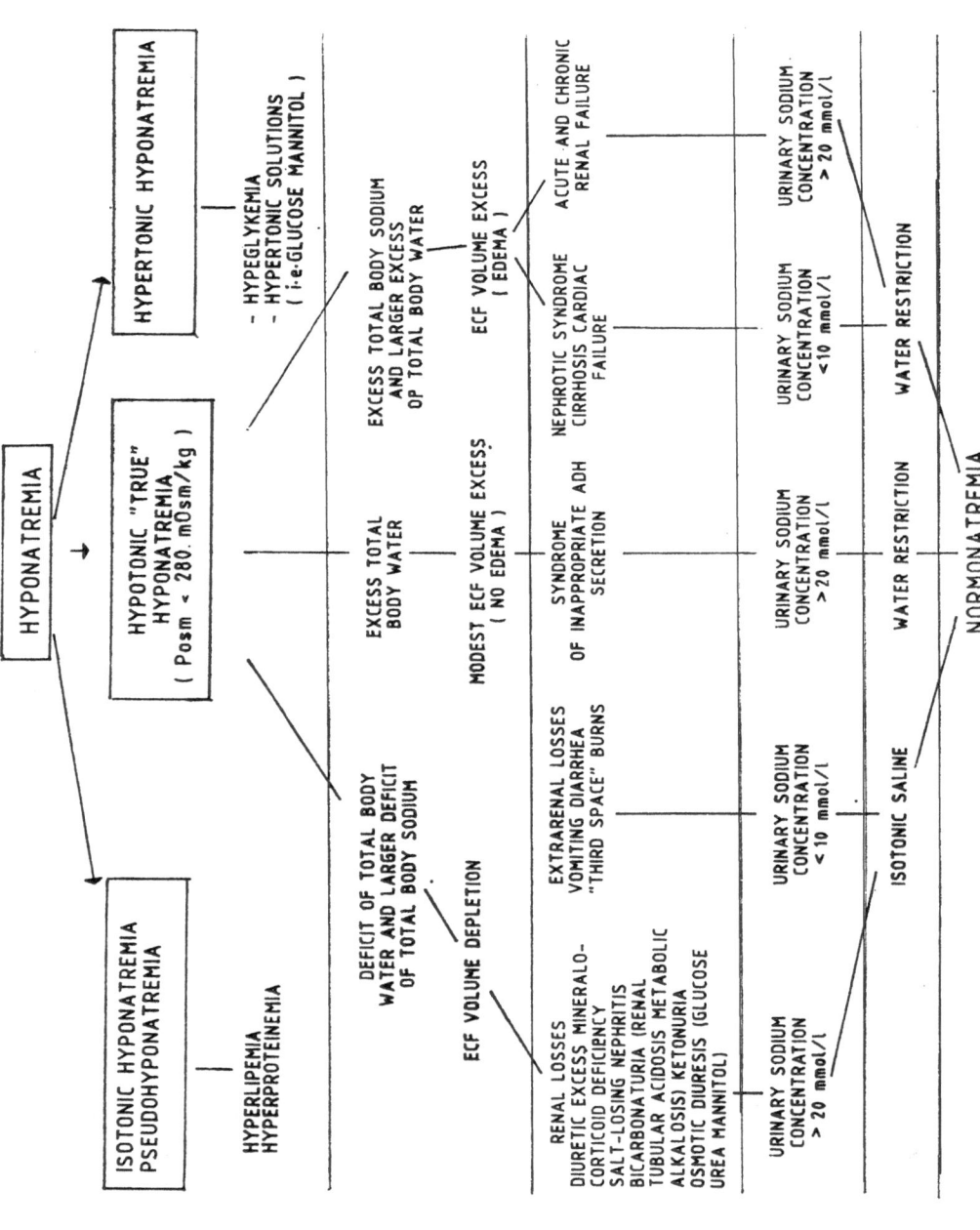

Fig. 20.1. Diagnostic and therapeutic approach to patients with hyponatremia.

primary or secondary hyperlipidemia (e.g. essential hyperlipidemia, familial hyperchylomicronemia or lipemias associated with poorly controlled diabetes mellitus, or with nephrotic syndrome) may cause pseudohyponatremia; their presence can be foreseen from gross lactescence (chylosity) of the serum observable by free eye. In severe hyperproteinemic states that produce pseudohyponatremia (most frequently in patients with multiple myeloma, less frequently in association with Sjogren's syndrome or macroglobulinemia), the serum or plasma are typically extremely viscid (in fact frequently in a gel state) compared to normal plasma. Multiplication of plasma lipids (mg/dl) by 0.002 and the increment of serum proteins above 8 g/dl by 0.25 yields the reduction (in mmol/l) in serum sodium caused by the accumulation of these solids (Narins et al. 1982).

20.1.2   REDISTRIBUTION OF BODY WATER

Low plasma sodium levels are found also when high concentrations of other osmotically active solutes are present in plasma. These solutes, at least initially, create osmotic gradients between the isotonic intracellular fluid and the now-hypertonic extracellular fluid. Solute-free water then moves from the cells to the extracellular compartment with subsequent dilution of the latter. It appears that 15—20% of all hyponatremias developed in hospitalized adults can be attributed to this mechanism (Anderson et al. 1985, Chung et al. 1986). This is most frequently observed in uncontrolled diabetic patients with hyperglycemia or during the administration of hypertonic glucose, mannitol or glycine solutions for therapeutical purposes. This osmotic shift of water has been estimated to lower plasma sodium concentration by 1.6 mmol/l for every 100 mg per 100 ml rise in blood glucose or blood mannitol, whereas upon increasing glycine concentration P_{Na} decreases by 3.8 mmol/l. Empirically it has been shown that in hyperglycemic states the corrected P_{Na} (i.e. P_{Na} estimated after blood glucose has been restored to normal) equals actual $P_{Na} \times 1/3$ glycemia in mmol/l (Goldberg 1981).

Although also urea and alcohol are occasionally considered to belong to this category, both penetrate cells rapidly, and prolonged excess of either of them is therefore unlikely to cause appreciable hyponatremia. Hence, hyponatremia associated with marked azotemia point to clinically important hypotonicity even though total P_{osm} measured is in normal range or exceeds it (Gennari 1984). In such cases it is better to calculate the effective plasma osmolality (equation 1.2), instead of directly measuring osmolality. Values obtained in this way, however, are valid only under normoglycemic conditions; if hyperglycemia is present (or with other osmotically active agents), 1 mOsm/kg has to be added to the calculated value of effective osmolality for each mmol/l glucose, mannitol or glycine, to obtain actual tonicity.

20.2 HYPOTONICITY AND THE CENTRAL NERVOUS SYSTEM

As plasma osmolality falls, an osmolal gradient is created across the cell membrane resulting in water movement into the cells. Two thirds of the extra water is sequestered intracellularly, making generalized cellular edema the hallmark of acute hypotonic states. Unlike extracranial tissues that expand freely as they swell, brain cell expansion is limited by the confines of the cranial vault, provoking the neurologic syndrome of cerebral edema. Thus the symptoms and signs of acute hypoosmolality are primarily due to cerebral overhydration.

The severity of the neurologic manifestations is related to the rapidity as well as to the degree of reduction in body fluid tonicity. In general, the patient begins to complain of nausea and malaise as P_{Na} falls below 125 mmol/l. Between 115 and 120 mmol/l headache, letargy and obtundation occur followed by abnormal sensorium, depressed deep-tendon reflexes, Cheyne-Stokes respiration, pseudobulbar palsy, generalized seizures and death with further progression of hypotonicity. In two prospective studies, the frequency of severe hyponatremia as the cause of significant CNS symptoms was thought to be 3% and 15% respectively, of all patients with hyponatremia (Baran and

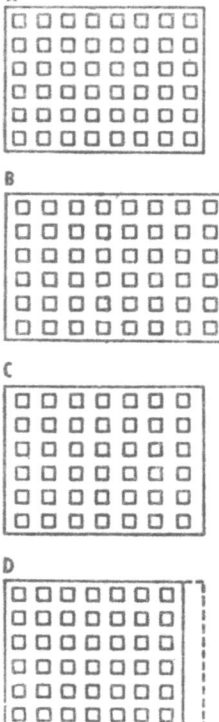

Fig. 20.2. Schematic representation of hypoosmolality induced alterations in volume and osmolality of brain cells. The normal state is depicted on panel (A). In this and subsequent panels, open squares represent the normally present impermeant solutes in ICF. The density of the symbols reflects solute concentration and their number total intracellular solute content. When hypotonicity develops abruptly, osmolality equalizes primarily by water movement no matter what the cell (panel B). Brain cells adapt to sustained ECF hypotonicity by decreasing their intracellular solute content (panel C), Overly rapid correction of the depressed plasma osmolality produces cerebral dehydration (panel D).

218

Hutchinson 1984, Anderson et al. 1985); death occurred in up to 50% of patients whose plasma sodium concentrations were reduced to less than 120 mmol/l over a period of 24 h (Arieff et al. 1976).

After 24 to 48 h of sustained hypotonicity, brain cells unlike other tissues adapt by profound decreases in brain electrolytes, amino acids (in particular taurine), and other unmeasured osmoles (chapter 1.4.2). The loss of intracellular solutes has been interpreted as having volume regulatory significance in returning brain volume to normal (Fig. 20.2). Perhaps, this adaptive response occurs only at the expense of the cell function, since solute loss must in some way reflect a change in physico-chemical makeup of the cell. The effects of chronic hyponatremia are similar to those in other metabolic encephalopathies, and most likely reflect disordered brain metabolism secondary to the electrolyte and amino-acid depletion of cells (Arieff et al. 1976, Thurston et al. 1987). The morbidity and mortality rates associated with chronic hypotonicity are lower than those of the acute disorder, and likely, they are largely determined by the nature and severity of the underlying disease process (Anderson 1986, Kovács et al. 1987b, Sterns 1987).

The very adaptation that permits survival in chronic hyponatremia makes the brain more susceptible to injury when the serum sodium concentration is suddenly increased or overcorrected. If serum osmolality is restored too quickly (i.e. before the cellular restoration of lost solute can be achieved) to normal values, a reverse osmotic gradient is created causing the adapted normovolemic brain cells shrink to volumes that may be less than normal (see Fig. 20.2). This noxious sequence may be the basis for a serious and often irreversible neurological damage, the central pontine myelinolysis syndrome. Since clinical findings may reflect pontine as well as extrapontine myelinolysis, the syndrome has recently been dubbed also as "the osmotic demyelination syndrome". The syndrome has been reported to occur more frequently in alcoholic and malnourished patients. Persons afflicted may have a fulminant neurologic disorder characterized by convulsions, quadriplegia, impaired swallowing (often with episodes of aspiration), hypoventilation and hypotension.

In a recent article Sterns et al. (1986) have cited eight cases of central pontine myelinolysis all associated with severe hyponatremia, and claimed that it is the speed of correction rather than hyponatremia per se which causes osmotic demyelination. They have claimed that neurological sequelae were never seen when plasma sodium levels were elevated by less than 12 mmol/l per day (0.5 mmol per hour). However, it should be said that not all investigators believe that chronic hyponatremia or its rapid correction bears any relation to central pontine myelinolysis (Arieff 1986, Narrins 1986). These opponents suggest that profound hyponatremia itself and/or its overcorrection is that which can lead to neurological damage. By this latter view chronic symptomatic hyponatremia should be corrected "rapidly" to mildly hyponatremic levels (120—125 mmol/l) with hypertonic saline at a rate of about 2 mmol/l per hour. This fourfold range (0.5 and 2 mmol/l per hour) of recommended rates of correction is perplexing to the practitioner. Considering the severity of the potential complications (death or permanent brain damage) it may be wise to err on the side of too slow rather than too rapid correction of hyponatremia. Perhaps the mean of these two extremes, a rate of about 1 to 1.5 mmol/l per hour would be most safe (Thurston et al. 1987).

20.3 HYPOTONIC ("TRUE") HYPONATREMIA

Hypotonic hyponatremia is probably the most common of all electrolyte disturbances. As it is currently encountered, it is often a hospital-acquired disorder occurring in elderly and pediatric patients with severe underlying disease and it is associated with substantial morbidity and mortality (Burrows et al. 1983, Baran and Hutchinson 1984, Gross et al. 1986). In a recent prospective study a daily incidence rate of hyponatremia ($P_{Na} < 130$ mmol/l) of approximately 1 per cent has been reported in hospitalized adult patients (mean age 58 years) on general medical-surgical wards; as much as two thirds of this hyponatremia was acquired in the hospital (Anderson et al. 1985). A similarly high, approximately 0.7 per cent, incidence rate of severe hyponatremia ($P_{Na} < 125$ mmol/l) has been documented in pediatric patients (with median age of 11 months) hospitalized in a general medical-surgical children's hospital; again, the prevailing majority of cases first arose or worsened in the hospital (Kovács et al. 1987c).

Because of the enormous capacity of the kidney to excrete water load (chapter 9.1.6), water retention resulting in hypotonic hyponatremia essentially occurs only when 1. there is a defect in renal water excretion and 2. the amount of free-water ingested or, more often, given nondipsogenically exceeds the actually compromised renal diluting ability. (A rare exception to this rule occurs in psychotic patients with primary polydipsia who drink a great deal of water in a hurry, and this may acutely overwhelm even a normal renal excretory capacity) (Kovács et al. 1984c, Anderson 1986).

The emphasis on the large capacity of the normal kidney to excrete solute-free water (see Fig. 8.1) is important, since still too often the cause of clinical hyponatremia is stated to be excessive intake of water. In relative terms, this statement must be true; however in absolute terms such an interpretation is an oversimplification. In fact in subjects with disturbed diluting capacity an intake of water not exceeding the usual daily needs of an age-matched healthy individual may result in excessive water retention in the organism, and in dilution of body fluids. It should be noted that the impairment of water excretion has not to be very severe. Supposing a patient with a daily solute intake of 400 mOsm/kg and a net water intake (intake minus insensible losses) of 2 l, the average U_{osm} will be 200 mOsm/kg to excrete this load and to remain in steady state. If the patient is unable to reduce U_{osm} below 222 mOsm/kg (a level still hypotonic to plasma), the solute load is excreted in only 1.800 ml water, and plasma sodium concentration will gradually fall. In this respect also the composition of ingested or given fluids is important. It is easy to appreciate that hyponatremia usually develops if fluids given to a patient with disturbed diluting capacity are hypotonic in relation to those that have been lost (Burrows et al. 1983, Chung et al. 1986).

Both AVP-dependent and AVP-independent mechanisms, and more often their various combinations, may contribute to disturbed renal diluting capacity in the course of various diseases (see Table 8.5). In fact, when vasopressin was specifically tested hypervasopressinism was found to be an essential variable in virtually all conditions associated with hyponatremia (Martinez-Maldonaldo 1980). The information concerning the causes of hypervasopressinism (chapter 19) was incorporated in the classification of clinical hyponatremia by Berl et al. (1976). According to their concept, hyponatremic states are distinguishable by different nonosmotic stimuli of AVP thought to be operative. Thus the hyponatremia of apparently "normovolemic" states could be separated from that of ECF volume depletion and from the hyponatremia of edematous states. Consequently, if "true" hypotonic hyponatremia has been diagnosed, the subsequent step should be clinical estimation of the volume status of the patient based on the patient's history, physical results (pulse rate, arterial pressure, skin turgor, sweating, ascites, edema, etc.), and laboratory tests (plasma sodium, glucose, urea and creatinine levels, and urine sodium levels). Such a diagnostic approach offers a rationale for the therapy of various forms of hyponatremia (see Fig. 20.1).

20.3.1 HYPOTONIC HYPONATREMIA ASSOCIATED WITH NORMAL BODY SODIUM ("NORMOVOLEMIC" HYPONATREMIA, SYNDROME OF INAPPROPRIATE SECRETION OF ANTIDIURETIC HORMONE, SIADH)

The true clinical significance of this problem has been clearly illustrated by recent reports undoubtedly worth of consideration that in just about 30 years of recognition (Schwartz et al. 1957), this syndrome has progressed from a rare occurrence to the commonest form of hyponatremia among hospitalized patients (Anderson 1986, Kovács et al. 1987b, d). Obviously the key to the genesis of this derangement is abnormal retention of water. SIADH will occur if an abudant hypotonic fluid supply exists and the kidney is under the influence of abnormally high levels of AVP. Because vasopressin is often elevated, albeit by a number of factors (chapter 19), in severely ill subjects the syndrome can be easily produced by regular intravenous administration or unchecked oral intake of hypotonic solutions ("isotonic" glucose infusion must be of special consideration. Although a 5 per cent solution of dextrose is roughly isotonic with plasma at the time of injection, the sugar is rapidly metabolized with a net effect of a plain water load.). Thus virtually all cases of acute SIADH in hospitalized patients are iatrogenic and may be characterized by the saying: "Nature did not know that we were going to invent the hollow needle and the intravenous fluids, thus it programmed AVP to be present in certain situations of stress" (Pestana 1977). This suggests, that SIADH is often preventable and it is to be hoped that acute hyponatremia of this kind will not occur in a good hospital, where fluid input, urinary output, body weight and plasma sodium concentration are more or less recorded. Chronic SIADH seen in patients with ectopic AVP secretion has apparently a different cause; why some patients with ectopic AVP release drink more water than seems appropriate to satiate thirst, is an interesting and still not resolved question.

20.3.1.1 Clinical features of SIADH

The main clinical features of the syndrome could have been predicted already on the basis of experiments designed to study the effects of exogenous AVP on normal individuals. Leaf et al. (1953) demonstrated that when pitressin was given to a normal person whose water intake had been restricted, no discernible effect ensued. If, on the other hand, fluid was not restricted, a reproducible series of events leading to water intoxication could be observed. These events (Table 20.1) are the cardinal features of "normovolemic" hyponatremia, and will be discussed.

Because of the hormone effect extra water is retained in the body with subsequent development of hypotonic hyponatremia. SIADH is usually associated with expansion of body water by 3—4 liters (as a rule of thumb, every liter of extra water lowers the plasma sodium by 3 mmol/l), but clinically apparent edema is usually absent. Since two thirds of body water and two

Table 20.1. Clinical criteria of syndrome of inappropriate secretion of antidiuretic hormone (SIADH)

1. Hyponatremia with corresponding hypoosmolality of the extracellular fluid.
2. Continued renal excretion of sodium, i.e. urine sodium typically matches intake.
3. Excretion of less than maximally diluted urine ($U_{osm} > 50$ mOsm/kg).
4. Hypouremia, hypouricemia, normal plasma creatinine value.
5. Weight gain.
6. Absence of other causes of decreased diluting ability (i.e. volume depletion and edematous disorders); normal renal and adrenal function
7. Improvement of hyponatremia and plasma hypoosmolality after water restriction.

thirds of any excess that may be retained reside within the cells, the interstitial fluid must expand by 4—5 l before edema becomes clinically manifest. Usually only an appreciable weight gain suggests that excess water has been retained. Nevertheless, some of the retained water (about 1/12th of its volume) remains in the intravascular compartment. Thus from a physiological perspective "normovolemic" hyponatremia is a modestly volume expanded state.

The other cardinal feature of the syndrome, natriuresis ($U_{Na} > 20$ mmol/l) cannot be attributed to hypervasopressinism per se since sodium excretion does not increase if fluid intake is restricted sufficiently to prevent weight gain. Rather, it reflects the attempt of the body to return ECF volume to normal; however, under the given conditions this is possible only by enhanced renal excretion of sodium (chapter 1.3.3). Acute expansion of the extracellular fluid volume causes sodium diuresis by increasing glomerular filtration rate and mainly by inhibiting tubular sodium reabsorption. In this setting humoral volume regulatory mechanisms probably play an important role in the development of natriuresis. The contribution of mineralocorticoids has not been fully elucidated: both low and high hormone levels have been reported (Martinez-Maldonaldo 1980). Many authors believe that sustained water retention may inhibit sodium reabsorption acting through the humoral natriuretic systems (the atrial natriuretic factor as well as the ouabain-like natriuretic hormone, see Table 1.2) (Lichardus 1978, Cogan et al., 1986, Wijdicks et al. 1987). It should be kept in mind that most patients with "normovolemic" hyponatremia soon reach a new steady state in which they no longer are in negative sodium balance, and urinary sodium excretion typically matches intake. Thus, despite hyponatremia, subjects on a usual salt diet have elevated sodium in urine. Confusion can arise, however, in an occasional patient with "normovolemic" hyponatremia who has little or no sodium in his urine. This issue can easily be resolved by increasing sodium intake. If sodium appears in urine, it can be assumed that its previous lack was due to a markedly restricted salt intake (Nolph and Schrier 1970).

The most common error in recognizing "normovolemic" hyponatremia is the failure to realize that urine osmolality needs only be inappropriately elevated (i.e. not maximally diluted, $U_{osm} > 50$—100 mOsm/kg) in the face of plasma hypoosmolality, and not necessarily greater than the corresponding plasma osmolality. Moreover, in chronic hyponatremia when a new steady state has been reached, urine becomes less concentrated though hypovasopressinism persists, and urinary water excretion matches water intake. This phenomenon is often referred to as renal "escape" from the antidiuretic action of vasopressin, and can only occur in the presence of positive water balance (Gross et al. 1983, Hall et al. 1986).

Hypouremia and hypouricemia as well as low plasma creatinine levels observed in these patients reflect the increased glomerular filtration rate and decreased net reabsorption of uric acid and urea that attends chronic volume expansion (Decaux et al. 1980, Schichiri et al. 1985). Although the retention of water lowers the plasma Na$^+$ concentration, it does not reduce either plasma bicarbonate or, in most cases, the plasma K$^+$ concentration (Martinez-Maldonaldo 1980).

20.3.1.2 Clinical patterns of vasopressin secretion in patients with SIADH

Zerbe et al. (1980) demonstrated four different patterns of AVP release in a group of patients with hyponatremia and presumed hypervasopressinism (Fig. 20.3). Type 1 pattern consists of large erratic oscillations of AVP secretion with apparently no relation to plasma osmolality; this pattern is most likely to result from intermittent secretion from an ectopic source or from rapid variation in a nonosmotic stimulus for neurohypophyseal vasopressin release. In type 2 pattern ("reset osmostat") changes in plasma vasopressin closely correlate with changes in plasma osmolality, the osmotic threshold however is set at abnormally low values of P_{osm}. A "reset" osmostat might occur, for example, if inhibitory afferent baroregulatory pathways are interrupted, resulting in false signals of intravascular volume depletion. In

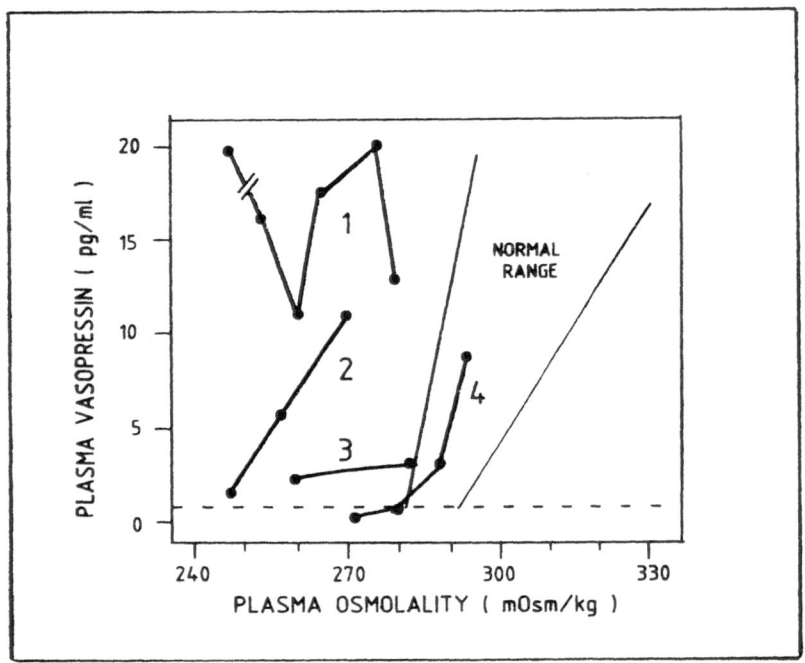

Fig. 20.3. The relationship between plasma AVP levels and plasma osmolality in patients with hypervasopressinism during osmotic challenge: (1) erratic release, (2) reset osmostat, (3) vasopressin leak, and (4) inappropriate antidiuresis with normally osmoregulated AVP (from Zerbe et al. 1980 with kind permission).

Table 20.2 Causes of the syndrome of inappropriate secretion of antidiuretic hormone (SIADH)

A. Increased hypothalamic production of vasopressin caused by nonosmotic secretory stimuli
Benign pulmonary diseases
— asthma
— pneumonia (viral, bacterial or fungal)
— lung abscess
— pneumothorax
— positive end-expiratory pressure (PEEP) ventilation
— acute respiratory failure
Neurological and neurosurgical conditions
— head trauma
— subarachnoid hemorrhage
— brain tumor (non-AVP producing)
— cerebral infarction
— brain abscess
— meningitis
— encephalitis
— Guillain-Barré syndrome
— acute intermittent porphyria
Postoperative patients
Psychiatric disorders
Endocrinopathies
— glucocorticoid deficiency
Preterm infants
— respiratory distress syndrome
— hypoxic-ischemic encephalopathy
— "late" hyponatremia

B. Ectopic (nonhypothalamic) production of vasopressin
— carcinoma (oat cell of lung, bronchogenic, duodenum, pancreas, thymus)
— Ewing's tumor
— Hodgkin's disease
Other sources
— tuberculous tissue (?)

C. Pharmacologic agents
Exogenous vasopressin, oxytocin or desmopressin
Potentiation of endogenous vasopressin secretion (carbamazepine, clofibrate, vincristine, cyclophosphamide, monoamine oxidase inhibitors, thioridazine, haloperidol, bromocriptine etc.)
Potentiation of vasopressin's tubular effect (chlorpropamide, carbamazepine)

---

these cases urine can be appropriately diluted after a water load and progressive hyponatremia does not occur. Type 3 pattern is characterized by slightly elevated plasma vasopressin at low levels of plasma osmolality, but when P_{osm} passes the normal threshold vasopressin concentrations start rising appropriately in response to further increase in tonicity. This nonsuppressible "leak" might be due to constant secretion of AVP from an ectopic source. Alternatively, it might be due to increased release of AVP at the median eminence in response to various stress stimuli; (chapter 11.1); this possibility, however has not been as yet specifically tested. Finally, there are few patients with decreased renal diluting ability but apparently normal increase and decrease in plasma vasopressin (type 4); in these cases the diluting effect is rather a consequence of increased renal sensitivity to the hormone, decreased generation of solute-free water or, alternatively, the production of some other antidiuretic factor may be considered (Smitz et al. 1985, Kern et al. 1986). It should be noted however that this classification has little, if any, clinical significance. In most clinical settings often more than one mechanism may be operative (Goldman et al. 1988) and thus the actual pattern found must not be indicative of the nature of the underlying disease process (Table 20.2).

20.3.1.3 Benign pulmonary diseases

A number of benign pulmonary processes have been reported to cause SIADH. Asthma is perhaps the best studied of them. During status asthmaticus AVP levels are high irrespective of the plasma osmolality, and AVP falls as the patient improves (Benfield et al. 1982, Rao et al. 1985). High levels of blood AVP associated with the clinical features of SIADH have been frequently reported in patients with bacterial and viral pneumonia (Rosenow et al. 1972, Nutman et al. 1981, Rivers et al. 1981, Kovács and Šoltés 1983), in a recent study the conventional criteria of the syndrome (Table 20.1) have been found in 45% of children admitted to hospital for pneumonia (Shann and Germer 1985).

Several nonosmotic stimuli may contribute to the development of hypervasopressinism in these pulmonary disorders. The most important of them seem to be hypoxia and hypercapnic acidosis, stress as well as regional hemodynamic abnormalities due to raised resistance to the blood flow through the lungs which results in decreased left atrial filling. Concomitant cardiac failure is frequently present in patients with severe lung disease and can, by hemodynamic mechanisms, induce AVP release. Also the central hemodynamic effects plus the associated increase in intracranial pressure are the major factors underlying nonosmotic AVP secretion during PEEP ventilation (Bar et al. 1980). Another hypothesis that has been advanced is that infected lung tissue may ectopically produce and liberate AVP in a fashion similar to that occurring in bronchogenic carcinoma. This frequently cited assumption however rests on a single report by Vorherr et al. (1970) who found bioassayable AVP in tuberculous lung tissue in a patient with hyponatremia.

20.3.1.4 Neurologic and neurosurgical conditions

SIADH has been described in association with various neurologic disorders. Although the danger of fluid overload in subjects with bacterial meningitis is well appreciated (Kaplan and Feigin 1978), "normovolemic" hyponatremia is still a frequent finding in patients with meningitis. The presence and duration of hyponatremia in meningitis appear to have a prognostic value: hyponatremia of long duration has been associated with neurologic abnormalities at three months follow up and with delayed development at one year (Shann and Germer 1985). A multitude of other neurologic conditions also occur with "normovolemic" hyponatremia, including acute intermittent porphyria, cerebrovascular disease, etc. (Lester and Nelson 1981). SIADH may occur with much greater frequency in neurosurgical patients than is generally appreciated. Clinical criteria of "normovolemic" hyponatremia have been found in nearly 10 per cent of 290 patients admitted because of subarachnoid hemorrhage, and almost in 5 per cent of 1808 patients treated for craniocerebral injuries (Dóczi et al. 1981, 1982).

Often it has been speculated that hypervasopressinism in these cases has a common etiology in increased intracranial pressure (chapter 5.4.7). However, other factors such as altered perfusion of the neurohypophysis or other brain areas, blood redistribution and relative central hypovolemia in patients confined to bed over long time (Segar and Moore 1969) and/or nonspecific stress, may likely contribute to its development as well.

"Cerebral salt wasting" due to a postulated cerebral natriuretic hormone might also play a contributory role, in some cases at least (Wijdicks et al. 1987). However, in a overwhelming majority of patients hypervasopressinism and excessive administration of hypotonic solutions can sufficiently explain hyponatremia and natriuresis (Bouzarth and Shenkin 1982).

A special group includes subjects with pituitary stalk disruption by trauma or surgery. These subjects may, after a delay to the primary insult, develop transient hypervasopressinism ("triphasic response" in Fig. 17.1) due to hormone release from in situ degenerating pituitary (Cusic et al. 1984).

20.3.1.5 Postoperative states

For long, postoperative conditions have been known to be characterized by avid renal sodium and water retention. This experience has dictated the principle of "keep the patient on the dry side". Nevertheless, "normovolemic" hyponatremia remains a frequent surgical problem sometimes seen preoperatively, and very frequently iatrogenically induced during the postoperative interval. A minimal estimate of the frequency of postoperative hyponatremia has been 4.4 per cent (Chung et al. 1986), but also much higher frequencies have been reported (20—50%) (Thomas and Morgan 1979, Burrows et al.

1983). In these studies, when the daily postoperative requirements for electrolytes were given in either an isotonic or hypotonic solution, hyponatremia occurred only in patients receiving hypotonic fluids.

Biossay and radioimmunoassay have shown high plasma AVP concentrations following anesthesia and surgery indicating that nonosmotic release of AVP was responsible for the enhanced renal water retention in these cases (Thomas and Morgan 1979, Chung et al. 1986). A number of factors contribute to the intraoperative and postoperative AVP release. Anesthesia lowers the threshold for AVP release by blocking the sympathetic reflexes, and it also seems to increase urine osmolality. Intubation and positive pressure breathing either during or after the surgery results in AVP release secondary to decreased intrathoracic blood flow. Finally, nonspecific stress and postoperative pain may also be significant stimuli for excessive AVP release.

20.3.1.6 Psychiatric disorders

Up to one third of chronically psychotic patients develop polydipsia and secondary polyuria (chapter 17.4) in 5 to 15 years from the onset of the psychotic symptoms (Vieweg et al. 1987). These patients usually have mild asymptomatic hyponatremia (Barlow and deWardener 1959, Cronin 1987) due to an associated abnormality in renal water excretion. Because of the apparently lower osmotic threshold for AVP secretion (reset osmostat) and the enhanced effect of vasopressin on urinary concentration such patients should be unable to have maximal water diuresis until plasma osmolality and plasma sodium levels drop to mildly abnormal values (Goldman et al. 1988).

However these abnormalities in vasopressin secretion and action are not sufficient to explain the patient's episodes of more severe hyponatremia and hypoosmolality, which is a frequent source of morbidity and mortality in chronic psychiatric disorders. Such episodes, characterized by diverse neurologic signs ranging from ataxia to irreversible coma might be associated with transiently aggravated defects in secretion and/or renal action of AVP, that sometimes coincide with exacerbation of psychosis (Rashkind et al. 1975, Singh et al. 1985). Alternatively, severe hyponatremia may develop in psychotic patients who ingest rapidly huge amounts of water from the tap or the shower, that acutely overwhelm the normal renal excreting capacity (Kovács et al. 1984c, Vieweg et al. 1985).

20.3.1.7 Endocrine disorders

In the original description of the syndrome of "inappropriate" secretion of AVP (Schwartz et al. 1957) normal adrenal function was one criterium for the diagnosis (see Table 20.1). However, AVP plays a role in the hyponatremia associated with adrenal cortical, anterior pituitary and thyroid insufficiency and low sodium plasma levels seen with this disorders may be regarded as special forms of the syndrome.

Glucocorticoid deficiency impairs renal water excretion, and it is now clear that both AVP-dependent and AVP-independent pathways are involved. Glucocorticoid deficiency has a deleterious effect on the cardiac function as reflected in a reduced stroke volume and cardiac output. The disordered cardiac function in turn stimulates release of vasopressin, probably by a baroreceptor-mediated pathway (Ishikawa and Schrier 1982). Now it has also become well known that if the anterior and the posterior lobe of the pituitary are both destroyed the manifestations of diabetes insipidus may be abolished; polyuria only occurs after ACTH or cortisol administration (Jamison 1983). Linas and coworkers (1980) found that rats with intact pituitary glands had an impaired ability to excrete water and to dilute urine after one day of glucocorticoid deficiency. Two weeks without glucocorticoid produced considerably more impairment. In glucocorticoid deficient Brattleboro rats excretion of an acute water load was normal after one day, but was reduced after two weeks of glucocorticoid depletion, as was urinary diluting ability. It was proposed that the AVP-independent pathway by which urinary dilution was impaired, was secondary to reduced cardiac output which decreased renal blood flow and GFR, and increased proximal sodium reabsorption.

Hyponatremia in the course of severe hypothyreoidism has been interpreted to represent a specific form of SIADH (Skowsky and Kikuchi 1978). This interpretation, however, has been challenged by the observation that severe hypothyroidism is accompanied by a decreased GFR (in SIADH, GFR is normal or elevated), decreased cardiac output and decreased effective circulating blood volume (Robinson 1985). Careful studies have also demonstrated that the decrease in free water clearance in these patients was directly related to urine volume and was therefore consistent with an effect due to decreased distal delivery of tubular fluid (DeRubertis et al. 1971).

20.3.1.8 Preterm infants

Sick preterm very low birthweight infants undergoing intensive care are at high risk of disturbances of water homeostasis (chapter 15.3). Nonosmotically stimulated AVP release associated with intracranial hemorrhage, hypoxic-ischemic encephalopathy, pneumothorax, atelectasis or acute deterioration of respiratory function during respiratory distress syndrome (hyaline membrane disease) is the most frequent, thought often unrecognized cause of hyponatremia in the first week of life (Paxson et al. 1977, Rees et al. 1984, Wiriyathian et al. 1986). However, when an event known to cause inappropriate release of arginine vasopressin is identified it should be possible to prevent body water accumulation by checking its effectiveness with regular weighing and repeated plasma sodium measurements and, when appropriate, by restricting the volume of the fluid administered.

It has been reported that also healthy preterm infants, when fed on pooled human milk or conventional "humanized" infant formulas, frequently become hyponatremic during the second-third week of life, while more mature newborns have no difficulty maintaining normal electrolyte values on the same diet (Sulyok et al. 1971, Roy et al. 1976). Although the long term clinical importance of this "late" hyponatremia is not clear, it is unlikely to be beneficial; its causes are therefore important subjects of further investigation.

Several groups have shown that in the first week of life urinary sodium excretion and, in particular, fractional sodium excretion is elevated and inversely proportional to the gestational and postconceptional age of the neonate (Sulyok et al. 1980, Al-Dahhan et al. 1983, Lichardus et al. 1986). The causes of the decreased renal tubular sodium reabsorption in preterm infants during the first week of life may be complex. It may be a physiological measure (i.e. volume-mediated natriuresis) resulting from the initially expanded extracellular fluid volume in preterm infants (Fig. 20.4.) or it may develop due to the inability of the immature kidney to maintain volume homeostasis by retaining sodium. In an attempt to elaborate this point several hormonal studies have been undertaken. The results obtained are schematically summarized in Fig. 20.5 (solid lines). As seen, the postnatal natriuresis in preterm infants appears to be promoted by both the atrial natriuretic factor and the natriuretic hormone (circulating inhibitor of Na^+, K^+-ATPase, considered to be expressed by endogenous digoxin-like immunoreactivity, EDLI). With advancing ECF volume contraction the activities of both natriuretic systems decrease. Simultaneously, the activities of the two major volume-conserving systems — the renin-angiotensin-aldosterone and the vasopressin systems — begin rising and after a few weeks they even predominate in the attempt to

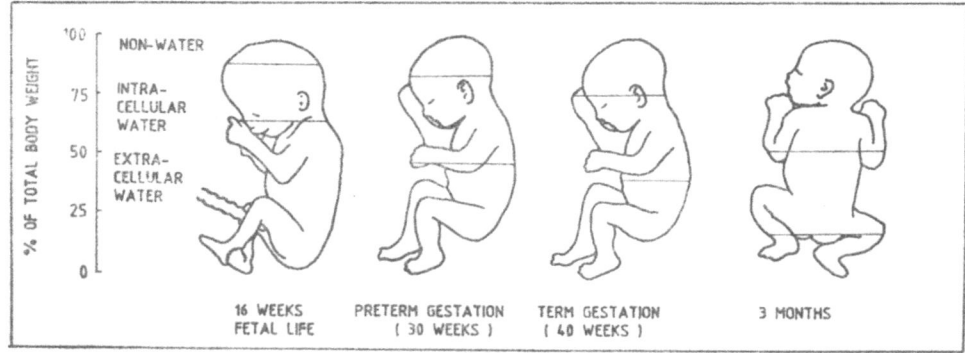

Fig. 20.4. Relative composition of body fluid compartments during transition from fetal to extrauterine life (data withdrawn from Friis—Hansen 1983).

prevent excessive volume losses (Sulyok et al. 1985, Tulassay et al. 1986, Kovács et al. 1987).

As a matter of fact, these humoral alterations seem to be identical with those which could be expected to occur in volume contracted states due to exaggerated renal sodium loss (see Fig. 1.3). Indeed, the late hyponatremia of preterm infants can be avoided and the secondary hormonal changes can be inversed by increasing the sodium intake to 4 to 5 mmol/kg/day from the 4th to the 14th postnatal day (see Fig. 20.5 broken lines). However, when sodium supplementation has been provided it caused a significant elevation in plasma ANP concentration and urinary EDLI excretion as well as in urinary sodium excretion (Sulyok et al. 1981, Tulassay et al. 1987, Kovács et al. 1988). Extracellular fluid volume was not determined in these studies, but one can speculate that these changes would occur as a consequence of expansion of ECF volume by this extra sodium.

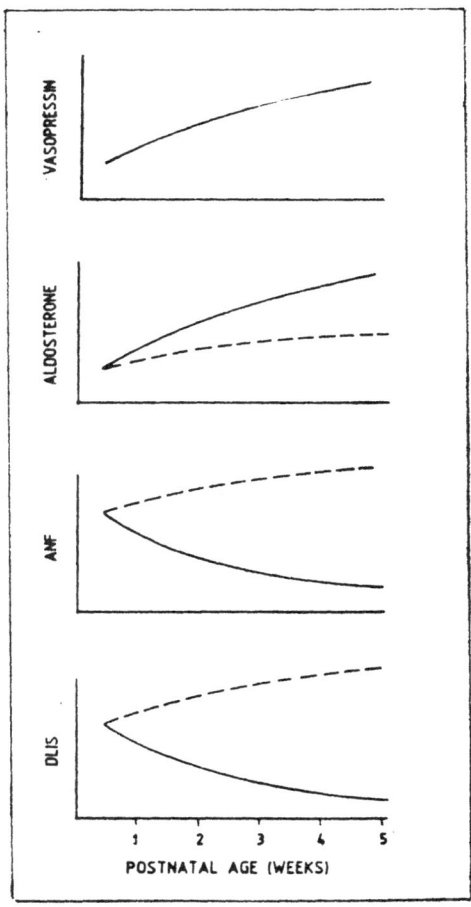

Fig. 20.5. Schematic summary of the changes in the activity of the major volume-regulatory systems in preterm infants fed donor milk (solid lines) or sodium supplemented infant formulas (broken lines) during first weeks of life (data from Sulyok et al. 1979, Kovács and Sulyok 1984, Tulassay et al. 1986, and Kovács et al. 1988) (ANF — atrial natriuretic factor, DLIS — digoxin-like immunoreactive substance)

231

Taken together, sodium diuresis and negative sodium balance seem to be self limiting physiological events which should not be taken on their own as a signal to increase sodium intake. It appears therefore that premature delivery is associated with a specific form of SIADH, in which the activity of volume retaining systems is stimulated by physiological contraction of the ECF volume. This view is further substantiated by findings suggesting that plasma sodium concentration in premature infants may be maintained in normal limits even with substantially lower fluid intake, provided the water is restricted more than sodium (Lorenz et al. 1982, Coulthard and Ney 1985).

The sodium concentration of "mature" donor milk and conventional "humanized" infant formulas is too low to match the composition of urinary losses. This factor may gain clinical importance and lead to water retention and hyponatremia at the time, when vasopressin secretion is stimulated by advancing physiological postnatal ECF volume contraction. In this respect, it is of interest how "nature" solved this enigma. It is well established that milk from mothers who have given birth to preterm infants has a higher sodium content than "mature" human milk (see Fig. 15.3), but lower than in sodium supplemented formulas. The cause of these differences is not known, but teleological considerations may suggest that the composition of the mother's milk is an important homeostatic variable that supports survival and normal development of infants even after preterm delivery. Indeed, during the first few weeks after delivery, the milk of the mother appears to meet the nutritional needs of the preterm infant better than "mature" donor's milk (Atkinson et al. 1983, Chessex et al. 1983). In order to prevent late hyponatremia preterm infants born before 34 weeks' gestation should therefore be fed their own mother's milk or formulas closely resembling its composition (Kovács et al. 1985, Lichardus et al. 1986).

20.3.1.9 Ectopic tumor production of AVP

Evidence reported by Odell and others (1977) has suggested that the intracellular production of polypeptide hormones which may be detected by radioimmunoassay may be a ubiquitous characteristic of malignant transformation. Ectopic production of vasopressin and ACTH in malignant tumors is well documented and usually occurs in relation to oat cell carcinoma of the lung although an association with several other malignant tumors has also been reported (Hansen et al. 1980, Osterman et al. 1986) (see Table 20.2). After a standard water load test abnormal AVP secretion, as defined by inappropriately elevated AVP levels relative to plasma osmolality, was detected in 40—70% of patients with oat cell carcinoma of the lung (Miller and Moses 1972, Odell et al. 1977, Hoeflinger et al. 1977). An observation worth comment and further investigation is that some of these subjects do continue drinking despite normovolemia which contributes to the development of hyponatremia. However it is necessary to bear in mind that many of these patients are severely ill with associated anorexia and decreased fluid consumption, thus preventing obvious signs of SIADH from becoming evident. In this circumstance, basal plasma osmolality may be entirely normal or even elevated although AVP secretion is excessive and after a standard water load severe hyponatremia may develop.

20.3.1.10 Drugs

Antidiuretic analogs of vasopressin, like dDAVP, obviously should also be included in the list of causes of impaired renal water excretion, althought only few cases of induced hyponatremia have been reported with this analog (Koskimes et al. 1984). In contrast, induced hyponatremia is a frequent complication in patients receiving oxytocin infusions for induction of labor in combination with prolonged administration of large volumes of hypotonic fluids. Transplacental hyponatremia associated with convulsions, increased risk of neonatal jaundice and transient tachypnoe has also been reported in infants of oxytocin-induced mothers (Singhi and Chookang 1984).

"Normovolemic" hyponatremia has been reported in association with drugs that stimulate endogenous release of AVP or produce AVP-like antidiuresis by potentiating the tubular effect of AVP (for example clofibrate and chlorpropamide respectively). The antineoplastic agents vincristine and cyclophosphamide stimulate AVP release by an unknown mechanism. The water retaining properties of vincristine and cyclophosphamide are particularly important as patients receiving these drugs may be encouraged to drink large volumes of water to prevent uric acid deposition and/or drug-related cystitis. This combination of enhanced AVP release and large water volumes can lead to severe, occasionally fatal, hyponatremia within 24 hours. This complication can be minimized by using isotonic saline instead of water (or 5 per cent glucose) to maintain a high urine output (Čáp et al. 1975, Lightwood and Smith 1984).

20.3.2 HYPOTONIC HYPONATREMIA ASSOCIATED WITH REDUCED BODY SODIUM (HYPOVOLEMIC HYPONATREMIA)

It should be emphasized that there are virtually no hypertonic fluids that can be lost from the body: the losses are generally isotonic or hypotonic. Consequently, hypovolemic hyponatremia in fact cannot occur as a primary condition (e.g. due to increased sodium losses). As a rule, the condition develops first as isotonic (more rarely hypertonic) hypovolemia, and turns hypotonic only because of replacement at a later stage with fluids which are hypotonic related to the losses. This pattern then is a sequential one: isotonic (more rarely hypertonic) ECF volume depletion first, and hypotonicity from partial replacement of sodium and water later (Pestana 1977).

Absolute extracellular fluid volume contraction may occur due to external losses via extrarenal or renal routes, by the intracorporeal rapid accumulation of fluid pools ("third space effect") or due to inadequate input of sodium. The clinical manifestations include weight loss, alterations of skin turgor, flat neck veins, tachycardia, orthostatic hypotension, oliguria, and "prerenal" azotemia (unless the production of urea is reduced). Acutely BUN will rise rapidly, whereas plasma creatinine will increase in this setting only when the degree of hypovolemia is severe enough to lower GFR. Extracellular fluid volume depletion in turn activates various volume (sodium) regulatory systems (see Fig. 1.3) including certain changes in renal hemodynamics. Thanks to these changes upon extrarenal sodium losses the kidneys can effectively retain sodium and excrete urine with typically low concentrations of sodium and chlorides (< 20 mmol/l). An exception to this rule are conditions associated with metabolic alkalosis; here, a large tubular supply of bicarbonates obligates the excretion of sodium, and hence it is only low chloride concentration in urine that suggests a deficiency in the circulating volume ($U_{Cl} < 20$ mmol/l). Certainly if hypovolemia is secondary to renal sodium losses in the first place, the urinary concentrations of sodium and chlorides will usually be higher than 20 mmol/l. Another special condition concerns proximal (type II) renal tubular acidosis; a more vivid resorption of chlorides as compared to bicarbonates (and sodium) frequently results in a dissociation of urinary levels of these parameters ($U_{Na} > 20$ mmol/l, $U_{Cl} < 20$ mmol/l) (Goldberg 1981).

The contraction of extracellular fluid volume simultaneously triggers another series of events which eventually result in the second set of alterations, i.e. changes in tonicity. Volume depletion can impair free-water clearance (C_{H_2O}) by both AVP-independent and AVP-dependent mechanisms (deFronzo and Thier 1980, Kovács et al. 1984a). First, the combination of a fall in GFR and an increase in proximal tubular sodium and water reabsorption, both induced by volume depletion, reduces the delivery of water to the diluting segments, thereby limiting the amount of free water that can be generated (see Fig. 8.8). Second, hypovolemia acting via left atrial, carotid and aortic baroreceptors, causes hypervasopressinism by lowering the threshold of the osmoregulatory system. Sustained AVP release has generally been considered a mechanism by which the body attempts maintaining the circulating volume via enhanced renal retention of water, even at the expense of tonicity. Unfortunately, "the sacrifice" of tonicity aimed at keeping the volume is not as effective as nature might have intended. Extra volume is required to replenish the deficiency of extracellular fluid; nevertheless, only one third of the retained water remains in this space and even less, some 1/12th, is distributed in the intravascular compartment. So, although this effort is very successfull in wrecking the tonicity, it does little alleviate the extracellular fluid deficit. Considerable ECF volume depletion continues to exist, while the cells are unnecessarily swollen with extra water. It may be therefore interesting to speculate about other functions potentially served by this hypervasopressinism. It is now well established that endogenous AVP, by virtue of its vasoconstrictor properties, increases total peripheral resistance, and thus plays a role in the maintenance of arterial pressure in hypotensive situations such as volume depleted states (chapter 9.4.1).

Volume depleted subjects are usually thirsty, probably because there is a parallel downward resetting of thresholds of vasopressin release and thirst (see Fig. 5.6, panel 3). If these subjects are allowed to ingest free water, they can "drink themselves" to slight hyponatremia. A serious hyponatremia however develops only if there are severe or sustained sodium losses which causing severe volume depletion reset the thresholds both for AVP and thirst to very low levels of plasma osmolality (as observed e.g. in children with serious gastroenteritis or in certain patients on diuretic therapy) or, more often, if patients receive nondipsogenic water (Gruskin et al. 1982, Ayus 1986).

20.3.2.1 Extrarenal losses

The extrarenal causes of extracellular fluid volume depletion include gastrointestinal losses and losses into a "third space" (e.g. burns, peritonitis, pancreatitis or traumatized muscle). The most common cause of hypovolemic hyponatremia in this setting is the loss of gastrointestinal fluids as a result of diarrhea. The clinical picture is dominated by symptoms of extracellular volume deficit; neurological signs of hyponatremia (chapter 20.2) are usually manifested at very low plasma sodium levels only (Gruskin et al. 1982). The seriousness of this problem, particularly in developing countries, is illustrated by a recent report which has documented a significantly higher incidence (20.8 versus 6.4 per cent) and tenfold case fatality rates of hypovolemic hyponatremia as compared with hypovolemic hypernatremia in malnourished children hospitalized for acute diarrhea (Samadi et al. 1983).

Volume loss with hypotonicity can be also produced by excessive sweating. Normally sweat contains less than 60 mmol/l of sodium (Quinton 1987). Pure sweat loss therefore is more likely to produce hypertonicity than hypotonicity. However, massive sweat loss with massive solute-free water ingestion can produce the opposite problem. The development of this form of hyponatremia which can occur upon significant physical exercise (for example approximately 30% of participants of the Hawaiian Ironman Triathlon World Championship have been reported to develop various degrees of hyponatremia) can be prevented by giving the individuals drink, during the exercise, hypotonic electrolyte solutions (see Table 14.1) instead of pure water (Hiller et al. 1986).

20.3.2.2 Diuretic treatment

Hyponatremia is a relatively common complication of diuretic therapy with either loop diuretics (furosemide, ethacrynic acid) or thiazides. Three mechanisms contribute to this tendency toward hyponatremia: 1. ECF volume depletion with its consequences as discussed above, 2. direct inhibition of NaCl reabsorption at the distal diluting sites of the nephron (by loop diuretics), and 3. potassium depletion. In patients in whom potassium depletion is of primary importance, the administration of KCl alone may be sufficient to raise the plasma sodium concentration toward normal (Fichman et al. 1971, Abramow and Cogan 1984).

Diuretics-induced hyponatremia usually begins within the first two weeks of therapy when urinary losses are maximal. After this time a new steady state is established: the ensuing activation of the sodium retaining mechanisms prevents further volume losses and thus limits the degree of hyponatremia. In edematous disorders both diuretics and the basic disease (which further reduce the effective circulating volume) contribute to the decrement in plasma sodium.

Generally, the degree of the diuretics-induced hyponatremia is modest, patients are asymptomatic, and plasma sodium levels normalize upon discontinuing the drug. Many subjects may have retained sufficient water to obscure the obvious physical finding of volume depletion, but seem to have an unusual sensitivity to volume stimuli for AVP release. Severe symptomatic hyponatremia, though not very frequent, constitutes however a medical emergency; when untreated the morbidity and mortality rates exceed 40%. The critical question is still why severe symptomatic hyponatremia develops only in a subgroup of elderly subjects (mainly in elderly women) receiving thiazides, despite the widespread use of saluretic agents. It is likely that an associated condition or illness potentiates the effect of the diuretic at one or another level of renal water handling (Ashouri 1986).

20.3.2.3 Renal disease

Hypovolemic hyponatremia in patients with renal disease (such as medullary cystic disease, polycystic disease, chronic interstitial nephritis, Bartter's syndrome, Fanconi syndrome or renal tubular acidosis) usually results from the inability of the renal tubule to conserve sodium. It is the sustained loss of sodium combined with the continued ingestion or infusion of hypotonic solutions which results in the generation of hyponatremia in renal patients.

236

20.3.2.4 Chronic mild sodium restriction

Prolonged reduced input of sodium may result in development of hyponatremia if water intake is not restricted. One example of a diminished oral solute input is that which occurred in healthy infants less than 6 months of age who were fed large quantities of solute-free fluids (either dilute milk, sugar water or plain water). Hypervasopressinism in this setting of feeding mismanagement may be an adaptive response to chronic ECF volume contraction. In addition the diminished solute load also impairs the infant's ability to excrete free water (e.g. in small infants receiving exclusively plain water the renal solute load derived solely from endogenous sources approximates 5 mOsm/kg/day) (Oh 1988). Supposing 5 kg of body weight the child would be able to produce not more than 500 ml of urine at minimal Uosm of 50 mOsm/kg. Because the fluid intake in such a child is usually more than 100 ml/kg, this extra water may be retained in the body, and cause hyponatremia. As the sodium depletion develops on chronic basis and the child may have retained sufficient water, there may be a striking absence of abnormalities other than signs from the nervous system on clinical examination. While the fully developed syndrome of hyponatremia and seizures occurs infrequently, mild cases manifested by irritability and lethargy may occur commonly (David et al. 1981, Borowitz and Rocco 1986).

Another example is seen in elderly patients who subsist on a tea-and-toast diet with very low solute loads. Because of a low solute load, these subjects may be unable to excrete ordinary amounts of water fast enough to avoid hyponatremia, in particular when they have additional slight intrinsic impairment of their diluting capacity.

20.3.3 HYPOTONIC HYPONATREMIA ASSOCIATED WITH INCREASED BODY SODIUM (HYPERVOLEMIC HYPONATREMIA)

Congestive heart failure, hepatic cirrhosis and the nephrotic syndrome represent conditions of effective circulating volume depletion even though the total ECF volume is markedly expanded. The body's response to the diminished effective circulating volume is essentially the same as it is to true volume depletion (see Fig. 1.3). Increased renal retention of sodium and water may be due both to a hypovolemia induced fall in GFR and, more importantly, an increase in tubular reabsorption of sodium and water. Thus, the urine sodium concentration usually is less than 10 mmol/l in these conditions.

Fluid retention in edematous states is usually isoosmotic. However, when sodium intake is restricted, but water intake is not, or only to a lesser degree, the avid water retention may lead to the development of hyponatremia.

As a rule, these patients have chronic mild hypotonicity and are not symptomatic from the hypotonicity unless they are iatrogenically water overloaded. In this later situation they may exhibit the syndrome of acute water intoxication.

Decreased intrarenal fluid delivery to loops of Henle as well as nonosmotically stimulated AVP release contribute to the disturbed renal diluting capacity and subsequent water-retaining tendency in edematous states (Schrier and Berl 1981). A major importance of hemodynamic alterations in the development of hypervasopressinism can be exemplified by analyses of plasma norepinephrine (NE) and plasma renin activity (PRA) and renal function in hyponatremic edematous patients. In a number of studies, it has been possible to grade into functional classes of impaired water metabolism which were then successfully correlated with corresponding abnormalities of NE, PRA, AVP as well as with the severity of the underlying disorder (Levine et al. 1982, Nicholls et al. 1986). Another mechanism, contributing to the enhanced retention of fluid by the kidney in edematous states is related to the inability to excrete the sodium and water that have been ingested; this most often occurs in patients with advanced acute or chronic renal failure.

It should be noted that the two mechanisms of renal sodium (and water) retention — the response to effective circulating volume depletion (i.e. "under-filling" of the vascular bed) and the primary renal dysfunction (i.e. fluid "over-flow") — are not mutually exclusive. This appears to be particularly true in hepatic cirrhosis. In some patients with this disorder, fluid accumulation in the dilated splanchnic venous system and in the peritoneum results in effective circulating volume depletion. However, cirrhosis may also directly promote sodium and water reabsorption independent of changes in volume (Better and Schrier 1983) (chapter 20.3.4.2).

20.3.3.1 Congestive heart failure (CHF)

Water is often retained in excess of sodium in severe congestive heart failure (Fig. 20.6) and therefore hyponatremia is frequently observed (Levine et al. 1982). Evidence in favor of the intrarenal mechanisms of impaired water excretion in cardiac failure has been provided by studies involving the administration of mannitol or the loop diuretic furosemide to patients with cardiac failure and hyponatremia; the administration of either of these agents has been found to convert the cardiac patient's hypertonic urine to a dilute urine (Schrier et al. 1973).

In addition, basal plasma arginine-vasopressin levels are often increased in patients with congestive heart failure with clinically stable condition. Szatalo-wicz et al. (1981), in a study of hospitalized patients with CHF, found that AVP levels, although not increased in absolute terms, were still inappropriate for the serum sodium concentration in 30 out of 37 patients with hyponatremia.

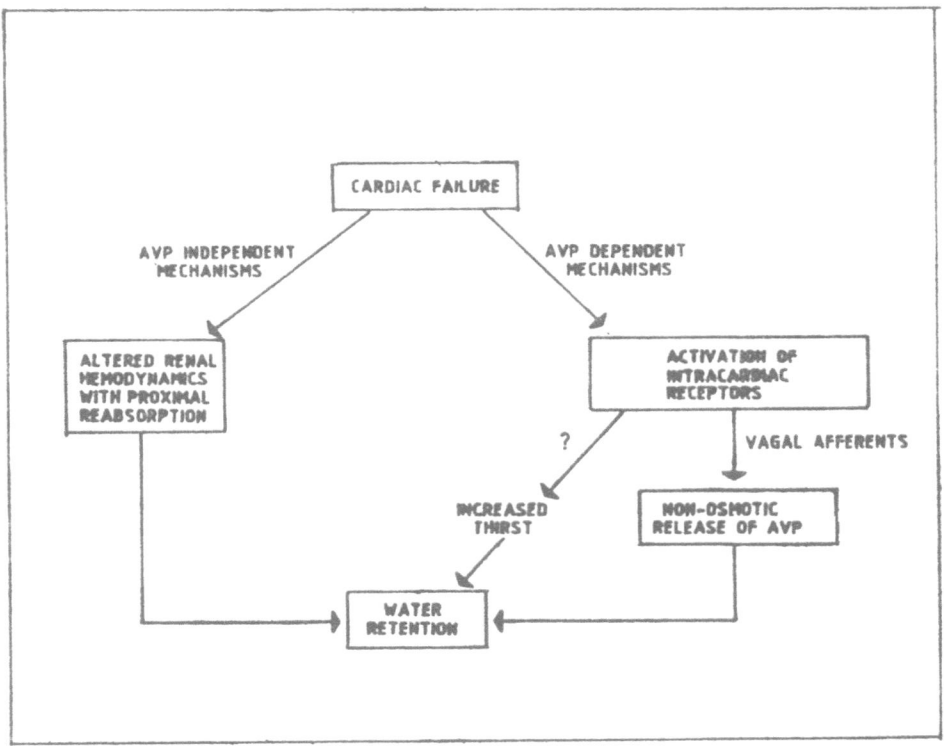

Fig. 20.6. Factors involved in disturbed water excretion in congestive heart failure.

Patients with detectable AVP had higher levels of blood urea nitrogen (BUN) and serum creatinine than those with undetectable levels of AVP. The presence of prerenal azotemia provided evidence for an intrarenal component of the impaired water excretion, but also suggested that lower cardiac outputs mediated the nonosmotic stimulation of vasopressin release. Administration of water load suppressed AVP secretion, however only in the presence of abnormally low values of P_{osm}, suggesting a "reset osmostat" in the genesis of hypovasopressinism in these patients. Subsequently it was demonstrated that enhancement of central blood volume hemodynamics as achieved by non-hypotensive afterload reduction suppressed plasma AVP and improved free-water clearance in hyponatremic cardiac failure (Bichet et al. 1986, Goldsmith et al. 1983, 1986).

Another important aspect relates to the hemodynamic significance of hypervasopressinism in CHF. Although the stimulated sympathetic nervous system, the renin-angiotensin system and the vasopressin system in CHF are probably under different control mechanisms, in this specific condition they facilitate each other's biologic activities and share the common properties

239

of vasoconstriction and antidiuresis. This suggests that they orchestrate a major defense system against inadequate perfusion from many causes, including inadequate cardiac output. The critical still unanswered question is whether these systems act to "overcompensate" in CHF resulting in circulatory congestion and heightened vascular impedance on a myocardium that is already operating under an imposed afterload stress. This may be the case since inhibition of norepinephrine release by bromocriptine and interruption of the renin-angiotensin system by converting enzyme blockade acutely improve the hemodynamic status of patients with CHF (Dzau 1987).

Recently it has been also shown that in relatively low plasma concentrations which are characteristic of clinical hyponatremia also vasopressin is capable of influencing hemodynamics in patients with CHF by further increasing the resistance to ejection of blood, reducing cardiac output, and thus leading to a condition in which cardiac output is lower and systemic vascular resistance is higher than optimal for the patient (Goldsmith et al. 1986). Although the available data concerning the effect of selective vasopressin antagonists are far from being conclusive (Nicod et al. 1985), with the renin-angiotensin system and converting enzyme inhibition as a precedent the therapy targeted at AVP-mediated vasoconstriction by selective V1 antagonists might prove to be another step in the rational design of specific vasodilator therapy for some patients with this disease.

20.3.3.2 Cirrhosis of the liver

Hyponatremia, the expression of the impaired capacity to excrete water, is a clinical problem commonly encountered in cirrhotic patients. Pronounced sodium and water retention is more characteristic for decompensated patients (i.e. those with ascites and/or edema), while cirrhotic patients without ascites or edema excrete water normally (Epstein 1985). The potentional mechanisms responsible for this defect in water excretion are probably similar to those present in cardiac failure. Numerous abnormalities encountered in cirrhosis could contribute to a diminished effective circulating blood volume in these patients, which in turn would stimulate the renal retention of salt and water in an effort to restore ECBV to normal (Table 20.3). Although this classic "underfilling" theory of sodium and water retention in cirrhosis has been challenged by observations proposing an alternative "overflow" hypothesis (see Table 20.3) it may be that "overflow" is primary early in the disease and that "underfilling" becomes more important with the development of severe hepatic cirrhosis (Better and Schrier 1983).

The results of recent studies have provided strong support for the traditional view that effective circulating blood volume in cirrhosis with ascites is contracted rather than expanded. These data have demonstrated a close correlation between high plasma norepinephrine levels, vasopressin and the capacity to excrete a water load. Patients, on the basis of their ability to excrete a standard water load could be subdivided into two groups. Patients excreting less than 80 % of the water load over a 5 hours period ("nonexcretors") had more pronounced ascites and hypoalbuminemia and exhibited significantly higher minimal urinary osmolality and lower plasma sodium levels as compared to patients excreting more than 80% of the water load over the same period ("excretors"). In addition, maneuvers that tend to increase effective blood volume — such as water immersion up to the neck or intravenous infusion of albumin, mannitol or ascitic fluid — were associated with a diminution in plasma renin activity, norepinephrine and vasopressin levels and also with an increase in the percentage of water load excreted. Thus, these maneuvers may overcome the circulatory disturbance without improving the function of the cirrhotic liver (Bichet et al. 1986, Nicholls et al. 1986).

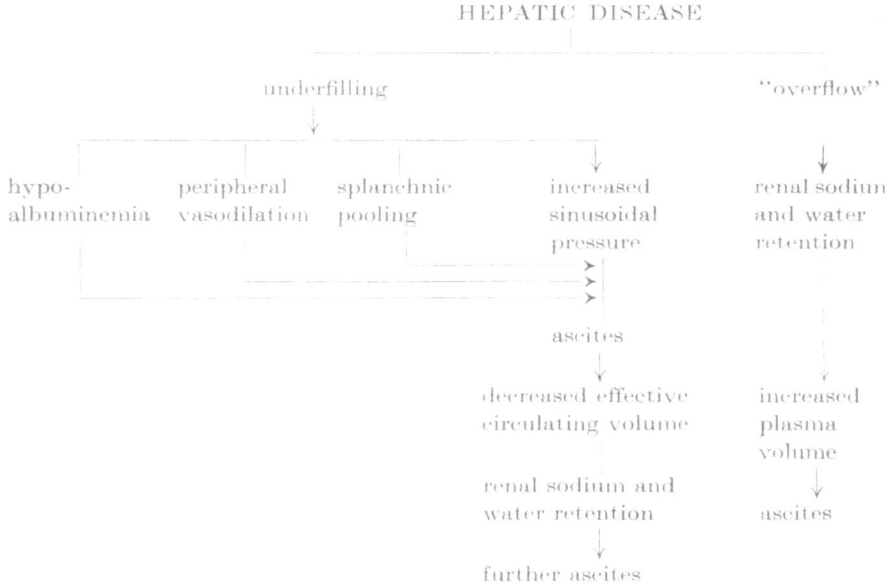

Table 20.3. Schematic illustration of main features of "underfilling" and "overflow" theories of the pathogenesis of fluid retention and ascites in hepatic disease. In some patients, both mechanisms may be operative.

20.3.3.3 Nephrotic syndrome

Patients with nephrotic syndrome are often oliguric with a low urinary concentration of sodium. This oliguric state is commonly attributed to an increase in tubular reabsorption of sodium. But hyponatremia and plasma hypoosmolality are also typical features of nephrotic syndrome (Usberti et al.

1984, Kovács et al. 1988a) suggesting that in this condition water is reabsorbed more avidly than sodium. (Because of the high serum lipid levels in many patients with the nephrotic syndrome, direct measurement of plasma osmolality is necessary to exclude pseudohyponatremia — chapter 20.1.1.)

Both "underfilling" and "overflow" may contribute to the increased sodium and water retention and to the development of edema in the nephrotic syndrome. The nephrotic syndrome can be produced by a variety of renal disorders and is characterized by an increase in the permeability of the glomerular capillary wall to proteins. Consequently, more albumin and globulins are filtered and then lost in the urine resulting in hypoalbuminemia. Hypoalbuminemia favors the movement of fluid out of the vascular space into the interstitium leading to effective volume depletion ("underfilling") and water retention. This sequence is most often seen when glomerular filtration rate is relatively normal. However, in some patients with more severe renal disease and glomerular involvement there may be primary fluid retention by the kidney either to a low GFR or perhaps to some direct effect of the kidney disease itself (Bichet and Schrier 1985).

Recently, central blood volume expansion (induced by head-out water immersion or by 20 % albumin infusion) has been used to ascertain the roles of intrarenal and extrarenal factors in the development of abnormal water excretion in hyponatremic children and adults with nephrotic syndrome. Both maneuvers resulted in profound natriuresis and diuresis as well as in a drop of plasma and/or urinary AVP levels with corresponding decrease in urine osmolality supporting the role of the "underfilling" mechanism in abnormal water excretion (Berlyne et al. 1981, Usberti et al. 1984, Kovács et al. 1987e, 1988a). The pathogenetic role of the decreased effective circulating blood volume is indirectly suggested also by the fact that expansion of the central blood volume induced by the above maneuvers simultaneously resulted in a decrease in the initially increased activity of the major vasoconstrictory systems (the sympathetic nervous system and the renin-angiotensin-aldosterone system), and a conspicuous elevation of the initially low concentrations of plasma atrial natriuretic factor could be observed following the administration of 20 % albumin (Rascher and Tulassay 1987). Intrarenal factors (decreased glomerular filtration rate, increased proximal tubular reabsorption) may undoubtely contribute to the problem, their partial significance in the reduction of renal water excretion is however difficult to estimate. In addition, these studies and simultaneous clinical observations allowed to draw conclusions that repeated head-out water immersion may be a useful tool in the treatment of gross nephrotic edemas, in particular in a subgroup of subjects who are resistant to the conventional therapy with diuretics (Kovács et al. 1988a).

20.3.3.4   Advanced acute and chronic renal failure

Hypervolemic hypotonic hyponatremia is not an infrequent finding in fluid overloaded patients with advanced acute (acute tubular necrosis) or chronic renal failure. These individuals are typically oliguric and excrete urine with high sodium concentrations ($U_{Na} > 20$ mmol/l).

Generally, in similar cases edema develops as a result of a dysbalance between the amounts of sodium and water ingested and those that can be filtered in the glomerules and potentially excreted in the definitive urine. For example, in a patient with a 20-fold reduction in GFR as compared to normal (i.e. 5 ml/min vs 100 ml/min) the daily filtered load drops proportionally and will make up but a fraction of the respective value for normal subjects (i.e. with a plasma sodium concentration of 140 mmol/l the daily filtered load will be 1008 mmol as compared to 20,160 mmol in a normal subject). In view of the markedly decreased GFR even an adaptively increased tubular sodium rejection is frequently insufficient to excrete the entire dietary load of this electrolyte which is then maintained in the extracellular fluid and induces expansion of the latter accompanied by the development of generalized edema.

The volume of fluid filtered and delivered to the diluting segments of the nephron is of paramount importance also for renal capacity to conserve and excrete water. For example, with a GFR value of 5 ml/min the daily filtrate will amount to approx. 7 l; thereof some 30% (slightly more than 2 l) delivered to the distal nephron can be excreted in urine. Hence, even under conditions of maximal suppression of AVP secretion, the intake of solute-free water in quantities not exceeding the compromised secretory capacity of the kidneys plus insensible losses will result in the development of hyponatremia.

20.4   TREATMENT OF HYPONATREMIA

There are two basic principles involved in the treatment of hyponatremia: 1. treatment directed toward correcting or positively modifying the basic disease and thereby eliminating the stimuli for enhanced renal water retention should begin whenever possible and 2. acute treatment of plasma hypotonicity should be considered only when the true serum sodium concentration is less than 120—125 mmol/l or when symptoms of brain edema are present (Gruskin et al. 1982, Kovács et al. 1984b). In general, hyponatremia is corrected by giving sodium to patients who are volume depleted and by restricting water intake in patients who are "normovolemic" or edematous (see Fig. 20.2). More vigorous therapy (usually requiring hypertonic saline infusions) should be considered when cerebral symptoms are present and/or the plasma sodium concentration is less than 110 to 115 mmol/l since in these settings irreversible neurological damage and death can occur.

The first aim of treatment in the latter cases is to raise the plasma sodium concentration to mildly hyponatremic values (120 to 125 mmol/l), a level at which the patient should be out of danger. In doing so one should however remember that too a rapid compensation, and chiefly overcompensation, of chronic (i.e. more than several hours of duration) hyponatremia carries the risk of permanent brain damage (chapter 20.2). The quantity of sodium necessary to raise the plasma sodium concentration, [Na$^+$] can be derived from the following formula:

$$[Na^+] \text{ required (mmol/l)} = (\text{desired } [Na^+] - \text{present } [Na^+]) \times$$
$$\text{total body water in liters} \qquad (\text{equation } 20.1)$$

The total body water is approximately 60 and 50 per cent of lean body weight in men and women respectively, but it should be realized that the actual amount of total body water may have been altered because of the disease. Thus, equation 20.1 is only an estimate and serial measurements of the plasma sodium concentration are necessary to assess the efficacy of treatment. The possible risk of overcorrection by hypertonic solutions can be minimized by switching to isotonic (0.9 per cent) saline infusion once the plasma sodium concentration reaches 120 mmol/l. Another point that deserves emphasis is that this formula does not include any isoosmotic losses which may also be present. The adequacy of volume repletion can be determined by following the skin turgor, the central venous pressure and urine sodium concentration. In hypovolemic subjects a rise of urine sodium above 20 mmol/l indicates that normovolemia probably has been achieved.

20.4.1 HYPOVOLEMIC HYPOTONIC HYPONATREMIA

True volume depletion due to gastrointestinal or renal losses (see Fig. 20.2) represents the main indication for the use of sodium in the treatment of hyponatremia. Not only will [Na$^+$] replace the lost solute, but volume repletion will increase fluid delivery to the diluting segments, inhibit volume-mediated AVP release and thus allow renal compensation of hyponatremia.

In mild asymptomatic hyponatremia, one third of the calculated sodium deficit (equation 20.1) can be given as isotonic saline in the first 4 to 6 hours, with the remainder being given over the ensuing 24 to 48 hours. Oral solutions containing electrolytes and glucose (see Table 14.1) constitute safe, reasonable and, as compared to intravenous treatment, equally effective alternatives in patients who are able to ingest fluids. The addition of glucose both provides extra calories and promotes small intestinal sodium reabsorption, since there is a coupled transport of sodium and glucose at this site. Correction of potassium depletion, if present, is another important component of therapy and in many cases will contribute to the restoration of plasma sodium concentration (Ashouri 1986).

20.4.2 NORMOVOLEMIC HYPOTONIC HYPONATREMIA (SYNDROME OF INAPPROPRIATE SECRETION OF ANTIDIURETIC HORMONE. SIADH)

Hyponatremia in the SIADH is due initially to water retention and then in part to renal sodium loss induced by volume expansion. In these patients with increased "effective" circulating volume most of the administered sodium will be excreted and the plasma sodium remains low unless ECF volume is simultaneously reduced. Effective volume may be reduced either by severe water restriction, i.e. 20 to 25 per cent of daily maintenance, or in symptomatic patients by the administration of loop diuretics and the replacement of a fraction of the measured urinary losses of water and sodium by sodium-containing solutions (Fig. 20.7) (Gruskin et al. 1982, Kovács and Šoltés 1983).

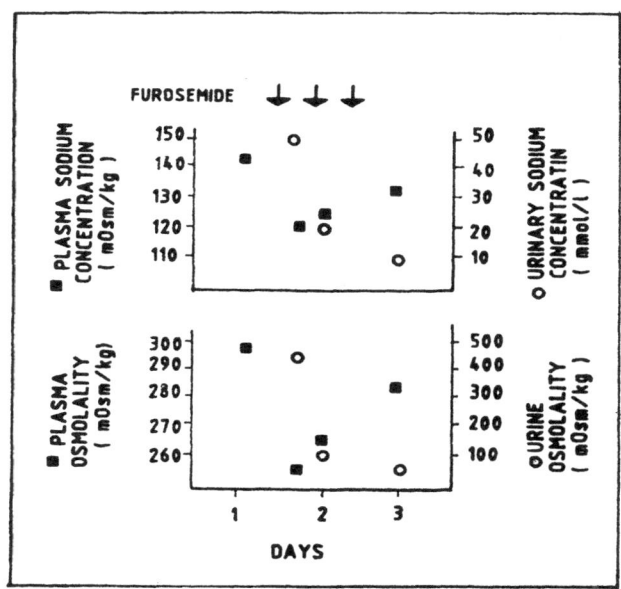

Fig. 20.7. Therapeutic effect of furosemide and replacement of urinary electrolyte losses in a child with pneumonia and SIADH (Kovács and Šoltés 1983).

If prolonged therapy for SIADH is required and continued water restriction is not possible, particularly in patients with ectopic hormone production, therapy must be aimed at increasing water excretion either by enhancing solute excretion or antagonizing the effect of AVP. An increase in solute output can be achieved by administering a high salt, high protein diet or, if available, by giving urea. As long as renal function is normal, urea has few side effects other than some gastrointestinal discomfort (Decaux et al. 1982, Rose 1984). As an alternative, SIADH can be treated by antagonizing the effect of vasopressin. This can be achieved by the administration of 40 to

80 mg furosemide per day in divided doses (with NaCl supplementation to prevent hypovolemia) or of demeclocycline or lithium (chapters 17.2.2.3 and 17.2.2.4) (Forrest et al. 1978, Decaux et al. 1981). Demeclocycline is more effective and better tolerated than lithium, although the latter is preferred in children since tetracyclines can interfere with bone development.

The development of effective V2 antagonists would be an interesting therapeutic advance in the treatment of patients with SIADH. The selective increase of water extretion by V2 receptor antagonists ("aquaretics") would make it possible to treat disorders of water balance without altering the electrolyte balance (chapter 7.3.4). Unfortunately, no suitable V2 antagonist is yet available for clinical use.

20.4.3 HYPERVOLEMIC HYPOTONIC HYPONATREMIA

In edematous patients in whom the extracellular fluid volume is increased and hyponatremia is truly a problem of water overload the therapy must be targeted at water removal since the administration of sodium will increase the severity of the edema. In patients with chronic mild hyponatremia negative water balance can be achieved by restricting water intake to a volume that is less than the output (assuming that the water content of food is approximately equal to the insensible water losses from the skin and respiratory tract). In patients in whom water restriction alone is ineffective loop diuretics in combination with hypertonic saline can be used.

In some subjects with severe heart failure or hepatic cirrhosis, the water retaining tendency is so great that water restriction and loop diuretics may be ineffective in maintaining safe plasma sodium levels. Since nonosmotically stimulated AVP secretion plays an important role in this setting, pharmacological induction of nephrogenic diabetes insipidus with demeclocycline (chapter 17.4.2.4) may be of therapeutical value in some cases (DeTroyer et al. 1976), but the drug's nephrotoxic effects preclude its wider use (Geheb and Cox 1980). Also repeated head-out water immersion can improve renal water excretion in edematous hyponatremic patients who are refractory to saluretic treatment (Kovács et al. 1987e). In addition, these edematous disorders represent another potentional field for therapeutical application of the long sought V2-antagonistic "aquaretic" agents (chapter 7.3.4).

In patients with severe or symptomatic hyponatremia, the plasma sodium concentration can be elevated more quickly by the use of loop diuretics in combination with hypertonic saline or by peritoneal dialysis (Miller and Finberg 1960).

LIST OF ABBREVIATIONS

ACTH	adrenocorticotropic hormone
ADH	antidiuretic hormone
AIDS	acquired immune-deficiency syndrome
ANP	atrial natriuretic peptide
A/P	antidiuretic/pressure ratio
AVP	arginine vasopressin
AVT	arginine vasotocin
AV3V	anteroventral third ventricle region
BNP	brain natriuretic peptide
BST	bed nucleus of the stria terminalis
BUN	blood urea nitrogen
cAMP	cyclic adenosine monophosphate
C_{creat}	endogenous creatinine clearance
CDI	central diabetes insipidus
CHF	congestive heart failure
C_{H_2O}	free water clearance
C_{Na}	renal clearance of sodium
CNS	central nervous system
CRF	corticotropin releasing factor
C_{osm}	osmotic clearance
dDAVP	1-deamino-8D arginine-vasopressin
dGAVP	deglycine arginine-vasopressin
DI	diabetes insipidus
DOCA	desoxycorticosterone acetate
dVDAVP	[1-deamino, 4-valine, 8-D-arginine] vasopressin
ECBV	effective circulating blood volume
EACA	epsilon aminocapronic acid
ECF	extracellular fluid
EDLI	endogenous digoxin-like immunoreactivity
EH	essential hypernatremia
FE_{Na}	fractional excretion of sodium
FE_{osm}	fractional excretion of osmotically active substances
FE_{H_2O}	fractional excretion of water
FVIII	factor VIII
GABA	gamma aminobutyric acid
GFR	glomerular filtration rate
GH	growth hormone
ICF	intracellular fluid
JGA	juxtaglomerular apparatus
LVP	lysine vasopressin

mRNA	messenger ribonucleic acid
Na^+, K^+- ATPase	sodium-potassium adenosine-triphosphatase
NDI	nephrogenic diabetes insipidus
NE	norepinephrine
NP	neurophysin
NTS	nucleus tractus solitarius
OT	oxytocin
OT-VT	oxytocin-vasotocin
OVLT	organum vasculosum of the lamina terminalis
P/A	pressor/antidiuretic
P_{creat}	plasma creatinine concentration
PDI	polydipsic diabetes insipidus
PGE_2	prostaglandin E2
$P_{glucose}$	plasma glucose concentration
P_{Na}	plasma sodium concentration
P_{osm}	plasma osmolality
P_{osm} eff	effective plasma osmolality
PRA	plasma renin activity
PRF	prolactin releasing factor
PVN	paraventricular nucleus
RIA	radioimmunoassay
SCN	suprachiasmatic nucleus
SFO	subfornical organ
SIADH	syndrome of inappropriate secretion of antidiuretic hormone
SON	supraoptic nucleus
$T^c_{H_2O}$	tubular reabsorption of solute free water
TRH	thyrotropin releasing hormone
TSH	thyroid stimulating hormone
U_{Cl}	urinary concentration of chloride
U_{creat}	urinary concentration of creatinine
U_{Na}	urinary concentration of sodium
U_{osm}	urine osmolality
U_{osm} min	minimal urine osmolality
V	urine flow rate, diuresis
V1	vasopressin receptor subtype (pressor)
V2	vasopressin receptor subtype (antidiuretic)
V3 (V1b)	vasopressin receptor subtype
VWD	von Willebrand's disease
VWF	von Willebrand's factor
VWF:RCo	von Willebrand's factor ristocetin cofactor
VWF:Ag	von Willebrand's factor antigen

REFERENCES

Abramow, M., Beauwens, R., Cogan, E.: (1987): Cellular events in vasopressin action. Kidney Int., 32 (suppl. 21): S56—S66

Abramow, M., Cogan, E.: (1984): Clinical aspects and pathophysiology of diuretic induced hyponatremia. Adv. Nephrol., 13: 1—28

Acher, R.,: (1980): Molecular evolution of biologically active polypeptides. Proc. R. Soc. Lond. [Biol] 210: 21—43

Acher, R., Chauvet, J., Chauvet, M. T., Levy, B., Miche, L. G., Roville, Y.: (1988): Stepwise processing of the neurohypophyseal hormone — neurophysin precursors: Variations during vertebrate evolution. Satellite symp. 8th Internat. Congress of Endocrinol. Kyoto, Japan

Akerlund, M., Stromberg, P., Forsling, M. L.: (1979): Primary dysmenorrhea and vasopressin. Br. J. Obstetr. Gynecol., 86: 484—487

Al-Dahhan, J., Haycock, G. B., Chantler, C., Stimmler, L.: (1983): Sodium homeostasis in term and preterm neonates. Arch. Dis. Child., 58: 335—342

Altura, B. M.: (1976a): dDAVP:A vasopressin analog with selective microvascular and RES actions for the treatment of circulatory shock in rats. Eur. J. Pharmacol., 37: 155—167

Altura, B. M.: (1976b): Microcirculatory approach to the treatment of circulatory shock with a new analog of vasopressin (2-phenylalanine, 8-ornithine) vasopressin. J. Pharmacol. Exp. Ther., 198: 187—196

Altura, B. M., Altura, B. T.: (1984): Actions of vasopressin, oxytocin and synthetic analogs on vascular smooth muscle. Fed. Proc., 43: 80—86

Amico, J. A.: (1985): Diabetes insipidus in pregnancy. In: Diabetes insipidus in man. (edit. Czernichow, P., Robinson, A. G.), Karger, Basel: 266—267

Amico, J. A., Ervin, M. G., Finn, F. M., Leake, R. D., Fisher, D. A., Robinson, A. G.: (1986): The plasma of pregnant women contains a novel oxytocin-vasotocin-like peptide. Metabolism, 35: 596—601

Anderson, L. T., David, R., Bonnet, R., Dancis, J.: (1979): Passive avoidance learning in Lesh-Nyhan disease: Effects of 1-desamino-8-D-arginine vasopressin. Life Sci., 24: 905—910

Anderson, R. J.: (1986): Hospital-associated hyponatremia. Kidney Int., 29: 1237—1247

Anderson, R. J., Chung, H. M., Kluge, R., Schrier, R. W.: (1985): Hyponatremia: A prospective analysis of its epidemiology and the pathogenetic role of vasopressin. Ann. Int. Med., 102: 164—168

Andersson, B.: (1978): Regulation of water intake. Physiol. Rev., 58: 582—603

Ang, V. T. Y., Jenkins, J. S.: (1982): Blood-CSF barrier to arginine vasopressin, desmopressin and desglycinamide arginine-vasopressin in the dog. J. Endocrinol., 93: 319—325

Anger, M. S., Berl, T.: (1986): Vasopressin and the concentrating mechanism. J. Cardiovasc. Pharmacol., 8 (suppl. 7): S50—S55

Antoni, F. A., Holmes, M. C., Jones, M. T.: (1983): Oxytocin as well as vasopressin potentiates ovine CRF in vitro. Peptides, 4: 411—415

Antoni, F. A., Holmes, M. L., Makara, G. B., Kárteszi, H., László, F. A.: (1984): Evidence that the effects of arginine-8-vasopressin (AVP) on pituitary corticotropin (ACTH) release are mediated by a novel type of receptor. Peptides, 5: 1—4

Aperia, A., Broberger, O., Herin, K., Thodenius, K., Zetterström, R.: (1983): Postnatal control of water and electrolyte homeostasis in pre-term and full term infants. Acta Paed. Scand., 305: 61—65

Aperia, A., Herin, P., Lundin, S., Zetterström, R.: (1984): Regulation of renal water excretion in newborn fullterm infants. Acta Paed. Scand., 73: 717—721

Applegate, R. J., Hasser, E. M., Bishop, U. S.: (1987): Vagal cold block in area postrema-lesioned dogs: Interaction of vasopressin and sympathetic nervous system. Am. J. Physiol., 252: H135—H141

Arant, B. S.: (1978): Developmental patterns of renal functional maturation compared in the human neonate. J. Pediatr., 92: 705—712

Arant, B. S.: (1982): Fluid therapy in the neonate — concepts in transition. J. Pediat., 101: 387—389

Arant, B. S.: (1987): Postnatal development of renal function during the first year of life. Pediat. Nephrol., 3: 308—313

Arawich, P. F., Sládek, L. D.: (1986): Vasopressin and glucoprivic feeding behavior. A new perspective on an "old" peptide. Brain Res., 385: 245—252

Arduino, F., Ferraz, F. P., Rodriguez, J.: (1966): Antidiuretic action of chlorpropamide in idiopathic diabetes insipidus. J. Clin. Endocrinol., 26: 1325—1328

Arieff, A. I.: (1984): Central nervous system manifestations of disordered sodium metabolism. Clin. Endocrinol. Metab., 13: 269—294

Arieff, A. I.: (1986): Hyponatremia, convulsions, respiratory arrest and permanent brain damage after elective surgery in healthy women. New Engl. J. Med., 314: 1529—1535

Arieff, A. I., Guisado, R.: (1976): Effects on the central nervous system of hypernatremic and hyponatremic states. Kidney Int., 10: 104—120

Arieff, A. I., Llach, F., Massry, S.: (1976): Neurological manifestations and morbidity of hyponatremia. Medicine (Baltimore) 55: 121—129

Aronson, A. S., Svenningsen, N. W.: (1974): dDAVP test for estimation of renal concentrating capacity in infants and children. Arch. Dis. Child., 49: 654—659

Ashouri, O. S.: (1986): Severe diuretic-induced hyponatremia in the elderly. Arch. Int. Med. 146: 1355—1357

Atkinson, S. A., Radde, I. L., Anderson, G. H.: (1983): Macromineral balances in premature infants fed on own mother's milk or formula. J. Pediatr., 102: 99—106

Ausiello, D. A., Skorecki, K. L., Verkman, A. S., Bonventre, J. V.: (1987): Vasopressin signaling in kidney cells. Kidney Int., 31: 521—529

Aycinena, P., Robertson, G. L.: (1983): Effects of hypercalcemia on secretion of the antidiuretic hormone, arginine vasopressin. (Abstract). Endocrinology, 112 (suppl. 142): 245

Ayus, J. C.: (1986): Diuretic-induced hyponatremia. Arch. Intern. Med., 146: 1295—1296

Baertschi, A. J., Massi, Y., Kwon, S.: (1985): Vasopressin responses to peripheral and central osmotic pulse stimulation. Peptides, 6: 1131—1135

Bahr, V., Hensen, J., Hader, O., Oelkes, W.: (1988): Effects of osmotically stimulated endogenous vasopressin on basal and CRH-stimulated ACTH release in man. Acta Endocrinol., 117: 103—108

Bakoš, P., Ponec, J., Lichardus, B.: (1984): Effect of lysine-vasopressin (LVP) and

1-deamino-8-D-arginine-vasopressin (dDAVP) upon electrical potential. Gen. Physiol. Biophys., 3, 297—305

Bar, H., LeRoith, D., Nyska, M., Glick, S. M.: (1980): Elevations in plasma ADH levels during PEEP ventillation in the dog: mechanisms involved. Am. J. Physiol., 239: E474—E481

Baran, T., Hutchinson, T. A.: (1984): The outcome of hyponatremia in a general hospital population. Clin. Nephrol., 22: 72—76

Barbour, G. L., Straub, K. D., O'Neal, B. L., Leatherman, J. W.: (1979): Vasopressin resistent nephrogenic diabetes insipidus. A result of amphotericin B therapy. Arch. Int. Med., 139: 86—89

Barchas, J. D., Akil, H., Elliott, G. R., Holman, R. B., Watson, S. J.: (1978): Behavioural neurochemistry: Neuroregulators and behavioural states. Science, 280: 964—973

Bargmann, W.: (1949): Über die Neurosecretorische Verknüpfung von Hypothalamus und Neurohypophyse. Z. Zellforsch. Mikroskop. Anat., 34: 610—634

Barlow, E. D., De Wardener, H. E.: (1959): Compulsive water drinking. Q. J. Med., 52: 235—258

Barnett, H. L.: (1966): Pediatric nephrology: Scientific study of kidneys and their diseases in infants and children. Am. J. Dis. Child., 41: 229—237

Barron, W. M.: (1987): Volume homeostasis during pregnancy in the rat. Am. J. Kidney Dis., 9: 296—302

Barron, W. M., Stamoutsos, B. A., Lindheimer, M. D.: (1984): Role of volume in the regulation of vasopressin secretion during pregnancy in the rat. J. Clin. Invest., 73: 923—932

Battle, D. D., VonRoitte, A. B., Graviria, M., Grupp, M.: (1985): Ameloriation of polyuria by amiloride in patients receiving long term lithium therapy. New Engl. J. Med., 312: 408—414

Baylis, P. H.: (1983): Posterior pituitary function in health and disease. Clin. Endocrinol. Metab., 12: 747—770

Baylis, P. H.: (1987): Osmoregulation and control of vasopressin secretion in healthy humans. Am. J. Physiol., 253: R671—R678

Baylis, P. H., Heath, D. A.: (1978): Water disturbances in patients treated with oral lithium carbonate. Ann. Int. Med., 88: 607—611

Baylis, P. H., Robertson, G. L.: (1980): Rat vasopressin response to insulin-induced hypoglycemia. Endocrinology, 107: 1975—1979

Baylis, P. H., Thompson, C. J.: (1988): Osmoregulation of vasopressin secretion and thirst in health and disease. Clin. Endocrinol. 29: 549—576

Baylis, P. H., Thompson, C., Burd, J., Tunbridge, W. M. G., Snodgrass, C. A.: (1986): Recurrent pregnancy-induced polyuria and thirst due to hypothalamic diabetes insipidus. Clin. Endocrinol., 24: 459—466

Baylis, P. H., Zerbe, R. L., Robertson, G. L.: (1981): Arginine-vasopressin response to insulin-induced hypoglycemia in man. J. Clin. Endocrinol. Metab., 53: 935—940

Beck, V., Yu, B. P.: (1982): Effects of aging on urinary concentrating mechanism and vasopressin dependent cAMP in rats. Am. J. Physiol., 243: F121—F125

Becker, D. J., Foley, T. P.: (1978): 1-deamino-8-D-arginine vasopressin in the treatment of central diabetes insipidus in childhood. J. Pediatr., 92: 1011—1015

Bell, E. F., Oh, W.: (1983): Water requirement of premature newborn infants. Acta Paed. Scand., Suppl. 305: 21—26

Bell, E. F., Warburton, D., Stonestreet, B. S., Oh, W.: (1979): High volume fluid intake predisposes premature infants to necrotizing enterocolitis. Lancet, ii: 90

Bell, E. F., Warburton, D., Stonestreet, B. S., Oh, W.: (1980): Effect of fluid administration of the development of symptomatic patient ductus arteriosus and congestive heart failure in premature infants. New Engl. J. Med., 302: 598—604

Bell, R. J., Congiu, M., Hardy, K. J., Wintour, E. M.: (1984): Gestation dependent aspects of the response of the ovine fetus to the osmotic stress induced by maternal water deprivation. Q. J. Exp. Physiol., 69: 108—112

Benfield, G. F. A., O'Doherty, K., Davies, B. H.: (1982): Status asthmaticus and the syndrome of inappropriate secretion of antidiuretic hormone. Thorax, 37: 147—148

Bennett, W. M.: (1981): Aminoglycoside nephrotoxicity: Experimental and clinical considerations. Miner. Electrolyte Metab., 6: 277—279

Berl, T.: (1987): The cAMP system in vasopressin sensitive nephron segments of the vitamin D treated rat. Kidney Int., 31: 1065—1071

Berl, T., Aisenbrey, G. A., Linas, S. L.: (1980): Renal concentrating defect in the hypokalemic rat is prostaglandin independent. Am. J. Physiol., 238: F37—F41

Berl, T., Anderson, R. J., McDonald, K. M., Schrier, R. W.: (1976): Clinical disorders of water metabolism. Kidney Int., 10: 117—126

Berl, T., Linas, S. L., Aisenbrey, G. A., Anderson, R. J.: (1977): On the mechanism of polyuria in potassium depletion. J. Clin. Invest., 60: 620—625

Berliner, R. W., Davidson, D. G.: (1957): Production of hypertonic urine in the absence of pituitary antidiuretic hormone. J. Clin. Invest., 36: 1 416—1 427

Berlyne, G. M., Braun, C., Adler, A., Feinroth, A., Feinroth, M., Horsch, S., Friedman, E. E. A.: (1981): Water immersion in nephrotic syndrome. Arch. Int. Med., 141: 1275—1280

Better, O. S., Schrier, R. W.: (1983): Disturbed volume homeostasis in patients with cirrhosis of the liver. Kidney Int., 23: 303—311

Bichet, D. G., Arthus, M. F., Barjon, J. N., Lonergan, M., Kortas, C.: (1987): Human platelet fraction arginine-vasopressin. Potential physiological role. J. Clin. Invest, 79: 881—887

Bichet, D. G., Kortas, C., Mettauer, B., Manzini, C., MarcAurele, J., Rouleau, J. L., Schrier, R. W: (1986): Modulation of plasma and platelet vasopressin by cardiac function in patients with heart failure. Kidney Int., 29: 1188—1196

Bichet, D. G., Schrier, R. W.: (1985): Role of vasopressin in abnormal water excretion in edematous disorders. In: Vasopressin (edit.: Schrier, R. W.) Raven Press, New York: 525—534

Bichet, D. G., Szatalowicz, V., Chaimowitz, C., Schrier, R. W.: (1986): Role of vasopressin in abnormal water excretion in cirrhotic patients. Ann. Int. Med., 96: 413—417

Birkášova, M., Birkaš, O., Flynn, M. J., Cort, J. H.: (1978): Desmopressin in the management of nocturnal enuresis in children: a double-blind study. Pediatrics, 62: 970—974

Bishop, V. S., Thanes, M. D., Schmid, P. G.: (1984): Effects of bilateral vagal cold block on vasopressin in conscious dogs. Am. J. Physiol., 246: R566—R569

Blachley, J. D., Hill, J. B.: (1981): Renal and electrolyte disturbances associated with cisplatin. Ann. Intern. Med., 95: 628—632

Blalock, T., Gerron, G., Quiter, E., Rudman, D.: (1977): Role of diet in the management of vasopressin responsive and resistent diabetes insipidus. Am. J. Clin. Nutr., 30: 1070—1075

Blessing, W. W., Willoughby, J. O.: (1987): Central neural pathways mediating baroreceptor-initiated secretion of vasopressin. In: Cardiogenic reflexes. Eds. R. Hainsworth, P. N. McWilliam, D. A. S. G. Mary, Oxford Univer. Press, Oxford: 301

Block, L. H., Furrer, J., Locher, R. A., Siegenthaler, W., Vetter, V.: (1981): Changes in tissue sensitivity to vasopressin in hereditary hypothalamic diabetes insipidus. Klin. Wochenschr., 59: 831—836

Boda, D.: (1986): Oral fluid and electrolyte support in clinical practice (Hung). Orv. Hetilap, 127: 1427—1433

Bode, H. H., Crawford, J. D.: (1969): Nephrogenic diabetes insipidus in North America — the Hopewell hypothesis. New Engl. J. Med., 280: 750—755

Bode, H. H., Harley, B. M., Crawford, J. D.: (1971): Restoration of normal drinking behaviour by chlorpropamide in patients with hypodipsia and diabetes insipidus. Am. J. Med., 51: 304—307

Bonnici, F.: (1973): Antidiuretic effect of clofibrate and carbamazepine in diabetes insipidus. Clin. Endocrinol., 2: 265—275

Borowitz, S. M., Rocco, M.: (1986): Acute water intoxication in healthy infants. Southern Med. J., 79: 1156—1158

Bouzarth, W. F., Shenkin, H. A.: (1982): Is "cerebral hyponatremia" iatrogenic? Lancet, i. 1061—1062

Boyle, W. A., Segel, L. D.: (1986): Direct cardial effects of vasopressin and their reversal by a vascular antagonist. Am. J. Physiol., 251: H734—741

Brackett, D. J., Schaefer, C. F., Wilson, M. F.: (1983): The role of vasopressin in the maintenance of cardiovascular function during early endotoxin shock. Adv. Shock Res., 9: 147—156

Braden, G. L., Singer, I., Cox, M.: (1985): Nephrogenic diabetes insipidus. In: Renal tubular disorders. (edit. Gonick, H. C., Buckaley, V. M. Jr), Marcel Dekker Inc.. New York: 387—456

Braverman, L. E., Mancini, J. P., McGoldrick, D. M.: (1965): Hereditary idiopathic diabetes insipidus: A case report with autopsy findings. Ann. Intern. Med., 63: 503—508

Brinton, R. E., Gehlert, D. R., Wamsley, J. K., Wang, Y. P., Yamamura, H. I.: (1986): Vasopressin metabolite AVP-(4—9) binding sites in brain: distribution distinct from that of parent peptide. Life Sci., 38: 443—452

Brody, M. J., Johnson, A. K.: (1980): Role of anteroventral third ventricle region in fluid and electrolyte balance, arterial pressure regulation and hypertension. In: Frontiers in Neuroendocrinology, (Ed.: Martini, L., Gannong, W. F.), Raven Press, New York: 220—245

Brommer, E. J. P., Barrett—Bergshoeff, M. D., Allen, R. A., Schiet, I., Bertina, R. M., Chalekamp: (1982): The use of desmopressin acetate (dDAVP) as a test of the fibrinolytic capacity of patients: Analysis of responders and nonresponders. Thrombosis and Haemostasis, 48: 156—161

Brooks, D. P., Shere, L., Crofton, J. T.: (1986): Central adrenergic control of AVP release. Neuroendocrinology, 42: 416—420

Brown, D., Shields, G. I., Valtin, H., Morris, J. F., Orci, L.: (1985): Lack of intramembranous particle clusters in collecting duct of mice with nephrogenic diabetes insipidus. Am. J. Physiol., 249: F582—589

Brown, W. W., Davis, B. B., Spry, L. A., Wongsurawat, N., Malone, D., Domoto, D. T.: (1986): Aging and the kidney. Arch. Int. Med., 146: 1790—1796

Brownstein, M. J., Russel, J. T., Gainer, H.: (1980): Synthesis, transport and release of posterior pituitary hormones. Science, 207: 373—379

Bruck, E., Abal, G., Aceto, T.: (1968): Pathogenesis and pathophysiology of hypertonic dehydration with diarrhea. Am. J. Dis. Child., 115: 122—144.

Brugnier, A., Poisson, D., Lestradet, H., Lebrune, B.: (1981): Diabète insipide familial d'origine centrale. Nouv. Presse. Med., 10: 897—899

Buijs, R. M., Swaab, D. F.: (1979): Immunelectron-microscopical demonstration of vasopressin and oxytocin synapses in the limbic system of the rat. Cell Tissue Res., 204: 355—365

Burbach, J. P. H., DeHoop, H. J., Schmale, H., Richter, D., Dekloet, E. R., denHaaf, J. A.: (1984a): Differential responses to osmotic stress of vasopressin-neurophysin mRNA in hypothalamic nuclei. Neuroendocrinology, 39: 582—584

Burbach, J. P. H., Kovács, G. L., DeWied, D., Nispen, J. W., Greven, H. M.: (1983): A major metabolite of arginine vasopressin in the brain is a highly potent neuropeptide. Science, 221: 1310—1312

Burbach, J. P. H., Wang, X. C., Ten Haaf, J. A., Dewied, D.: (1984b): Substances resembling C-terminal vasopressin fragments are present in the brain but not in the pituitary gland. Brain Res., 306: 384—387

Baurroughs, A. K., Matthews, K., Qadiri, M., Thomas, N., Kernoff, P., Tuddenham, E., McIntyre, N.: (1985): Desmopressin and bleeding time in patients with cirrhosis. Br. Med. J., 291: 1377—1381

Burrow, G. N., Wassenaar, W., Robertson, G. L., Seal, H.: (1981): dDAVP treatment of diabetes insipidus during pregnancy and the post-partum period. Acta Endocrinol., 9: 23—25

Burrows, F. A., Shutack, J. G., Crone, R. K.: (1983): Inappropriate secretion of antidiuretic hormone in a postsurgical pediatric population. Crit. Care Med., 11: 527—532

Butler. W. T., Bennett, J. E., Alling, D. W., Wertlake, P. T., Utz, J. P., Hill, G. J.: (1964): Nephrotoxicity of amphotericin B: Early and late effects in 81 patients. Ann. Intern. Med., 61: 175—179

Cacabelos, R.: (1986): Sistema vasopresinergico I. Medicina Clin., 88: 160—168

Čáp, J., Mišíková, Z., Kováč, R.: (1975): Vincristine neurotoxicity (Slov). Čs. Pediat. 30: 565—567

Cataldi—Betcher, E. L., Seltzer, H. H., Slocum, B. A., Jones, K. W.: (1983): Complications occurring during enteral nutrition support: a prospective study. J. Parent. Enteral. Nutr., 7: 546—552

Chan, D. K. O.: (1977): Comparative physiology of the vasomotor effects of neurohypophyseal peptides in the vertebrates. Am. Zool., 17: 751—762

Chauvet, M. T., Hurpet, D., Chauvet, J., Acher, R.: (1980): Phenypressin (Phe2-Arg8)-vasopressin, a new neurohypophyseal peptide found in marsupials. Nature, 287: 640

Chessex, P., Reichman, B., Verellen, G.: (1983): Quality of growth in premature infants fed their own mother's milk. J. Pediat., 102: 107—112

Chevalier, J., Bourguet, J., Hugon, J. S.: (1974): Membrane associated particles: Distribution in frog urinary bladder epithelium at rest and after oxytocin treatment. Cell Tissue Res., 152: 129—140

Chu, P., Staff, W. G., Morris, J. A., Polak, J. M.: (1986): DIDMOAD syndrome with megacystis and megaureter. Postgrad. Med. J., 62: 859—863

Chung, H. M., Kluge, R., Schrier, R. W., Anderson, R. J. M: (1986): Postoperative hyponatremia. A prospective study. Arch. Int. Med., 146: 333—336

Claybaugh, J. R., Sato, A. K.: (1985): Factors influencing urinary vasopressin concentration. Fed. Proc., 44: 62—65

Clements, J. A., Funder, J. W.: (1986): Arginine-vasopressin (AVP) and AVP-like immunoreactivity in peripheral tissues. Endocrine Reviews, 7: 449—460

Cody, R. J., Atlas, S. A., Laragh, J. H.: (1987): Physiologic and pharmacologic studies of atrial natriuretic factor: a natriuretic and vasoactive peptide. J. Clin. Pharmacol., 27: 927—936

Cogan, E., Abramov, M.: (1986): Inhibition by lithium of the hydroosmotic action of vasopressin in the isolated perfused cortical collecting tubule of the rabbit. J. Clin. Invest., 77: 1507—1514

Cogan, E., Debieve, M. F., Philipart, I., Pepersack, T., Abramow, M.: (1986): High plasma levels of atrial natriuretic factor in SIADH. New Engl. J. Med., 314: 1258—1259

Coggins, C. H., Leaf, A.: (1967): Diabetes insipidus. Am. J. Med., 42: 807—813

Constantini, M. G., Pearlmutter, A. F.: (1984): Properties of the specific binding site for arginine-vasopressin in rat hyppocampal synaptic membranes. J. Biol. Chem., 259: 11739—11745

Cooper, K. E., Kasting, N. W., Lederis, K., Veale, W. L.: (1979): Evidence supporting a role for endogenous vasopressin in natural suppresion of fever in the sheep. J. Physiol., 295: 33—45

Coulthard, M. G., Ney, E. N.: (1985): Effect of varying water intake on renal function in healthy preterm babies. Arch. Dis. Child., 60: 614—620

Cowley, A. W.: (1982): Vasopressin and cardiovascular regulation. In: Cardiovascular Physiology IV. Baltimore, University Park Press, Baltimore 1982: 189—242

Cowley, A. W., Liard, J. F.: (1987): Cardiovascular actions of vasopressin. In: Vasopressin (edit. Gash, D. M. and Boer, Gy.), Plenum Publ. Corp., New York: 389—433

Cowley, A. W., Merril, D. C., Osborn, J., Barber, B. J.: (1984a): Influences of vasopressin and angiotensin on baroreflexes in the dog. Circ. Res., 54: 163—172

Cowley, A. W., Merril, D. C., Quillen, E. W., Skelton, M. M.: (1984b): Long-term blood pressure and metabolic effects of vasopressin with servo-controlled fluid volume. Am. J. Physiol., 247: R537—R545

Cowley, A. W., Monos, E., Guyton, A. C.: (1974): Interaction of vasopressin and the baroreceptor reflex system in the regulation of arterial blood pressure in the dog. Circ. Res., 34: 505—514

Cowley, A. W., Switzer, S. J., Guinn, M. M.: (1980): Evidence and quantification of the vasopressin arterial pressure control system in the dog. Circ. Res., 46: 58—67

Crawford, J. D., Kennedy, G. C., Hill, L. E.: (1960): Clinical results of treatment of diabetes insipidus with drugs of the chlorothiazide series. New Engl. J. Med., 262: 737—743

Creager, M. A., Faxon, D. P., Cutler, S. S., Kohlmon, O., Ryan, T. J., Gaurits, M.: (1986): Contribution of vasopressin to vasoconstriction in patients with congestive heart failure. J. Am. Coll. Cardiol., 7: 758—765

Cronin, R. E.: (1987): Psychogenic polydipsia with hyponatremia: Report of eleven cases. Am. J. Kidney Dis., 9: 410—416

Cserr, H. F., DePasquale, M., Patlak, C. S.: (1987): Volume regulatory influx of electrolytes from plasma to brain during acute hyperosmolality. Am. J. Physiol., 253: F530—F537

Cusic, J. F., Hagen, T. C., Findling, J. W.: (1984): Inappropriate secretion of antidiuretic hormone after transsphenoidal surgery for pituitary tumors. New Engl. J. Med., 311: 36—38

Czernichow, P., Pomarade, R., Brauner, R., Rappaport, R.: (1985): Neurogenic diabetes insipidus in children. In: Diabetes insipidus in man. (edit. Czernichow, P., Robinson, A. G.), Karger, Basel: 190—209

Czernichow, P., Robinson, A. G. (Edit): (1985): Diabetes insipidus in man. Karger, Basel: 1—320

Daniel, S. S., Stark, R. I., Husain, M. K., Baxi, L. V., James, L. S.: (1982): Role of arginine vasopressin in fetal homeostasis. Am. J. Physiol., 242: F740—F744

Daniel, S. S., Stark, R. I., Husain, M. K., Sanocka, U. M., James, S. J.: (1984): Excretion of vasopressin in the hypoxic lamb: comparison between fetus and newborn. Pediat. Res., 18: 227—231

David, R., Ellis, D., Gartner, J. C.: (1981): Water intoxication in normal infants: role of antidiuretic hormone in pathogenesis. Pediatrics, 68: 349—353

Davidson, J. M., Gilmore, E. A., Durr, J., Robertson, G. L., Lindheimer, M. D.: (1984): Altered osmotic threshold for vasopressin secretion and thirst in human pregnancy. Am. J. Physiol., 246: F105—109

Davies, D. P., Ansari, B. M., Mandal, B. K.: (1979): The declining incidence of infantile hypernatremic dehydration in Great-Britain. Am. J. Dis. Child., 133: 148—150

Day, T. A., Renaud, L. P.: (1984): Electrophysiological evidence that noradrenergic afferents selectively facilitate the activity of supraoptic vasopressin neurons. Brain Res., 303: 233—240

DeBold, A. J., Borenstein, H. B., Veress, A. T., Sonnenberg, H.: (1981): A rapid and potent natriuretic response to intravenous injection of atrial myocardial extracts in rats. Life Sci., 28: 89—94

DeFronzo, R. A., Thier, S. O.: (1980): Pathophysiologic approach to hyponatremia. Arch. Int. Med., 140: 897—902

DeJong, P. E., Statius VanEps, L. W.: (1985): Sickle cell nephropathy. Kidney Int., 27: 711—717

DeKloet, F. R., Voorhuis, T. A. M., Burbach, J. P. H., DeWied, D.: (1985): Autoradiographic localization of binding sites for the arginine-vasopressin (VP) metabolite VP4-9 in rat brain. Neurosci. Lett., 56: 7—11

DeLaFuente, B., Danek, S., Hoyer, L. W.: (1985): The effect of 1-deamino-8-D-arginine vasopressin (dDAVP) in a nonhaemophilic patient with an acquired type II. factor VIII inhibitor. Br. J. Haematol., 59: 127—131

DeRouffignac, C., Elalouf, J. M., Roinel, N.: (1987): Physiological control of the urinary concentrating mechanism by peptide hormones. Kidney Int., 31: 611— 620

DeRubertis, F. R., Michelis, M. F., Davis, B. B.: (1974): Essential hypernatremia. Arch. Int. Med., 134: 889—895

DeSousa, R. C.: (1986): Effects of vasopressin on epithelium transport. J. Cardiovasc. Pharmacol., 8 (suppl. 7): S23—S28

DeWane, G. W., Porter, J. C.: (1980): An apparent stress-induced release of arginine vasopressin by human neonates. J. Clin. Endocrinol. Metab., 51: 1412—1416

DeWardener, H. E., Herxheimer, A.: (1965): The effect of a high water intake on the kidney's ability to concentrate urine in man. J. Physiol., 139: 42 —52

DeWardener, H. E., MacGregor, G. A.: (1983): The relationship of a circulating sodium transport inhibitor (the natriuretic hormone?) to hypertension. Medicine, 62: 310—326

DeWardener, H. E., Mills, I. H., Clapham, W. F., Hayter, C. J.: (1961): Studies on efferent mechanism of sodium diuresis which follows administration of intravenous saline in dog. Clin. Sci. 21: 249—258

DeWied, D.: (1976): Behavioral effects of intraventricularly administered vasopressin and vasopressin fragments. Life Sci., 19: 685—690

DeWied, D.: (1984): The neuropeptide concept. Maturitas, 6: 217—223

DeWied, D., Jolles, J.: (1982): Neuropeptides derived from pro-opiocortin: behavioral, physiological and neurochemical effects. Physiol. Rev., 62: 976—1059

DeWied, D., Greven, H. M., Lande, S., Witter, A.: (1972): Dissociation of the behavioral and endocrine effects of lysine vasopressin by tryptic digestion. Br. J. Pharmacol., 45: 118—122

Decaux, G., Genette, F., Mockel, J.: (1980): Hypouremia in the syndrome of inappropriate secretion of antidiuretic hormone. Ann. Int. Med., 93: 716—717

Decaux, G., Unger, J., Brimioulle, S., Mockel, J.: (1982): Hyponatremia in the syndrome of inapropriate secretion of antidiuretic hormone. Rapid correction with urea, sodium chloride and water restriction. JAMA, 247: 471—474

Decaux, G., Waterlot, Y., Genette, F., Mockel, J.: (1981): Treatment of inappropriate secretion of antidiuretic hormone with furosemide. New Engl. J. Med., 304: 329—330

DeRubertis, F. R., Michelis, M. F., Bloom, M. E., Mintz, D. H., Field, J. B., Davis, B.B.: (1971): Impaired water excretion in myxedema. Am. J. Med. 51: 41—51

DeTroyer, A., Pilloy, W., Bioechaert, I.: (1976): Demeclocycline treatment of water retention in cirrhosis. Ann. Int. Med. 85: 336—337

Dicker, S. E., Eggleton, M. G.: (1963): Nephrogenic diabetes insipidus. Clin. Sci., 24: 81—89

Dimson, S. B.: (1986): dDAVP and urine osmolality in refractory enuresis. Arch. Dis. Child., 61: 1104—1107

Dlouhá, H.: (1982): The postnatal development and kidney function. Academia, Praha

Dlouhá, H., Kreček, J., Zicha, J.: (1982): Postnatal development and diabetes insipidus in Brattleboro rats. Ann. N.Y. Acad. Sci., 394: 10—20

Dóczi, T., Bende, J., Huszka, E., Kis, J.: (1981): Syndrome of inappropriate secretion of antidiuretic hormone after subarachnoid hemorrhage. Neurosurgery, 9: 394—397

Dóczi, T., Lászlo, F. A., Szerdahelyi, P.: (1984): Involvement of vasopressin in brain edema formation. Neurosurgery, 14: 436—441

Dóczi, T., Tarjanyi, J., Huszka, E., Kiss, J.: (1982): Syndrome of inappropriate secretion of antidiuretic hormone after head injury. Neurosurgery, 10: 685—688

Dogterom, J., Van Wimersma Greidanus, T., Swaab, D. F.: (1977): Evidence for the release of vasopressin and oxytocin into cerebrospinal fluid: Measurements in plasma and CSF of intact and hypophysectomized rats. Neuroendocrinology, 24: 108—118

Dousa, T. P., Barness, L. D.: (1974): The effect of colchicine and vinblastine on the cellular action of vasopressin in mammalian kidney. A possible role for microtubulus. J. Clin. Invest., 54: 252—256

DuVigneaud, V., Gish, D. T., Katsoyannis, P. G.: (1954a): A synthetic preparation possessing biological properties associated with arginine-vasopressin. J. Am. chem. Soc., 76: 4751—4752

DuVigneaud, V., Ressler, C., Swan, J. M., Katsoyannis, P. G., Roberts, C. W.: (1954b): The synthesis of oxytocin. J. Am. chem. Soc., 76: 3115—3121

Dunger, B. B., Lightman, S., Williams, M., Preece, M. A., Grant, D. B.: (1985): Lack of thirst, osmoreceptor dysfunction, early puberty and abnormally aggressive behavior in two boys. Clin. Endocrinol., 22: 469—478

Dunger, D. B., Seckl, J. R., Grant, D. B., Yeoman, L., Lightman, S. L.: (1988): A short water deprivation test incorporating urinary arginine vasopressin estimations for the investigation of posterior pituitary function in child. Acta Endocrinol., 117: 13—18

Dunn, F. L., Brennan, T. J., Nelson, A. E., Robertson, G. L.: (1973): The role of blood osmolality and volume in regulating vasopressin secretion in the rat. J. Clin. Invest., 52: 3212—3215

Durr, J. A., Hoggard, J. G., Hunt, J. M.: (1987): Diabetes insipidus in pregnancy associated with abnormally high circulating vasopressinase activity. N. Engl. J. Med., 316: 1 070

Dutton, A., Dyball, R. E. J.: (1979): Phasic firing enhances vasopressin release from the rat neurohypophysis. J. Physiol. (Lond.) 290: 433—440

Dyer, R. G.: (1988): Oxytocin and parturition — new complications. J. Endocrinol., 116: 167—168

Dzau, V. J.: (1987): Renal and circulatory mechanisms in congestive heart failure. Kidney Int., 31: 1402—1415

Earnest, D. J., Sladek, C. D.: (1986): Circadian rhythms of vasopressin release from individual rat suprachiasmatic explants in vitro. Brain Res., 382: 129—133

257

Edelmann, C. H., Spitzer, A.: (1969): The maturing kidney: A modern view of well balanced infants with imbalanced nephrons. J. Pediatr., 75: 509—519

Edelmann, L. E., Barnett, H. L., Troupkov, V.: (1960): Renal concentrating mechanism in newborn infants—effects of dietary protein and water content, role of urea and responsiveness to antidiuretic hormone. J. Clin. Invest, 39: 1062—1069

Emsley, R. A., Potgieter, A., Taljaard, J. J. F., Coetzee, D., Joubert, G., Gledhill, R. F.: (1987): Impaired water excretion and elevated plasma vasopressin in patients with alcohol-withdrawal symptoms. Quart. J. Med., 244: 671—678

Engel, W. D., Baumgart, S., Schwartz, J. G., Fox, W. W., Polin, R. A.: (1981): Insensible water loss in the critically ill neonate. Am. J. Dis. Child., 135: 516—520

Engle, W. D., Arant, B. S.: (1983): Renal handling of beta-2-microglobulin in the human neonate. Kidney Int. 24: 360—364

Epstein, F. H., Kleeman, C. R., Pursel, S.: (1957): The effect of feeding protein and urea on renal concentrating process. J. Clin. Invest., 36: 635—639

Epstein, F. H., Rosa, R. M., Bunn, H. F.: (1984): Treatment of sickle cell anemia with dDAVP. In: The Neurohypophysis. Physiological and clinical aspects. Plenum Med. Book Comp. New York—London: 191

Epstein, M.: (1978): Renal effects of head-out water immersion in man: Implications for an understanding of volume homeostasis. Physiol. Rev., 58: 529—581

Epstein, M: (1985): Derangements of water handling in liver disease. Gastroenterology, 89: 1415—1425

Epstein. M., Hollenberg, N. K.: (1976): Age as a determinant of renal sodium concentration in normal man. J. Lab. Clin. Med., 87: 411—417

Epstein. M., Preston, S., Weitzman, R. E.: (1981): Isoosmotic central blood volume expansion suppresses plasma arginine vasopressin in normal man. J. Clin. Endocrinol. Metab., 52: 256—262

Errington, M. L., Rocha e Silva, M.: (1974): On the role of vasopressin and angiotensin in the development of irreversible haemorrhagic shock. J. Physiol. (Lond.), 242: 119—141

Ervin, M. G., Amico, J. A., Leake, R. D., Ross, M. G., Robinson, A. G., Fisher, D. A.: (1988): Arginine-vasotocin and a novel oxytocin-vasotocin-like material in plasma of human newborns. Biol. Neonate, 53: 17—22

Ervin, M. G., Leake, R. D., Ross, M. G., Calvario, G. C., Fisher, D. A.: (1985): Arginine vasotocin in ovine fetal blood, urine and amniotic fluid. J. Clin. Invest., 75: 1696—1701

Ervin, M. G., Ross, M. G., Leake, R. D., Fisher, D. A.: (1986): Changes in steady state plasma arginine vasotocin levels affect ovine fetal renal and cardiovascular function. Endocrinology, 118: 759—765

Farini, F.: (1913): Diabete insipido ed opoterapia. Gass. Osped. Clin., 34: 1135—1139

Faye. H., Payne, R. B.: (1986): Rapid measurement of serum water to assess pseudo-hyponatremia. Clin. Chem., 32: 983—986

Fehm—Wolfsdorf, G., Bork, J., Voigt, K. H., Fehm, H. L.: (1984): Human memory and neurohypophyseal hormones: Opposite effects of vasopressin and oxytocin. Psychoneuroendocrinology, 9: 285—292

Feig, P. V.: (1981): Hypernatremia and hypotonic syndromes. Med. Clin. North. Am., 65: 271—290

Feig, P. V., Mc Curdy, D. K.: (1977): The hypertonic state. New Engl. J. Med., 297: 1444—1454

Fejes—Toth, G., Naray, A., Ratge, D.: (1985): Evidence against role of antidiuretic hormone in support of blood pressure during dehydratation. Am. J. Physiol., 249: H42—H48

Felsl, I., Gottsmann, M., Eversmann, T., Jehle, W., Uhlich, E.: (1978): Influence of various stress situations on vasopressin secretion in man. Acta Endocrinol., 215: 122—123

Ferguson, D. W., Abboud, F. H., Mark, A. L.: (1984): Selective impairment of baro-reflex-mediated vasoconstrictor responses in patients with ventricular dysfunction. Circulation, 69: 451—460

Fichman, M. P., Brooker, G.: (1972): Deficient renal cyclic adenosine 3'—5'-mono-phosphate production in nephrogenic diabetes insipidus. J. Clin. Endocrinol. Metab., 35: 35—47

Fichman, M. P., Vorherr, H., Kleeman, C. R.: (1971): Diuretic induced hyponatremia. Ann. Int. Med., 75: 853—863

Finberg, L.: (1973): Hypernatremic dehydratation in infants. New Engl. J. Med., 289: 196—201

Finberg, L.: (1980): The role of oral electrolyte-glucose solutions in hydration of children: international and domestic aspects. J. Pediat., 96: 51—55

Finberg, L., Kiley, J., Luttrell, L. N.: (1963): Mass accidental salt poisoning in infancy: a study of a hospital disaster. JAMA, 184: 187—190

Fisher, A. W. F., Price, P. G., Leceris, K.: (1979): A 3-dimensional reconstruction of the hypothalamo-neurohypophyseal system of the rat. Cell. Tiss. Res., 204: 343—354

Fisher, B. M., Baylis, P. H., Frier, B. M.: (1987): Plasma oxytocin, arginine vaso-pressin and atrial natriuretic peptide responses to insulin-induced hypoglycemia in man. Clin. Endocrinol., 26: 179—185

Fisher, D. A.: (1986): The unique endocrine milieu of the fetus. J. Clin. Invest., 78: 603—611

Fitzsimons, J. T.: (1985): Physiology and pathology of thirst and sodium appetite. In: The Kidney: Physiology and Pathophysiology. Raven Press, New York: 885—901

Fjellestad, A., Czernichow, P.: (1986): Central diabetes insipidus in children. V. Oral treatment with a vasopressin hormone analogue (dDAVP). Acta Paediatr. Scand., 75: 605—610

Fliers, E., Swaab, D. F., Pool, C. W., Verwer, R. W. H.: (1985): The vasopressin and oxytocin neurons in the human supraoptic and paraventricular nucleus: changes with aging and senile dementia. Brain Res., 342: 45—53

Forrest, J. N., Cox, M., Hong, C., Morrison, G., Bia, M., Singer, I.: (1973): Demeclo-cycline induced nephrogenic diabetes insipidus. In vivo and in vitro studies. Ann. Int. Med., 79: 679—684

Forrest, J. N., Cox, M., Hong, C., Morrison, G., Bia, M., Singer, I.: (1978): Superiority of demeclocycline over lithium in the treatment of chronic syndrome of inappropriate secretion of ADH. N. Engl. J. Med., 298: 173—179

Forsling, M. L., Stromberg, P., Akerlund, M.: (1982): Effect of ovarian steroids on vasopressin secretion. J. Endocrinol., 95: 147—151

Fressinaud, P., Corvol, P., Mentard, J., Allegrini, J.: (1974): Radioimmunoassay of urinary antidiuretic hormone in man: Stimulation — suppression tests. Kidney Int., 6: 184—190

Friedman, A. L., Segar, W. E.: (1979): Antidiuretic hormone excess. J. Pediat., 94: 521—526

Friis-Hansen, B.: (1983): Water distribution in the fetus and newborn infant. Acta Paed. Scand., Suppl. 305: 7—11

Fromter, E.: (1987): Cellular handling of water. Kidney Int., 32 (suppl. 21): S2—S7

Fuchs, A. E., Periyasamy, S., Alexandrova, M., Sollof, M. S.: (1983): Correlation between oxytocin receptor concentration and responsiveness to oxytocin in pregnant rat myometrium: effect of ovarian steroids. Endocrinology, 113: 742—749

Fujiwara, P., Berry, M., Hauger, P., Cogan, M.: (1985): Chicken-soup hypernatremia (letter). N. Engl. J. Med., 313: 161—1162

Gaffney, P. R., Jenkins, D. H.: (1983): Vasopressin: Mediator of the clinical signs of fetal distress. Br. J. Obstetr. Gynecol., 90: 987

Galla, J. H., Brooker, B. B., Luke, R. G.: (1986): Role of the loop segment in the urinary concentrating defect of hypercalcemia. Kidney Int., 29: 977—982

Ganguly, A., Robertson, G. L.: (1980): Elevated threshold for vasopressin release in primary aldosteronism (abstract). Clin. Res., 28: 330A

Garcia, H., Kaplan, S. L., Feigin, R. D.: (1981): Cerebrospinal fluid concentration of arginine vasopressin in children with bacterial meningitis. J. Pediat., 98: 67—70

Garcia, M., Miller, M., Moses, A. M.: (1971): Chlorpropamide induced water retention in patients with diabetes mellitus. Ann. Intern. Med., 75: 549—553

Garcia-Perez, A., Smith, W. L.: (1984): Apical-basolateral membrane asymmetry in canine cortical collecting tubular cells. J. Clin. Invest. 74: 63—74

Gardiner, S. M., Bennett, T.: (1983): The cardiovascular and renal responses to short-term isolation in Brattleboro rats. Clin. Sci., 64: 377—382

Gauer, O. H., Henry, J. P.: (1963): Circulatory basis of fluid volume control. Physiol. Rev., 43: 423—481

Gauer, O. H., Henry, J. P., Behn, C.: (1970): The regulation of extracellular fluid volume. Ann. Rev. Physiol., 32: 547—595

Gauflin, L., Skowsky, W. R., Goodman, S. J.: (1977): Release of ADH during mass-induced elevation of intracranial pressure. J. Neurosurg., 46: 627—638

Geheb, M., Cox, M.: (1980): Renal effect of demeclocycline. JAMA, 234: 2514—2519

Gellai, M., Silverstein, J. H., Hwang, J. C., La Rochelle, F. T., Valtin, H.: (1984): Influence of vasopressin on renal hemodynamics in conscious Brattleboro rats. Am. J. Physiol., 246: F819—F827

Gennari, F. J.: (1984): Serum osmolality: uses and limitations. New Engl. J. Med., 310: 102—105

Gennari, F. J., Kassirer, J. P.: (1974): Osmotic diuresis. New Engl. J. Med., 291: 714—720

George, C. P. L., Messerli, F. H., Genest, J., Nowaczynski, W., Boucher, R., Kuchel, O., Rojo-Ortega: (1975): Diurnal variation of plasma vasopressin in man. J. Clin. Endocrinol. Metab., 41: 332—338

Gill, J. R., Bartter, F. C.: (1961): On the impairment of renal concentrating ability in prolonged hypercalcemia and hypercalciuria in man. J. Clin. Invest., 40: 716—722

Gill, G., Baylis, B., Burn, J.: (1985): A case of "essential" hypernatremia due to resetting of the osmostat. Clin. Endocrinol., 22: 545—551

Godard, C., Geering, J. M., Geering, K., Vallotton, M. B.: (1979): Plasma renin activity related to sodium balance, renal function and urinary vasopressin in the newborn infant. Pediatr. Res., 13: 742—745

Godard, C., Vallotton, M. B., Favre, L.: (1982): Urinary prostaglandins, vasopressin and kallikrein excretion in healthy children from birth to adolescence. J. Pediatr., 100: 898—902

Goetz, K. L.: (1988): Physiology and pathophysiology of atrial peptides. Am. J. Physiol., 254: E1—E15

Gold, P. W., Goodwin, F. K., Baccanger, J. C., Post, R. M., Weingartner, M., Robertson, G. L.: (1981): Central vasopressin function in affective illness. Int. J. Ment. Menth, 9: 91—107

Gold, P. W., Keye, W., Robertson, G. L., Ebert, M.: (1983a): Abnormalities in plasma and cerebrospinal fluid arginine vasopressin in patients with anorexia nervosa. New Engl. J. Med., 308: 1117—1123

Gold, P. W., Robertson, G. L., Ballanger, J. C., Kaye, W., Chen. J., Rubinson, D. R., Goodwin, F. K.: (1983b): Carbamazepine diminishes the sensitivity of the plasma arginine vasopressin response to osmotic stimulation. J. Clin. Endocrinol. Metab., 57: 952—957

Gold, P. W., Robertson, G. L., Post, R. M., Kaye, W., Ballenger, J., Rubinow, D., Goodwin, F. K.: (1983c): The effect of lithium on the osmoregulation of arginine vasopressin secretion. J. Clin. Endocrinol. Metab., 56: 295—299

Goldberg, M.: (1981): Hyponatremia. Med. Clin. North Amer., 65: 251—269

Goldfarb, S., Agus, Z. S.: (1984): Mechanism of the polyuria of hypercalcemia. Am. J. Nephrol., 4: 69—76

Goldman, M. B., Luchnis, D. J., Robertson, G. L.: (1988): Mechanism of altered water metabolism in psychotic patients with polydipsia and hyponatremia. New Engl. J. Med., 318: 397—403

Goldsmith, S. R., Dodge, D., Cowley, A. W.: (1987): Nonosmotic influences on osmotic stimulation of vasopressin in humans. Am. J. Physiol., 252: H85—H88

Goldsmith, S. R., Francis, G. S., Cowley, A. W.: (1986a): Arginine-vasopressin and renal response to water loading in congestive heart failure. Am. J. Cardiol., 58: 295—299

Goldsmith, S. R., Francis, G. S., Cowley, A. W., Goldenberg, I. F., Cohn, J. N.: (1986b): Hemodynamic effects of infused arginine vasopressin in congestive hearth failure J. Am. Coll. Cardiol., 8: 779—783

Goldsmith, S. R., Francis, G. S., Cowley, A. W., Levine, T. B., Cohn, J. N.: (1983): Increased plasma arginine vasopressin in patients with congestive heart failure. JACC, 1: 1385—1390

Goldstein, R.: (1984): The involvement of arginine-vasotocin in the maturation of the kitten brain. Peptides, 5: 25—28

Goodnick, P. J., Fieve, R. R.: (1985): Plasma lithium level and interepisode functioning in bipolar disorder. Am. J. Psychiatry, 142: 761—762

Graves, S. W., Williams, G. H.: (1987): Endogenous digitalis-like natriuretic factors. Ann. Rev. Med. 38: 433—444

Green, J. R., Buchan, T. L., Alvord, E., Svanson, A. G.: (1967): Hereditary and idiopathic types of diabetes insipidus. Brain, 90: 707—713

Greger, N. G., Kirkland, R. T., Clayton, G. W., Kirkland, J. L.: (1986): Central diabetes indipidus: 22 year's experience. Am. J. Dis. Child., 140: 551—554

Grigoriev, A. I., Lichardus, B., Lobachik, V. I., Michajlovskij, N., Zhidkov, V. V., Sukhanov, Yu. V: (1983): Regulation of man's hydratation status during gravity-induced blood redistribution. The Physiologist, 26: 528—529

Gross, P. A., Ketteler, M., Hausmann, C., Ritz, E.: (1987): The charted and uncharted waters of hyponatremia. Kidney Int., 33: (suppl. 21) S67—S75

Gross, P. A., Kim, K. J., Anderson, R. J.: (1983): Mechanisms of escape from desmopressin in rat. Circ. Res., 53: 794—804

Gross, P. A., Pehrisch, H., Rascher, W., Hackenthal, E., Schomig, A., Ritz, E.: (1986): Vasopressin in hyponatremia: what stimuli? J. Cardiovasc. Pharmacol., 8: (suppl. 7) S92—S95

Grossman, S. H., Davis, D., Gunnells, J. C., Shand, D. G.: (1982): Plasma norepinephrine in the evaluation of baroreceptor function in humans. Hypertension, 4: 566—571

Groszman, R. J., Kravetz, D., Bosch, J., Glickman, M., Bruix, J., Bredfeldt, J., H. Conn, Rodes, J.: (1982): Nitroglycerin improves the hemodynamic response to vasopressin in portal hypertension. Hepatology, 2: 757—762

Gruber, K. A., Wilkin, L. D., Johnson, A. K.: (1986): Neurohypophyseal hormone release and biosynthesis in rats with lesions of the anteroventral third ventricle (AV3V) region. Brain Res., 378: 115—119

Gruskin, A. B., Baluarte, H. J., Prebis, J. W., Polinsky, M. S., Morgenstern, B. Z., Perlman, S. A.: (1982): Serum sodium abnormalities in children. Pediat. Clin. North Am., 29: 907—932

Guignard, J. P., Torrado, A., Da Cunna, O., Gautier, E.: (1975): Glomerular filtration rate in first three weeks of life. J. Pediatr., 87: 268—272

Guillon, G., Balestre, M. N., Roberts, J. M., Bottari, S. P.: (1987): Oxytocin and vasopressin: distinct receptors in myometrium. J. Clin. Endocrinol. Metab., 64, 1129—1135

Gutsche, H. V., Peterson, L. N., Levine, D. Z.: (1984): In vivo evidence of impaired solute transport by the thick ascending limb in potassium depleted rats. J. Clin. Invest., 73: 908—916

Hadeed, A. H., Leake, R. D., Weitzman, R. E., Fisher, D. A.: (1979): Possible mechanisms of high blood levels of vasopressin during the neonatal period. J. Pediatr., 94: 805—808

Hall, J. E., Montani, J. P., Woods, L. L., Mizelle, H. L.: (1986): Renal escape from vasopressin: role of pressure diuresis. Am. J. Physiol., 250: F907—F916

Halter, J. B., Goldberg, A. P., Robertson, G. L., Porte, D.: (1977): Selective osmoreceptor dysfunction in the syndrome of chronic hypernatremia. J. Clin. Endocrinol., 44: 609—616

Hamburger-Bar, R., Eisenberg, J., Belmaker, R. H.: (1987): Animal and clinical studies of vasopressin effects on learning and memory. Isr. J. Med. Sci., 23: 12—18

Hammond, D. N., Moll, G. W., Robertson, G. L., Chelmicka-Schorr, E.: (1986): Hypodipsic hyponatremia with normal osmoregulation of vasopressin. New Engl. J. Med., 315: 433—436

Handelmann, G. E., Russel, J. T.: (1983): Vasopressin administration to neonatal rats reduces antidiuretic response in adult kidneys. Peptides, 4: 827—832

Hansell, P., Goranson, A., Leppälouto, J., Arjamaa, O., Vakkuri, O., Ulfendahl, H. R.: (1987): CNS-induced natriuresis is not mediated by the atrial natriuretic factor. Acta Physiol. Scand. 129: 222—227

Hansen, M., Hammer, M., Hummer, L.: (1980): Diagnostic and therapeutic implications of ectopic hormone production in small cell carcinoma of the lung. Thorax, 35: 101—106

Harmanci, M. C., Stern, P., Kachodorian, W. A., Valtin, H., DiScala, V. A.: (1980): Vasopressin and collecting duct intramembranous particle clusters: A dose-response relationship. Am. J. Physiol., 239: F560—564

Hays, R. M., Ding, G., Franki, N.: (1987): Morphological aspects of the action of ADH. Kidney Int., 32 (suppl. 21): S51—S55

Hebert, E.: (1981): Discovery of pro-opiomelanocortin, a cellular polyprotein. Trends Biochem. Sci., 6: 184—188

Hedge, G. A., Huffman, L. J.: (1987): Vasopressin and endocrine function. In: Vasopressin. Principles and properties. (Edit.: Gash, D. M., Boer, G. J.) Plenum Press, New York, 435—475

Helderman, J. H., Vestal, R. E., Rowe, J. W., Shock, N. W.: (1978): The response of arginine vasopressin to intravenous ethanol and hypertonic saline in man: the impact of aging. J. Gerontol., 33: 39—47

Heller, J., Stulc, J., Roth, Z.: (1959): The physiology of the antidiuretic hormone. I. A simple titration method. Physiol. bohemoslov., 8: 558—564

Hiller, W. D. B., O'Toole, M. L., Laird, R. H.: (1986): Hyponatremia and ultramarathons (letter). JAMA 256: 213

Hime, M. C., Richardson, J. A.: (1978): Diabetes insipidus and pregnancy: Case report, incidence and review of the literature. Obstetr. Gynecol. Surv., 33: 375—385

Himmelstein, D. U., Jones, A. A., Woolhandler, S.: (1983): Hypernatremic dehydration in nursing home patients: an indicator of neglect. J. Am. Geriatr. Soc., 31: 466 — 471

Hoeflinger, J. M., Dubied, M. G., Vallotton, M. B.: (1977): Urinary excretion of AVP in various forms of lung cancer. Clin. Res., 25: 295—301

Hofbauer, K. G., Seng Chin Mah: (1987): Vasopressin antagonists: present and future. Kidney Int., 32 (suppl. 21): S76—S82

Hogan, G. R., Dodge, P. R., Gill, S. R., Pickering, L. K., Master, S.: (1984): The incidence of seizures after rehydration of hypernatremic rabbits with intravenous or ad libitum oral fluids. Pediat. Res., 18: 340—345

Hollinshead, W. H.: (1964): The interphase of diabetes insipidus. Mayo Clin. Proc., 39: 92—100

Holmberg, L., Nilsson, M., Borge, L., Gunnarsson, M., Sjorin, E.: (1983): Platelet aggregation induced by 1-desamino-8-D-arginine vasopressin (dDAVP) in type II.B. von Willebrand's disease. New Engl. J. Med., 309: 816—821

Horký, K., Šrámková, J., Widimský, J., Dvořáková, J.: (1981): Concentrations of arginine vasopressin in plasma and urine in healthy subjects with differential states of hydration (Czech). Čas. Lék. Čes., 120: 665—670

Hussey, K. P.: (1985): Vasopressin therapy for upper gastrointestinal tract hemorrhage. Has its efficacy been proven? Arch. Int. Med., 145: 1263—1267

Jkkos, D., Luft, R., Olivecrona, H.: (1955): Hypophysectomy in man: Effect on water excretion during the first two postoperative months. J. Clin. Endocrinol. Metab., 15: 553—567

Imai, Y., Nolan, P. L., Johnston, C. I.: (1983): Restoration of suppressed baroreflex sensitivity in rats with hereditary diabetes insipidus (Brattleboro rats) by arginine vasopressin and dDAVP. Circ. Res., 43: 140—145

Ishikawa, S., Schrier, R. W.: (1982): Effect of arginine vasopressin antagonist on renal water excretion in glucocorticoid and mineralocorticoid deficient rats. Kidney Int., 22: 587—593

Ivanova, L. N., Solyenov, A. B., Zelenina, M. N., Khegam, I. I.: (1987): Decrease in the response to ADH of the rat kidney as a result of early postnatal tratment with cortison. Pflüger's Arch., 408: 328—332

Ivell, R., Schmale, H., Kirsch, B., Nahke, P., Richter, D.: (1986): Expression of a mutant vasopressin gene: differential polyadenylation and read-through of the mRNA 3'end in a frameshift mutant. EMBO J., 5: 971—977

Iwamoto, H. S., Rudolph, A. M., Keil, L. C., Heymann, M. A.: (1979): Hemodynamic responses of the sheep fetus to vasopressin infusion. Circ. Res., 44: 430—436

Jamison, R. L.: (1983): A patient with polyuria and hyponatremia. Kidney Int., 24: 256—267

Jamison, R. L.: (1987): Short and long loop nephrons. Kidney Int., 31: 597—605

Jamison, R. L., Kriz, W.: (1982): Urinary concentrating mechanism: Structure and function. Oxford University Press, New York—Oxford

Jamison, R. L., Oliver, R. E.: (1982): Disorders of urinary concentration and dilution. Am. J. Med., 72: 308—323

Janda, J., Blahová, K., Marek, V., Eliášek, J.: (1988): Untersuchung des Konzentrationsvermögens bei nierengesunden Kindern und Jugendlichen. Kinderarztl. Prax. 56: 133—137

Jard, S.: (1983a): Vasopressin isoreceptors in mammals: relation to cyclic AMP dependent and cyclic AMP independent transduction mechanisms. Curr. Top. Membr. Transp. 18: 255—285

Jard, S.: (1983b): Vasopressin: Mechanism of receptor activation. Prog. Brain Res., 60: 383—394

Jard, S., Elands, J., Schmidt, A., Tribollet, E., Barberis, C.: (1988): Vasopressin and oxytocin receptors. 8th International Congress of Endocrinology, Kyoto 1988, Abstracts S—167

Jard, S., Guillon, G., Gaillard, J. M. R., Schoenenberg, P., Muller, A. F., Manning, M., Sawyer: (1986): Vasopressin antagonists facilitate the discrimination of a novel vasopressin receptor sub-type in the rat adenohypophysis. Mol. Pharmacol., 30: 171—177

Jespersen, B., Danielsen, H., Pedersen, E. B.: (1987): Effect of chronic hypokalemia on renal concentrating ability and secretion of arginine vasopressin. Scand. J. Clin. Lab. Invest., 47: 5—9

Jewell, P. A., Verney, E. B.: (1957): An experimental attempt to determine the site of neurohypophyseal osmoreceptors in the dog. Philos. Trans. R. Soc. London Ser. B., 240: 197—324

Johnson, A. K.: (1985): Role of the periventricular tissue surrounding the anteroventral third ventricle (AV3V) in the regulation of body fluid homeostasis. In: Vasopressin (edit. Schrier, R. W.), Raven Press, New York: 319—331

Johnston, C. I.: (1985): Vasopressin in circulatory control and hypertension. J. Hypertension, 3: 557—569

Jolles, J.: (1986): Cognitive, emitional and behavioural dysfunctions in aging and dementia. Prog. Brain. Res., 70: 15—39

Joppich, R., Haberle, D. A., Weber, P. C.: (1981): Studies on the immaturity of the ADH-dependent cAMP system in conscious newborn piglets— possible inpairing effects of renal prostaglandins. Pediat. Res., 15: 278—281

Kamoi, K., Robertson, G. L.: (1985): Opiates and vasopressin secretion. In: Vasopressin (Edit. by Schrier, R. W.), New York, Raven Press: 259—264

Kaplan, S. L., Feigin, R. D.: (1978): The syndrome of inappropriate secretion of antidiuretic hormone in children with bacterial meningitis. J. Pediatr., 92: 758—761

Kasson, B. G., Adashi, E. Y., Hsveh, A. J. W.: (1986): Arginine vasopressin in the testis: An intragonadal peptide control system. Endocrine Rev., 7: 156 —168

Kasting, N. W.: (1986): Characteristics of body temperature, vasopressin and oxytocin responses to endotoxin in the rat. Can. J. Physiol, Pharmacol., 64: 1575—1578

Kern, P. A., Robbins, R. J., Bichet, D., Berl, T., Verbalis, J. G.: (1986): Syndrome of inappropriate antidiuresis in the absence of arginine vasopressin. J. Clin. Endocrinol. Metab., 62: 148—152

Kerpel-Fronius, E.: (1959): Pathologie und Klinik des Salz- und Wassserhaushaltes. Akademia, Budapest

Khokhar, A. M., Ramage, C. M., Slater, J. D. H.: (1978): Radioimmunoassay of arginine-vasopressin in human urine and its use in physiological and pathological states. J. Endocrinol., 79: 375—389

Kim, J. K., Summer, S. N., Berl, T.: (1984): Studies on the cyclic AMP system in the inner medullary collecting duct of the potassium depleted rat. Kidney Int., 26: 384—391

Kinter, L. B., Huffman, W. F., Stassen, F. L.: (1988): Antagonists of the antidiuretic activity of vasopressin. Am. J. Physiol., 254: F165—177

Kiss, J. Z., Williams, T. H., Palkovits, M.: (1984): Distributions and projections of cholecystokinin immunoreactive neurons in the hypothalamic paraventricular nucleus of the rat. J. Comp. Neurol., 227: 173—181

Kobrinsky, N. L., Israels, E. D., Cheang, M. S., Doyle, J. J., Winter, J. S. D., Walker,

R. D., Bishop, A. J.: (1985): Absent factor VIII response to synthetic vasopressin analogue (dDAVP) in nephrogenic diabetes insipidus. Lancet, i: 1293—1294

Kobrinsky, N. L., Israels, E. D., Gerrard, J. M.: (1984): Shortening of the bleeding time by 1-deamino-8-D-arginine vasopressin in various bleeding disorders. Lancet, i: 145—148

Kobrinsky, N. L., Letts, R. M., Patel, L. R., Israels, E. D., Monson, R. C., Schwetz, N., Cheang, M. S.: (1987): 1-deamino-8-D-arginine vasopressin (desmopressin) decreases operative blood loss in patients having Harrington rod spinal fusion surgery. Ann. Int. Med., 107: 446

Kokko, J. P.: (1987): The role of collecting duct in urinary concentration. Kidney Int., 31: 606—610

Kokko, J. P., Rector, F. C.: (1972): Countercurrent multiplication system without active transport in inner medulla. Kidney Int., 2: 214—223

Kopta, G. A., Valocik, R. E.: (1985): Antagonism of vasopressin induced coronary artery constriction by the vasopressin antagonist d(CH2)5 Tyr (Me) AVP. J. Cardiovasc. Pharmacol., 7: 958—963

Korányi, A. V.: (1897): Physiologische und klinische Untersuchungen über den osmotischen Druck thierischer Flüssigkeiten. Z. Klin. Med., 33: 1

Kortas, C., Bichet, D. G., Rouleau, J. L., Schrier, R. W.: (1986): Vasopressin in congestive heart failure. J. Cardiovascular. Pharmacol. 8 (suppl. 7): S107—S110

Koskimes, O., Pylkkanen, J., Vilska, J.: (1984): Water intoxication in infants caused by urine concentration test with vasopressin analog, dDAVP. Acta Paed. Scand, 73: 131—132

Kosten, T. R., Forresst, J. N. Jr.: (1986): Treatment of severe lithium-induced polyuria with amiloride. Am. J. Psychiatry, 143: 1563—1568

Kovács, G. L., Bohus, B., Versteeg, D. H. G., De Kloet, E. R., De Wied, D.: (1979): Effect of oxytocin and vasopressin on memory consolidation. Brain Res., 175: 303—314

Kovács, G. L., Telegdy, G.: (1982): Role of oxytocin in memory and amnesia. Pharmacol. Ther., 18: 375—395

Kovács, L.: (1985): Renal regulation of water homeostasis in infants and children. Doctor of Science Thesis, Bratislava. Comenius University

Kovács, L., Birčák, J., Lichardus, B.: (1987a): Endogenous digoxin-like substance in the urine of preterm infants (letter). Eur. J. Pediat., 146: 622

Kovács, L., Huttová, E., Melicherčik, O., Gucalová, Y., Lichardus, B., Michaličkova, J.: (1985a): Breast feeding and sodium level in human milk (Slov). Čs. Pediat., 39: 214—217

Kovács, L., Kerekes, L., Lichardus, B., Sulyok, E.: (1988): Salt supplementation increases urinary excretion of endogenous digoxin-like immunoreactivity in preterm infants. (abstr). 5th Internat. Congress of Pediat. Nephrol. of Socialist. Countries, Warsawa

Kovács L., Lehotská, V., Némethová, V.: (1984a): Hyponatremic states I. Pathophysiologic mechanisms (Slov). Čs. Pediat., 39: 214—217

Kovács, L., Lehotská, V., Némethová, V., Lichardus, B.: (1984b): Hypotonic syndrome (Hung). Orvosképzés, 59: 466—479

Kovács, L., Lehotská, V., Némethová, V., Lichardus, B.: (1985): Diagnosis of disturbances of water homeostasis in infants and children (Hung). Orv. Hetilap, 126: 255—258

Kovács, L., Lehotská, V., Némethová, V., Michajlovskij, N., Benko, J., Lichardus, B.: (1984): Syndrome of inappropriate secretion of antidiuretic hormone (Hung). Gyermekgyógyászat, 35: 493—498

Kovács, L., Lehotská, V., Némethová, V., Michajlovskij, N., Michaličková, J., Lichar-

dus, B.: (1985b): Simple diagnosis of diabetes insipidus and vasopressin excess. Exp. Clin. Endocrinol., 85: 228—234

Kovács L., Lichardus, B., Birčák, J., Michajlovskij, N., Némethová, V., Lehotská, V.: (1987b): Normovolemic hyponatremia in hospitalized children (Slov). Čs. Pediat., 42: 326—331

Kovács, L., Lichardus, B., Michajlovskij, N., Lehotská, V., Birčák, J.: (1987): Hospital acquired hyponatremia in infants and children (Hung). Orv. Hetilap, 128: 1027—1031

Kovács, L., Lichardus, B., Michajovskij, N., Lehotská, V., Šašinka, M., Birčák, J.: (1987): Severe euvolemic hyponatremia (abstr.). Int. J. Pediat. Nephrol., 8: 114

Kovács, L., Lichardus, B., Ponecová, M., Mašurová, A., Birčák, J., Sulyok, E.: (1988): Endogenous digoxin-like immunoreactivity in preterm infants with late hyponatremia. Contr. Nephrol. vol. 67 (Edit.: Boda, D., Turi, S.), Karger, Basel, pp. 145—148.

Kovács, L., Šašinka, M., Lichardus, B., Tulassay, T., Michajlovskij, N., Birčák, J.: (1987): Renal salt and water handling and urinary vasopressin response during water immersion in nephrotic syndrome (abstr.). Int. J. Pediat. Nephrol., 8: 108

Kovács, L., Šašinka, M., Lichardus, B., Tulassay, T., Michajlovskij, N., Birčák, J.: (1988a): Effect of water immersion on renal function and vasopressin secretion in children with nephrotic syndrome (Russian). Pediatria (Moscow), № 5: 38—41

Kovács, L., Šoltés, L.: (1983): Syndrome of inappropriate secretion of antidiuretic hormone in infants with acute respiratory infection (Slov). Čs. Pediat., 38: 164—166

Kovács, L., Sulyok, E.: (1984): Hyponatremia in preterm infants. Arginine vasopressin secretion (letter). Arch. Dis. Child., 59: 1107

Kovács, L., Sulyok, E., Lichardus, B., Michajlovskij, N., Birčák, J.: (1986): Renal response to arginine-vasopressin in premature infants with late hyponatremia. Arch. Dis. Child., 61: 1030—1032

Kramer, H. J.: (1985): Mechanismen der postobstructiven Polyurie. Klin. Wochenschr., 63: 934—943

Kramer, H. J., Lichardus, B.: (1986): Atrial natriuretic hormones — thirty years after the discovery of atrial volume receptors. Klin. Wochensch., 64: 719—731

Kramer, J. H., Lichardus, B.: (1987): Regulation of body fluid volume and disorders of sodium homeostasis. Curr. Nephrol., 10, Year Book Medical Publishers, Inc., Chicago, USA, 221—266

Kramer, H. J., Lichardus, B., DeWardener, H. E.: (1989): Natriuretic hormones and disorders of sodium homeostasis. Curr. Nephrol., 12, Year Book Medical Publishers, Inc. Chicago, USA, 39—86.

Kregenow, F. M.: (1981): Osmoregulatory salt transporting mechanisms: Control of cell volume in an isotonic media. Ann. Rev. Physiol., 43: 493—505

Kuhn, W., Ryffel, K.: (1942): Herstellung konzentrierter Lösungen aus verdünnten durch blosse Membranwirkung. Ein Modellversuch zur Function der Niere. Hoppe-Seylers Z. Physiol. Chem., 276: 145—178

Kvetňanský, R., Lichardus, B., Ježová, D., Opršalová, Z., Makara, G. B.: (1988): Vasopressin and dDAVP reduce elevated plasma catecholamine levels in rats with hypothalamic deafferentation. Cell. Molec. Neurobiol., 8: 225—234

Laczi, F., Van Ree, J. M., Wagner, G., Szilárd, J., László, F. A., De Wied, D.: (1983b): Effects of desglycinamide-arginine vasopressin (DGAVP) on memory processes in diabetes insipidus patients and in non-diabetic subjects. Acta Endocrinol., 102: 205—212

Laczi, F., Van Ree, J. M., Balogh, L., Szász, A., Jandaházy, I., Wagner, A., Gáspár, R.: (1983c): Lack of effect of DGAVP on memory in patients with Korsakoff syndrome. Acta Endocrinol., 104: 177—182

Lang, R. E., Heil, J. W. E., Ganten, D., Hermann, K., Unger, T., Rascher, W.: (1983): Oxytocin unlike vasopressin is a stress hormone in the rat. Neuroendocrinology, 37: 314—316

László, F. A., Baláspiri, L.: (1986): Experimental water intoxication induced by dDAVP in rat, and its prevention with the vasopressin antagonist d(CH_2) $_5$Tyr(Et) AVP. Acta Med. Hung., 43: 333—339

Laycock, J. F., Penn, W., Shirley, D. G., Walter, S. J.: (1979): The role of vasopressin in blood pressure regulation immediately following acute haemorrhage in the rat. J. Physiol. (Lond.), 296: 267—275

LeMoal, M., Dantler, R., Nemede, P., Badulel, A., Lebrun, C., Ettenberg, A., VanDerKooy, D.: (1984): Behavioral effects of peripheral administration of arginine vasopressin: A review of our search for a mode of action and hypothesis. Psychoneuroendocrinology, 9: 319

Leaf, A., Bartter, F. C., Santos, R. F., Wrong, O.: (1953): Evidence in man that urinary electrolyte loss induced by pitressin is a function of water retention. J. Clin. Invest., 53: 868—878

Leaf, A., Frazier, H. S.: (1961): Some recent studies on the action neurohypophyseal hormones. Prog. Cardiovasc. Dis., 4: 47—64

Leaf, A., Mamby, A. R.: (1952): Antidiuretic mechanism not regulated by extracellular fluid tonicity. J. Clin. Invest., 31: 60—71

Leake, R. D., Stegner, H., Palmer, S. M., Oaks, G. K., Fisher, D. A.: (1986): Arginine vasopressin and arginine vasotocin inhibit ovine fetal/maternal water transfer. Pediat. Res., 17: 583—586

Leake, R. D., Weitzman, R. E., Effros, R. M., Siegal, S. R., Fisher, D. A.: (1979): Maternal fetal osmolar homeostasis: fetal posterior pituitary autonomy. Pediat. Res., 13: 841—844

Legros, J. J.: (1979): The neurohypophyseal peptides. Triangle 18: 17—26

Lehotská, V., Kovács, L., Gucalová, Y., Škultétyová, M.: (1981a): Glomerular filtration rate in newborns and small infants (Slov). Čs. Pediat., 36: 570—573

Lehotská, V., Kovács, L., Némethová, V., Lichardus, B.: (1984): Effects of prolonged administration of dDAVP on the frequency of nocturnal enuresis (Hung). Gyermekgyógyászat, 35: 499—504

Lehotská, V., Lichardus, B., Némethová, V., Škultétyová, M.: (1981b): Adiuretin (dDAVP) test for evaluation of renal concentrating ability in infants (Slov). Čs. Pediat., 36: 324—327

Leimbach, W. N., Schmid, P. G., Mark, A. L.: (1984): Baroreflex control of plasma arginine-vasopressin in humans. Am. J. Physiol., 247: H638—H644

Lester, M. C., Nelson, P. B.: (1981): Neurological aspects of vasopressin release and the syndrome of inappropriate secretion of antidiuretic hormone. Neurosurgery, 8: 735—740

Levi, M., Peterson, L., Berl, T.: (1983): Mechanism of concentrating defect in hypercalcemia. Role of polydipsia and prostaglandins. Kidney Int., 23: 489—497

Levine, S. D., Schlondorff, D.: (1984): The role of calcium in the action of vasopressin. Semin. Nephrol., 4: 144—158

Levine, T. B., Francis, G. S., Goldsmith, S. R., Simon, A. B., Cohn, J. N.: (1982c): Activity of the sympathetic nervous system and renin of the angiotensin system assessed by plasma hormone levels in congestive heart failure. Am. J. Cardiol., 49: 1659—1666

Levine, T. B., Francis, J. A., Vrobel, T., Conh, J. N.: (1982b): Hyponatremia as a marker for high renin heart failure. Br. Heart J., 47: 161—166

Liard, J. F.: (1987): Vasopressin in cardiovascular regulation. In: Vasopressin analogues and portal hypertension. Eds. Lebrec. D., Blei. A. T., John Libbey Eurotext, Paris

Liard, J. F.: (1986): Cardiovascular effects of vasopressin: Some recent aspects. J. Cardiovasc. Pharmacol., 8 (suppl. 7): S61—S65

Libber, S., Harrison, H., Spector, D.: (1986): Treatment of nephrogenic diabetes insipidus with prostaglandin synthesis inhibitors. J. Pediatry, 108: 305—311

Lichardus, B.: (1978): Mechanisms of acute renal regulation of extracellular fluid volume (Slov). Veda, Bratislava 1978: 1—154

Lichardus, B., Albrecht, I., Ponec, J., Linhart. L.: (1977): Water deprivation for 24 hours increases selectively blood flow in posterior pituitary of conscious rats. Endocrinologia exp., 11: 99—104

Lichardus, B., Kvethanský, R., Makara, G., Opršalová. Z., Michajlovskij, N., Földeš, O., Ježová. D.: (1988): Circulating vasopressin attenuates the increased activity of the sympathetic nervous system induced by anterolateral deafferentation of the hypothalamus. In: Progress in Neuropeptide Research (edit.: Döhler, K.-D., Pawlikovski, M.). Borkhauser Verlag. Basel –Boston, 91—97.

Lichardus, B., Mitro, A., Cort, J. H.: (1965): Size of cell nuclei in the hypothalamus of the rat as a function of salt loading. Amer. J. Physiol., 208: 1075—1077

Lichardus, B., Okoličany, J., McKinley, M. J., Denton, D. A., Ponec, J.: (1987): Brain involvement in the regulation of renal sodium excretion. Klin. Wochenschr., 65: Suppl. VIII. 33—39

Lichardus, B., Pearce, J. W.: (1966): Evidence for a humoral natriuretic factor released by blood volume expansion. Nature, 209: 407—409

Lichardus, B., Pliška, V., Uhrín, V., Barth. T.: (1968): The cow as a model for investigating natriuretic activity. Lancet, i: 127—129

Lichardus, B., Ponec, J.: (1981): The past and the presence of a natriuretic hormone. Adv. Physiol. Sci., 22. Kidney and Body Fluids, Akadémia Kiadó-Pergamon Press, Budapest: 631—635

Lichardus, B., Sulyok, E., Kovács, L., Michajlovskij, N., Lehotská, V., Némethová, V., Ertl. T.: (1986): Renal salt wasting increases vasopressin excretion in preterm infants. In: Systemic hormones, neurotransmitters and brain development (ed. Dörner, G., McCann. S.) Karger, Basel: 179—184

Lichardus, B., Szaboová, A., Földeš, O., Ponec, J., Horký, K., Šrámková, J.: (1983): The impairment of osmoregulation in the rat offsprings of hyperadiuretic mothers is probably of renal nature. Exp. Clin. Endocrinol., 82: 107—110

Lichardus, B., Vigaš, M.: (1968): The effect of triglycyl-vasopressin on survival time of rats after traumatic shock. Endocrinologia exp., 2: 237—241

Lightwood, T. J., Smith, A. P.: (1984): SIADH due to treatment of lung cancer with cis-platin. Thorax, 39: 636—637

Lima, A., Lolait, S., Barlow, J., Avtelitano, D., Toh, B., Boublick, J., Abraham, J.: (1984): Immunoreactive arginine-vasopressin in Brattleboro rat ovary. Nature, 310: 61—64

Linas, S. L., Berl, T., Robertson, G. L., Aisenbray, G. A., Schrier, R. W., Anderson, R. J.: (1980): Role of vasopressin in the impaired water excretion of glucocorticoid deficiency. Kidney Int. 23: 58—67

Lindheimer, M. D., Barron, W. M., Davidson, J. M.: (1985): Water metabolism and vasopressin secretion in pregnancy. In: Vasopressin (edit.: Schrier, R. W.) Raven Press, New York. 229—240

Lorenz, J. M., Kleinman, L. L., Kotagal, V. R., Reller, M. D.: (1982): Water balance in very low-birth-weight infants: relationship to water and sodium intake and effect on outcome. J. Pediat., 101: 423—432

Ludlam, C. A., Peake. I. R., Allen, N.: (1980): Factor VIII and fibrinolytic response to deamino-8-D-arginine vasopressin in normal subjects and dissociate response in some patients with hemophilia. Br. J. Haematol., 45: 499—511

Luerssen, T. G., Robertson, G. L.: (1980): Cerebrospinal fluid vasopressin and vasotocin in health and disease. In: Neurobiology of cerebrospinal fluid (edit. Wood, B.) Plenum Publ. Corp. New York, 613—623

Lumpkin, M. D.: (1987): Arginine vasopressin as a thyreotropin-releasing hormone. Science, 235: 1070—1073

Lusher, J. M., Warrier, A. I.: (1984): dDAVP in von Willebrand's disease and in moderately severe hemophilia A. In: The Neurohypophysis (edit. Reichlin, S.), Plenum Medical Book Co, New York

Magee, G., Williams. M. H.: (1982): Treatment of massive hemoptysis with intravenous pitressin. Lung, 160: 165—169

Maggi, M., Malozowski, S., Kassis, S., Guardabasso, V., Rodbard, D.: (1987): Identification and characterization of two classes of receptors for oxytocin and vasopressin in porcine tunica albuginea, epididymis and vas deferens. Endocrinology, 120: 986—994

Mahowald, J. M., Himmelstein, D. U.: (1981): Hypernatremia in the elderly: relation to infection and mortality. J. Am. Geriatr. Soc., 29: 177—180

Majzoub, J. A., Carrazana, E. J., Shulman, J. S., Baker, K. J., Emanuel, R. L.: (1987): Defective regulation of vasopressin gene expression in Brattleboro rats. Am. J. Physiol. 252: E637—E642

Makara, G. B.: (1985): Mechanisms by which stressful stimuli activate the pituitary adrenal system. Fed. Proc., 44: 149—153

Mann, F. D.: (1987): Is loss of body water a factor of aging? Postgrad. Med., 81: 182—183

Manning, M., Sawyer. W. H.: (1986): Synthesis and receptor specifities of vasopressin antagonists. J. Cardiovasc. Pharmacol., 8 (suppl. 7): S29—S35

Manning, M., Bankowski, K., Sawyer, W. H.: (1987): Selective agonists and antagonists of vasopressin. In: Vasopressin (edit: Gash, M., Boer, G. J.) Plenum Press, New York, 335—368

Mannucci, P. M., Aberg, M., Nilsson, I. M., Robertson, B.: (1975): Mechanism of plasminogen activator and factor VIII increase after vasoactive drugs. Br. J. Hematol., 30: 81—93

Mannucci, P. M., Canciani, M. T., Rota, L., Donovan, B. S.: (1981): Response of factor VIII/vonWillebrand factor to dDAVP in healthy subjects and patients with hemophilia A and von Willenbrand's disease. Br. J. Haematol., 47: 283—293

Mannucci, P. M., Ruggeri, Z. M., Pareti, F. I.: (1977): 1-deamino-8-D-arginine vasopressin: A new pharmacologic approach to the management of hemophilia and von Willebrand's disease. Lancet, i: 869—872

Marek, J., Loutocky, A., Pacovsky, V., Zaoral, M.: (1978): Ten year experience with dDAVP in treatment of diabetes insipidus. Endokrinologie, 72: 188—194

Markwick, A. J., Lolait, S. J., Funder, J. W.: (1986): Immunoreactive arginine vasopressin in the rat thymus. Endocrinology, 119: 1690—1696

Markwick, C.: (1983): New ways to boost factor VIII in hemophilia: dDAVP for mild hemophilia A, Von Willebrand's disease. JAMA. 249: 3278—3279

Martinek, J., Heller, S., Čadek, K.: (1964): Renal functions in early postnatal life in human (Czech). Čs. Fyziol., 13: 441—460

Martinez-Maldonaldo, M.: (1980): Inappropriate antidiuretic hormone secretion of unknown origin. Kidney Int., 17: 554—567

Martinez-Maldonaldo, M., Stauroulaki-Tsapara, A., Tasparas, N., Suki, W. N., Eknoyan, G.: (1975): Renal effects of lithium in rats: Alterations in water and electrolyte metabolism and the response to AVP and cAMP during prolonged administration. J. Lab. Clin. Med., 8

Matsuo, H.: (1988): Two families of natriuretic peptide: ANP and BNP. 8th International Congress of Endocrinology, Kyoto 1988, Abstracts, s17

Mattar, J. A., Weil, H. H., Shubin, H., Stein, L.: (1974): Cardiac arrest in the critically ill: Hyperosmolal states following cardiac arrest. Am. J. Med., 56: 162—165

Mattle, H.: (1985): Neurologische Manifestationen der gestörten Osmolalität. Schweiz. Med. Wochenschr., 115: 882—889

Matulay, D., Watson, M.: (1967): Hypernatremia as a cause of brain damage. Arch. Dis. Child., 42: 485—491

McKinley, M. J.: (1987): An important region for osmoregulation: The anterior wall of the third ventricle. NIPS, 2: 13—16

McKinley, M. J., Congiu, M., Denton, D. A., Lichardus, B., Park, R. G., Tarjan, E., Weisinger, R. S.: (1985): Cerebrospinal fluid composition and homeostatic responses to dehydratation. In: Vasopressin (Ed. Schrier, R. W.), Raven Press, New York 1985: 299—309

McNeil, J. R.: (1983): Role of vasopressin in the control of arterial blood pressure. Can. J. Physiol. Pharmacol., 61: 1226—1235

Michajlovskij, N., Lichardus, B., Kvetňanský, R., Ponec, J.: (1988): Effect of acute and repeated immobilization stress on food and water intake, urine output and vasopressin changes in rats. Endocrinol. experiment. 22: 143—157

Mikaelsson, M., Nilson, I. M., Cedergreen, B., Jonsson, S., Rydberg, L., Wiechel, B.: (1984): The use of desmopressin (dDAVP) in the preparation of improved factor VIII concentrate. Scand. J. Haematol., 33: (suppl. 40): 93—101

Miller, M. (1987): Increased vasopressin secretion: an early manifestation of aging in the rat. J. Gerontol., 42: 3—7

Miller, M., Moses, A. M.: (1972): Urinary antidiuretic hormone in polyuric disorders and in inappropriate ADH syndrome. Ann. Int. Med., 77: 715—721

Miller, M., Dalakos, T., Moses, A. M., Fellerman, H., Streeten, D. H. P.: (1970): Recognition of partial defects in antidiuretic hormone secretion. Ann. int. Med., 73: 721—729

Miller, N. L., Finberg, L.: (1960): Peritoneal dialysis for salt poisoning. New Engl. J. Med., 263: 1347—1350

Milsom, S. R., Conaglen, J. V., Donald, R. A., Espiner, E. A., Nichols, E. A., Livesey, J. H.: (1985): Augmentation of the response to CRF on man: Relative contributions of endogenous angiotensin and vasopressin. Clin. Endocrinol., 22: 623—628

Miselis, R. R.: (1981): The efferent projections of the subfornical organ of the rat: a circumventricular organ within the network subserving water balance. Brain Res., 230: 1—23

Mitchell, R. H., Kirk, C. J., Billah, M. M.: (1979): Hormonal stimulation of phosphatidyl-inositol breakdown with particular reference to the hepatic effects of vasopressin. Biochem. Soc. Trans., 415: 81—147

Möhring, J., Glanzer, K., Maziel, J. A., Dusing, R., Kramer, H. J., Arbogast. R., Koch-Weser, J.: (1980a): Vasopressor effect of antidiuretic hormone in two patients with idiopatic orthostatic hypotension. J. Cardiovasc. Pharmacol., 2: 367—376

Möhring, J., Glanzer, K., Maciel, J. A., Dusing, R., Kramer, H. J., Arbogast, R., Koch-Weser, J.: (1980b): Greatly enhanced pressor response to ADH in patients with impaired cardiovascular reflexes due to idiopathic orthostatic hypotension. J. Cardiovasc. Pharmacol.

Montani, J. P., Liard, J. F., Schoun, J., Möhring, J.: (1980): Hemodynamic effects of exogenous and endogenous vasopressin at low plasma concentrations in conscious dogs. Circ. Res., 47: 346—355

Morel, F.: (1981): Sites of hormone action in the mammalian nephron. Am. J. Physiol., 240: F159—F164

Morel, F., Imbert-Teboul, M., Chabardes, D.: (1987): Receptors to vasopressin and other hormones in the mammalian kidney. Kidney Int., 31: 512—520

Morton, J. J., Padfield, P. L.: (1986): Vasopressin and hypertension in man. J. Cardiovasc. Pharmacol., 8: suppl. 7: S101—106

Moses, A. M.: (1964): Synthetic lysine vasopressin nasal spray in the treatment of diabetes insipidus. Clin. Pharmacol. Ther., 5: 422—427

Moses, A. M.: (1985): Clinical and laboratory observations in the adult with diabetes insipidus and related syndromes. Front. Horm. Res., 13: 156—175

Moses, A. M., Numann, P., Miller, M.: (1973): Mechanism of chlorpropamide-induced antidiuresis in man: Evidence for release of ADH and enhancement of peripheral action. Metabolism, 22: 59—64

Nagy, Gy., Mulchachey, J. J., Smyth, D. G., Neil, J. D.: (1988): The glycopeptide moiety of vasopressin—neurophysin precursor is neurohypophyseal prolactin releasing factor. Biochem. Biophys. Res. Comm., 151: 524—529

Narrins, R. G.: (1986): Therapy of hyponatremia. Does haste make waste? New Engl. J. Med., 314: 1573—1575

Narrins, R. G., Jones, E. R., Stom, M. C., Rudnick, M. R., Bastl, C. P.: (1982): Diagnostic strategies in disorders of fluid, electrolyte and acid-base homeostasis. Am. J. Med., 72: 496—521

Nash, M. A., Edelmann, C. H. Jr.: (1973): The developing kidney: immature function or inappropriate standard? Nephron, 11: 71—90

Natochin, Yu., Shakhmatova, E. I., Bakoš, P.: (1987): Water and sodium transport: Effect of calcium channel blocker and calmodulin antagonists on the apical and basolateral membrane of amphibian epithelia. Gen. Physiol. Biophys., 6: 35—44

Némethová, V., Lichardus, B.: (1974): Clinical experience with dDAVP (1-deamino-8-D-arginine vasopressin) in the treatment of diabetes insipidus in children. Endokrinologie, 63: 137—141

Némethová, V., Lichardus, B., Lehotská, V.: (1974): Evaluation of renal concentrating ability in children with synthetic analog of vasopressin, dDAVP (Slov). Bratisl. lek. Listy, 61: 229—236

Némethová, V., Lichardus, B., Lehotská, V.: (1977): Erfahrungen mit einem dDAVP-Schnelltest zur Bestimmung der Konzentrationsfähigkeit der Niere. Monatschr. Kinderheilk., 125: 165—168

Némethová, V., Lichardus, B., Lehotská, V.: (1979): Long term clinical experience with 1-deamino-8-D-arginine-vasopressin (dDAVP) in children with central diabetes insipidus (Slov). Bratisl. lek. Listy, 71: 217—224

Némethová, V., Lichardus, B., Michajlovskij, N., Kolena, J., Lehotská, V., Kovács, L.: (1985): Diabetes insipidus renalis (Slov). Čs. Pediat. 39: 525—527

Niaudet, P., Dechaux, M., Leroy, D., Broyer, M.: (1985): Nephrogenic diabetes insipidus in children. In: Diabetes insipidus in man. (edit. P. Czernichow, A. G. Robinson), Karger, Basel: 224—231

Nicholls, K., Shapiro, M. D., Groves, B. S., Schrier, R. W.: (1986): Factors determining renal response to water immersion in nonexcretor cirrhotic patients. Kidney Int., 30: 417—421

Nicod, P., Goy, J., Weaber, B.: (1985): Acute hemodynamic effect of a vascular antagonist of vasopressin in patients with congestive heart failure. Am. J. Cardiol., 55: 1043—1047

271

Nieuwenhuis, H. K., Sixma, J. J.: (1988): 1-desamino-8-D-arginine vasopressin (desmopressin) shortens the bleeding time in storage pool deficiency. Ann. Int. Med., 108: 65—67

Nolph, K., Schrier, R. W.: (1970): Sodium, potassium and water metabolism in the syndrome of inappropriate secretion of antidiuretic hormone. Am. J. Med., 49: 534—545

Nordgaard, J. P., Pedersen, E. B., Djurhuus, J. C.: (1985): Diurnal antidiuretic hormone levels in enuretics. J. Urol., 134: 1029—1031

Norman, L. J., Challis, J. R. G.: (1987): Synergism between systemic CRF and arginine vasopressin on ACTH release in vivo varies as a function of gestational age in the ovine fetus. Endocrinology, 120: 1052—1057

Nussey, S. S., Ang, V. T. Y., Bevan, D. H., Jenkins, J. S.: (1986a): Human platelet argivasopressin. Clin. Endocrinol, 24: 427—433

Nussey, S., Ang, V., Jenkins, J., Chondrey, H., Bisset, G.: (1984): Brattleboro rat adrenal contains vasopressin. Nature, 310: 64—66

Nussey, S., S., Bevan, D. H., Ang, V. T. Y., Jenkins, J. S.: (1986b): Effects of arginine vasopressin (AVP) infusions on circulating concentrations of platelet AVP, factor VIII: C and von Willebrand factor. Thrombosis and Haemostasis, 55: 34—36

Nussey, S. S., Hawthorn, J., Page, S. R., Ang, V. T. Y., Jenkins, J. J.: (1988a): Responses of plasma oxytocin and arginine vasopressin to nausea induced by apomorphine and ipecacuanha. Clin. Endocrinol., 28: 297—304

Nussey, S. S., Page, S. R., Ang, V. T. Y., Jenkins, J. S.: (1988b): The response of plasma oxytocin to surgical stress. Clin. Endocrinol., 28: 277—282

Nussey, S. S., Prysor-Jones, R. A., Taylor, A., Ang, V. T. Y., Jenkins, J. S.: (1987): Arginine vasopressin and oxytocin in the bovine adrenal gland. J. Endocrinol., 115: 141—149

Nutman, J., Wilunsky, E., Avni, A., Reisner, S. H.: (1981): Syndrome of inappropriate antidiuretic hormone secretion in newborn infants with respiratory problems. Isr. J. Med. Sci., 17: 1009—1013

Odell, W., Wolfsen, A., Yoshimoto, Y., Weitzman, R.: (1977): Ectopic peptide synthesis: a universal concomitant of neoplasia. Clin. Res., 25: 525—531

Oh, W.: (1981): Renal functions and clinical disorders in the neonate. Clin. Perinatol., 8: 215—223

Oh, W.: (1988): Renal function and fluid therapy in high risk infants. Biol. Neonates, 53: 230—236

Ohilbin, D. M., Coggins, C. H.: (1978): Plasma antidiuretic hormone levels in cardiac surgical patients during morphine and halothane anesthesia. Anesthesiology, 49: 95—98

Ohnishi, K., Saito, M., Nakayama, T., Matano, M., Okuda, K.: (1987): Effects of vasopressin on portal hemodynamic in patients with portal hypertension. Am. J. Gastroenterol, 82: 135—138

Ohzeki, T., Igarashi, T., Okamoto, A.: (1984): Familial cases of congenital nephrogenic diabetes insipidus type II: remarkable increment of urinary adenosine 3—5 monophosphate in response to ADH. J. Pediat., 104: 593—595

Oiso, Y., Robertson, G. L.: (1985): Effect of ethanol on vasopressin secretion and the role of endogenous opioids. In: Vasopressin (edit. Schrier, R. W.), New York, Raven Press, 265—269

Oliver, G., Schäffer, E. A.: (1895): On the physiological action of extract of pituitary body and certain other glandular organs. J. Physiol., 18: 277—279

Oliver, R. E., Jamison, R. L.: (1980): Diabetes insipidus. A physiologic approach to diagnosis. Postgrad. Med., 66: 120—131

Onrot, J., Goldberg, M. R., Hollister, A. S., Biaggioni, I., Robertson, R. M., Robertson, D.: (1986): Management of chronic orthostatic hypotension. Am. J. Med., 80: 454—464

Oravec, D., Lichardus, B.: (1972): The management of diabetes insipidus in pregnancy. Br. med. J., 4: 114

Orloff, J., Handler, J.: (1962): The similarity of effects of vasopressin, adenosine 3', 5'-monophosphate (cyclic AMP) and theophylline in the toad bladder. J. Clin. Invest., 41: 702—709

Os, I., Kjeldsen, E., Aakesson, I., Skjoto, J., Eide, I., Hjermann, I., Leren, P.: (1985): Evidence of age related variation in plasma vasopressin of normotensive men. Scand. J. Clin. Lab. Invest., 45: 263—268

Osterman, J., Calhoun, A., Dunham, M., Culum, U. X., Clark, R. M., Stewart, D. D., Scheithauer, B. W.: (1986): Chronic SIADH and hypertension in a patient with olfactory neuroblastoma. Arch. Int. Med., 146: 1731—1735

Oyama, S. N., Kagan, A., Glick, S. M.: (1971): Radioimmunoassay of vasopressin: Application to unextracted human urine. J. Clin. Endocrinol. Metab., 33: 739—744

Padfield, P. L., Brown, J. J., Lever, A. F., Morton, J. J., Robertson, J. I. S: (1981): Blood pressure in acute and chronic vasopressin excess. Studies of malignant hypertension and the syndrome of inappropriate antidiuretic hormone secretion. New Engl. J. Med., 304: 1067—107

Page, M., Asmal, A. C., Edwards, C. R. W.: (1976): Recessive inheritance of diabetes. The syndrome of diabetes insipidus, diabetes mellitus optic atrophy and deafness. Am. J. Med., 45: 505—520

Parry, H. B., Livett, B. G.: (1973): A new hypothalamic pathway to the median eminence containing neurophysin and its hypertrophy in sheep with natural scrapie. Nature, Lond. 242: 65—95

Patel, K. P., Schmid, P. G.: (1987): The role of central adrenergic pathways in the action of vasopressin on baroreflex control of circulation. In: Brain Peptides and Catecholamines in Cardiovascular Regulation, Raven Press, New York, 1987: 53—64

Pavel, S.: (1980): Presence of relatively high concentrations of arginine vasotocin in the cerebrospinal fluid of newborns and infants. J. Clin. Endocrinol. Metab. 50: 271—273

Paxson, C. L., Stoener, J. W., Denson, S. E., Adcock, E. W., Morris, F. H.: (1977): ISADH in neonates with pneumothorax or atelectasis. J. Pediat., 91: 459—463

Peake, I. R.: (1984): The nature of factor VIII. Clin. Sci., 67: 561—567

Pepys, J., Jenkins, P. A., Lachman, P. J.: (1965): An iatrogenic autoantibody: Immunological responses to "pituitary snuff" in patients with diabetes insipidus. J. Endocrinol., 33: 8—12

Pestana, C.: (1977): Fluids and electrolytes in the surgical patient. Williams nad Wilkins, Baltimore

Phillips, P. A., Rolls, B. J., Legingham, J. G. G., Forsling, M. L., Morton, J. J., Crowe, M. J.: (1984): Reduced thirst after water deprivation in healthy elderly men. New Engl. J. Med., 311: 753—759

Pliska, V.: (1985): Pharmacology of deamino-D-arginine vasopressin. (In: Diabetes insipidus in man (edit.: Czernichow, P. and Robinson, A. G.) Karger, Basel. 278—291

Pochard, J. L., Lutz-Bucher, B.: (1986): Vasopressin and oxytocin levels in human neonates. Acta Paediatr. Scand., 75: 774—778

Pohjavuori, M.: (1983): Obstetric determinants of plasma vasopressin concentrations and renin activity at birth. J. Pediatr., 103: 966—968

Polaček, E., Vocel, J., Neugebauerová, L., Sebková, M., Vechetová, E.: (1965): The osmotic concentrating ability in healthy infants and children. Arch. Dis. Child., 40: 291—295

Pollock, A. S., Arieff, A. I.: (1980): Abnormalities of cell volume regulation and their functional consequences. Am. J. Physiol., 239: F195—F205

Ponec, J., Lichardus, B.: (1977): Failure to demonstrate natriuretic effect of neurophysin in rats. Endocrinologia experiment., 11: 235—240

Ponec, J., Lichardus, B.: (1980): Decreased free water excretion after indomethacin in the absence of ADH in saline loaded hypophysectomized Wistar and hydropenic Brattleboro rats. Endokrinologie, 75: 67—76

Post, E. M., Richman, R. A., Blackett, P. R., Duncan, K. P., Miller, K.: (1983): Desmopressin response of enuretic children. Am. J. Dis. Child., 137: 962—964

Puri, V. N.: (1980): Urinary levels of antidiuretic hormone in nocturnal enuresis. Indian Pediatr., 17: 675—676

Quillen, E. W., Cowley, A. W.: (1983): Influence of volume changes on osmolality-vasopressin relationship in conscious dogs. Am. J. Physiol., 244: H73—H79

Quinton, P. M.: (1987): Physiology of sweat secretion. Kidney Int., 32 (suppl. 21): S102—S108

Radetzki, H. M., Hughes, J. R., Radetzki, J. E.: (1972): Differences between serum and plasma osmolalities and their relationship to lactic acid values. Proc. Soc. Exp. Biol. Med. 139: 315—317

Radó, J. P., Borbély, L.: (1975): Inhibition of the antidiuretic effect of 1-deamino-8-D-arginine vasopressin (dDAVP) by glybenclamide in water loaded healthy subjects. Endocrinologie, 66: 88—93

Radó, J. P., Szende, L., Marosi, J.: (1974): Influence of glycoside on the antidiuretic response induced by 1-deamino-8D-arginine vasopressin (DDAVP) in patients with pituitary diabetes insipidus. Metabolism., 23: 1057—1063

Raichle, M. E., Grubb, R. L.: (1978): Regulation of brain water permeability by centrally released vasopressin. Brain Res., 143: 191—194

Rajerison, R. M., Butlen, D., Jard, S.: (1977): Effects of in vivo treatment with vasopressin and analogues on renal adenylate cyclase responsiveness to vasopressin. Endocrinology, 101: 1—12

Ramsay, D. J., Thrasher, T. N., Keil., L. C.: The organum vasculosum laminae terminalis: a critical area for osmoreception. Progr. Brain. Res., 60: 91—98

Rao, M., Mitchell, M., Cohen, S., Kravath, R., Steiner, P.: (1985): Antidiuretic hormone (ADH) response in severe status asthmaticus. Am. Rev. Resp. Dis., 131: A623

Ruscher, W., Tulassay, T.: (1987): Hormonal regulation of water metabolism in children with nephrotic syndrome. Kidney Int., 32 (suppl. 21): S83—S89

Raskind, M. A., Orenstein, H., Christopher, T. G.: (1975): Acute psychosis increased water ingestion and inappropriate antidiuretic hormone secretion. Am. J. Psychiatry, 132: 907—910

Rasmussen, H., Kojima, I., Apfeldorf, W., Barrett, P.: (1986): Cellular mechanism of hormone action in the kidney: messenger function of calcium and cyclic AMP. Kidney Int., 29: 90—97

Raymond, K. H., Lifschitz, M. D.: (1986): Effect of prostaglandins on renal salt and water excretion. Am. J. Med., 80 (suppl 1A): 22—33

Raymond, K. H., Davidson, K. K., McKinley, M. J.: (1985): In vivo and in vitro studies of urinary concentrating ability in potassium depleted rabbits. J. Clin. Invest., 76: 561—566

Reeder, R. F., Nattie, E. E., North, W. G.: (1986): Effect of vasopressin on cold induced brain edema in rats. J. Neurosurg., 64: 941—950

Rees, L., Brook, C. D. G., Forsling., M. L.: (1983): Continuous urine collection in the study of vasopressin in the newborn. Horm. Res., 17: 134—140

Rees, L., Brook, C. G. D., Shaw, J. C. L., Forsling, M. L.: (1984): Hyponatremia in the first week of life in preterm infants: Arginine-vasopressin secretion. Arch. Dis. Child., 59: 414—422

Reppert, S. M., Artman, H. G., Swaminathan, S., Fisher, D. A.: (1981): Vasopressin exhibits a rhythmic daily pattern in cerebrospinal fluid but not in blood. Science, 213: 1256—1257

Reppert, S. M., Schwartz, W. J., Uhl, G. R.: (1987): Arginine-vasopressin: a novel peptide rhythm in cerebrospinal fluid. Trends Neurosci. (TINS), 10: 76—80

Reppert, S. M., Uhl, G. R.: (1987): Vasopressin messenger ribonucleic acid in supraoptic and suprachiasmatic nuclei: appearance and circadian regulation during development. Endocrinology, 120: 2483—2487

Reuss, A. L., Rosenthal, I. M.: (1963): Intelligence in nephrogenic diabetes insipidus Am. J. Dis. Child., 105: 358—364

Richards, S. J., Morris, R. J., Raisman, G.: (1985): Solitary magnocellular neurons in the homozygous Brattleboro rat have vasopressin and glycopeptide immunoreactivity. Neuroscience, 16: 617—623

Richardson, D. W., Robinson, A. G.: (1985): Desmopressin. Ann. Int. Med., 103: 228—239

Richman, R. A., Post, E. M., Notman, D. D., Hochberg, Z., Moses, A. M.: (1981): Simplifying the diagnosis of diabetes insipidus in children. Am. J. Dis. Child., 135: 839—841

Richter, D.: (1985): Biosynthesis of vasopressin. In: Current Topics in Neuroendocrinology, 4. 1985, 1—16. (edit: Ganten, D. and Pfaff, D.) Springer Verlag, Berlin—Heidelberg, 1985

Riphagen, C. L., Pittman, Q. J.: (1986): Arginine-vasopressin as a central neurotransmitter. Fed. Proc., 45: 2318—2322

Rivers, R. P. A., Forsing, M. L., Oliver, R. P.: (1981): Inappropriate secretion of antidiuretic hormone in infants with respiratory infections. Arch. Dis. Child., 56: 558—563

Robertson, G. L.: (1977): The regulation of vasopressin function in health and disease. Recent Proc. Horm. Res., 33: 333—385

Robertson, G. L.: (1980): Control of the posterior pituitary and antidiuretic hormone secretion. Contr. Nephrol., 21: 33—40

Robertson, G. L.: (1983): Thirst and vasopressin function in normal and disordered states of water balance. J. Lab. Clin. Med., 101: 351—371

Robertson, G. L.: (1984): Abnormalities of thirst regulation. Kidney Int., 25: 460—469

Robertson, G. L.: (1985a): Diagnosis of diabetes insipidus. In: Diabetes insipidus in man (Ed. Czernichow, P., Robinson. A. G.). S. Karger, Basel 1985: 176—189

Robertson, G. L.: (1985b): Osmoregulation of thirst and vasopressin secretion: functional properties and the relationship to water balance. In: Vasopressin (Ed. Schrier, R. W.), Raven Press, New York 1985: 203—212

Robertson, G. L.: (1987): Physiology of ADH secretion. Kidney Int., 32 (suppl. 21.): S20—S26

Robertson, G. L.: (1988): Dipsogenic diabetes insipidus: A variant of primary polydipsia caused by a selective defect in the osmoregulation of thirst (abstr.). 8th Int. Cong. Endocrinol., Satellite Symp., Kyoto, Japan, 31: 49

Robertson, G. L., Aycinena, P., Zerbe, R. L.: (1982): Neurogenic disorders of osmoregulation. Am. J. Med., 72: 339—351

Robertson, G. L., Mahr, E. A., Athar, S., Sinha, T.: (1973): Development and clinical application of a new method for the radioimmunoassay of arginine vasopressin in human plasma. J. Clin. Invest., 52: 2340—2352

Robertson, G. L., Shelton, R. L., Athar, S.: (1976): The osmoregulation of vasopressin. Kidney Int., 10: 25—37

Robillard, J. E., Nakamura, K. T.: (1988): Hormonal regulation of renal function during development. Biol. Neonate, 53: 201—211

Robillard, J. E., Weitzman, R. E.: (1980): Developmental aspects of the fetal renal response to exogenous arginine vasopressin. Am. J. Physiol., 238: F407—F414

Robillard, J. E., Weitzman, R. E., Fischer, D. A., Smith, F. G. Jr: (1979): The dynamics of vasopressin release and blood volume regulation during fetal hemorrhage in the lamb fetus. Pediatr. Res., 13: 606—610

Robinson, A. G.: (1984): The contribution of measured secretion of neurophysins to our understanding of neurohypophyseal function. In: The Neurohypophysis (edit. Reichlin, S.) Plenum Medical Book Company, New York, 65—93

Robinson, A. G.,: (1985): Neurohypophyseal function in hypothyreoidism. In: Vasopressin (edit.: Schrier, R. W.) Raven Press, New York, 507—516

Robinson, A. G., Loeb, N.: (1971): Ethanol ingestion: commonest cause of elevated plasma osmolality? New Engl. J. Med., 284: 1253—1255

Robinson, A. G., Verbalis, J. G.: (1985): Treatment of central diabetes insipidus. In: Diabetes insipidus in man. (Czernichow, P., Robinson, A. G.). Karger, Basel: 292—303

Robinson, B. G., Clifton-Bligh, P., Posen, S., Morris, B. J.: (1983): Plasma vasopressin in hypercalcemic states. Aust. NZ. J. Med., 13: 5—7

Rodbard, D., Munson, P. J.: (1978): Is there an osmotic threshold for vasopressin release? Am. J. Physiol., 234: E339—E342

Rodbell, M.: (1980): The roles of hormone receptors and GTP-regulatory proteins in membrane transduction. Nature, 284: 17—22

Rodriguez-Soriano, J., Vallo, A., Castilio, G., Oliveros, K.: (1981): Renal handling of water and sodium in infancy and childhood: A study using clearance methods during hypotonic saline diuresis. Kidney Int. 20: 700—704

Rodriguez-Soriano, J., Vallo, A., Oliveros, R., Castillo, G.: (1983): Renal handling of sodium in premature and full term neonates: A study using clearance methods during water diuresis. Pediat. Res., 17: 1013—1016

Ronnholm, K. A. R., Perheentupa, I., Siihes, M. A.: (1986): Supplementation with human milk protein improves growth of small premature infants fed human milk. Pediatrics, 77: 649—653

Rosa, R. M., Bierer, B. E., Thomas, R.: (1980): A study of induced hyponatremia in the prevention and treatment of sickle-cell crisis. N. Engl. J. Med., 303: 1138—1143

Rose, B. D.: (1984): Clinical physiology of acid-base and electrolyte disorders. McGraw-Hill, New York.

Rose, C. E., Anderson, R. J., Carey, R. M.: (1984): Antidiuresis and vasopressin release with hypoxemia and hypercapnia in conscious dogs. Am. J. Physiol., 247: R127—R134

Rose, J. C., Meis, P. S., Morris, M.: (1981): Ontogeny of endocrine (ACTH, vasopressin, cortisol) response to hypotension in lamb fetuses. Am. J. Physiol., 240: E656—E661

Rosenberg, G. A., Kyner, W. T., Fenstermacher, J. D., Patlak, C. S.: (1986): Effect of vasopressin on ependymal and capillary permeability to tritiated water in cat. Am. J. Physiol., 251: F485—F489

Rosenbloom, A. A., Sack, J., Fisher, D. A.: (1975): The circulating vasopressinase at pregnancy: species comparison using radioimmunoassay. Am. J. Obstetr. Gynecol., 121: 316—319

Rosenow, E. L., Segar, W. E., Zehr, J. E.: (1972): Inappropriate antidiuretic hormone secretion in pneumonia. Mayo Clin. Proc., 47: 169—174

Ross, M. G., Ervin, M. G., Leake, R. D., Fisher, D. A.: (1984): Fetal lung fluid regulation by neuropeptides. Am. J. Obstet. Gynecol., 150: 421—425

Ross, M. G., Ervin, M. G., Leake, R. D., Humme, J. A., Fisher, D. A.: (1986): Continuous ovine fetal hemorrhage: sensitivity of plasma and urine arginine vasopressin response. Am. J. Physiol., 251: E464—469

Rowe, J. W., Shelton, R. L., Helderman, J. H., Vistal, R. E., Robertson, G. L.: (1979): Influence of the emetic reflex on vasopressin release in man. Kidney Int., 16: 729—735

Rowe, J. W., Kilgore, A., Robertson, G. L.: (1980): Evidence in man that cigarette smoking induces vasopressin release via an airway specific mechanism. J. Clin. Enodcrinol. Metab., 51: 170—172

Rowe, J. W., Minaker, K. L., Sparrow, W. D., Robertson, G. L.: (1982): Age-related failure of volume-pressure mediated vasopressin release. J. Clin. Endocrinol. Metab., 54: 661—664

Roy, R. N., Chance, G. W., Radde, I. C., Hill, D. E., Willis, D. M., Sheepers, I.: (1976): Late hyponatremia in very low birthweight infants (< 1.3 kilogram). Pediat. Res., 10: 526—531

Rubini, M.: (1961): Water excretion in potassium-deficient man. J. Clin. Invest., 40: 2215—2221

Rubinstein, A. M., Steiner, D. F.: (1971): Proinsulin. Ann. Rev. Med., 22: 1—17

Ruggeri, Z. M., Manucci, P. M., Lombardi, R., Federici, A. B., Zimmerman, T. S.: (1982): Multimeric composition of factor VIII (von Willebrandt factor) following administration of dDAVP: Implications for pathophysiology and therapy. Blood, 59: 1272—1278

Ruppert, S., Scherer, G., Schutz, G.: (1984): Recent gene conversion involving bovine vasopressin and oxytocin precursor genes suggested by nucleotide sequence. Nature, 308: 554—557

Rurak, D. W., Gruber, N. C.: (1984): The effect of vasopressin on fetal oxygenation in sheep. Can. J. Physiol. Pharmacol., 62: 27—30

Sachs, H., Tabatake, Y.: (1964): Evidence for a precursor in vasopressin biosynthesis. Endocrinology, 75: 943—948

Sack, R. B., Pierce, N., Hirschhorn, N.: (1978): The current status of oral therapy in the treatment of acute diarrhoea illness. Am. J. Clin. Nutr., 31: 2251—2258

Salata, R., Klein, I.: (1987): Effects of lithium on the endocrine system. J. Lab. Clin. Med., 110: 130—136

Salzman, E. W., Weinstein, M. J., Weintraub, R. M.: (1986): Treatment with desmopressin acetate to reduce blood loss after cardiac surgery: A double-blind randomized trial. New Engl. J. Med., 314: 1402—1406

Samadi, A. R., Wahed, M. A., Islam, M. R., Ahmed, S. M.: (1983): Consequences of hyponatremia and hypernatremia in children with acute diarrhoea in Bangladesh. Br. Med. J., 286: 671—673

Sandler, L. M., Burrin, J. M., Joplin, G. F., Bloom, S. R.: (1986): Combined use of vasopressin and synthetic hypothalamic releasing factors as a new test of anterior pituitary function. Br. Med. J., 292: 511—514

Sands, J. M., Novoguchi, H., Knepper, M. A.: (1987): Vasopressin effects on urea and H_2O transport in inner medullary collecting duct subsegments. Am. J. Physiol., 253: F823—F832

Sarifstein, R., Miller, P., Dikman, S., Lyman, N., Shapiro, C.: (1981): Cisplatin nephrotoxicity in rats: Defect in papillary hypertonicity. Am. J. Physiol., 241: F175—179

Sato, S., Uchigata, Y., Uwadana, N., Kita, K., Suzuki, Y., Hayashi, S.: (1982): A syndrome of periodic adrenocorticotropin and vasopressin discharge. J Clin. Endocrinol. Metab., 54: 517—522

Saunders, N., Balle, J. N., Laski, B.: (1976): Severe salt poisoning in an infant. J. Pediatr., 88: 258—260

Sausville, E., Carney, D., Battey, J.: (1985): The human vasopressin gene is linked to the oxytocin gene and is selectively expressed in a lung cancer cell line. J. Biol. Chem., 260: 10236—10241

Sawchenko, P. E.: (1987): Adrenalectomy induced enhancement of CRF and vasopressin immunoreactivity in parvocelular neurosecretory neurons. J. Neurosci., 7: 1093—1106

Scharrer, E., Scharrer, B.: (1954): Neurosecretion. Physiol. Rev., 25: 171—181

Scherbaum, W. A., Wass, J. A. H., Besssr, G. M., Bottazzo, G. F., Doniach, D.: (1986): Autoimmune cranial diabetes insipidus: its association with other endocrine diseases and with histiocytocis X. Clin. Endocrinol., 25: 411—420

Schmale, H., Fehr, S., Richter, D.: (1987): Vasopressin biosynthesis: from gene to peptide hormone. Kidney Int., 32 (suppl. 21): S8—S13

Schmale, H., Richter, D.: (1984): Single base deletion in the vasopressin gene is the cause of diabetes insipidus in Brattleboro rats. Nature, 308: 705—709

Schmitt, B. D.: (1982): Nocturnal enuresis: An update on treatment. Pediat. Clin. North A., 29: 21—36

Schoen, E. J.: (1960): Renal diabetes insipidus. Pediatrics, 26: 808—810

Schreiber, V.: (1979): Pathophysiology of endocrine glands (Czech). Avicenum, Praha

Schreiber, V.: (1985): Endogenous digitalis-like factors revisited 1981—1985. Cor Vasa 27: 92—100

Schrier, R. W., Berl, T.: Nonosmolar factors affecting renal water excretion. New Engl. J. Med., 293: 81—88

Schrier, R. W.. Berl, T.: (1980): Disorders in water metabolism. In: Renal and electrolyte disorders (edit. R. W. Schrier), Little Brown and Co., Boston 1980: 1—64

Schrier, R. W., Bichet, D. G.: (1981): Osmotic and nonosmotic control of vasopressin in the pathogenesis of impaired water excretion in adrenal, thyroid and edematous disorders. J. Lab. Clin. Med., 98: 1—16

Schrier, R. W., Kim, J. K.: (1987): Water metabolism in historical perspectives: its research in the past and present. Kidney Int., 32 (suppl. 21): S113—S16

Schrier, R. W., Lehman, D., Zacherle, B., Early, L. E.: (1973): Effect of furosemide on free water excretion in patients with hyponatremia. Kidney Int. 3: 30—34

Schubert, F., George, J. M., Rao, M. B.: (1981): Vasopressin and oxytocin content of human fetal brain at different stages of gestation. Brain Res., 213: 111—117

Schück, O.: (1984): Examination of kidney function. Martinus Nijhoff Publ., Boston/ Avicenum, Praha

Schwartz, G. J., Feld, L. G., Langford, D. J.: (1984): A simple estimate of glomerular filtration rate in full term infants during the first year of life. J. Pediatr., 104: 849—853

Schwartz, J., Vale, W.: (1988): Dissociation of the adrenocorticotropin secretory responses to corticotropin-releasing factor (CRF), vasopressin and oxytocin. Endocrinology, 122: 1695—1700

Schwartz, W. B., Bennett, W., Curelop, P., Bartter, F. C.: (1957): A syndrome of renal sodium loss and hyponatremia probably resulting from inappropriate secretion of antidiuretic hormone. Am. J. Med., 23: 529—542

Sczepanska-Sadowska, E., Gram, D., Simon-Oppermann, C.: (1983): Vasopressin in blood and third ventricle CSF during dehydratation, thirst and hemorrhoe. Am. J. Physiol., 245: R549—R555

Seckl, J. R., Dunger, D. B., Huen, K., Lightman, S. L.: (1987): The plasma arginine vasopressin response to insulin-induced hypoglycemia in children with short stature is related to age and the onset of puberty. Clin. Endocrinol., 26: 347—353

Seckl, J. R., Williams, T. D. M., Lightman, S. L.: (1986): Oral hypertonic saline causes transient fall of vasopressin in humans. Am. J. Physiol., 251: R214—R217

Segar, W. E., Moore, W. W.: (1968): The regulation of antidiuretic hormone release in man. Effects of change in position and ambient temperature on blood ADH levels. J. Clin. Invest., 47: 2143—2151

Serros, E. R., Kirschenbaum, M. A.: (1981): Prostaglandin-dependent polyuria in hypercalcemia. Am. J. Physiol., 241: F243—F239

Shaffer, S. G., Brandt, S. K., Hall, R. T.: (1986): Postnatal changes in total body water and extracellular volume in preterm infants with respiratory distress syndrome. J. Pediat., 109: 509—514

Shann, F., Germer, S.: (1985): Hyponatremia associated with pneumonia or bacterial meningitis. Arch. Dis. Child., 60: 963—966

Share, L., Crofton, J. T.: (1984): The role of vasopressin in hypertension. Fed. Proc., 43: 103—106

Sherlock, K. S.: (1987): Vasopressin and vasopressin analogues in liver disease. J. Hepatology, 5: 232—234

Shichiri, M., Sinoda, T., Kijima, Y., Shiigai. T., Kanayama, M.: (1985): Renal handling of urate in the syndrome of inappropriate secretion of antidiuretic hormone. Arch. Int. Med., 145: 2045—2047

Shirley, D. G., Walter, S. J., Laycock, J. F.: (1982): The antidiuretic effect of chronic hydrochlorothiazide treatment in rats with diabetes insipidus: renal mechanisms. Clin. Sci., 63: 533—535

Silverman. A. J. Zimmerman, E. A.: (1983): Magnocellular neurosecretory system. Annu. Rev. Neurosci., 6: 357—380

Simmons, M. A., Adcock, E., Bard, H., Battageia, F.: (1974): Hypernatremia, intracranial hemorrhage and NaHCO₃ administration in neonates. New Engl. J. Med., 291: 6—10

Simon, N. M., Garber, E., Arieff, A. J.: (1977): Persistant nephrogenic diabetes insipidus after lithium carbonate. Ann. Int. Med., 86: 446—447

Sims, D. G.: (1977): Histiocytosis X. Follow up of 43 cases. Arch. Dis. Child., 52: 433—440

Singer, I.: (1981): Differential diagnosis of polyuria and diabetes insipidus. Med. Clin. North. Am., 65: 303—320

Singer, I., Forrest, J. N. Jr: (1976): Drug induced states of nephrogenic diabetes insipidus. Kidney Int., 10: 82—95

Singh, S., Padi, M. N., Bullard, H., Freeman, M.: (1985): Water intoxication in psychiatric patients. Br. J. Psychiatry, 146: 127—131

Singhi, S. C., Chookang, E.: (1984): Maternal fluid overload during labour: transplacental hyponatremia and risk of transient neonatal tachypnoea in term infants. Arch. Dis. Child., 59: 1155—1158

Skowsky, W. R., Fisher, D. A.: (1977): Fetal neurohypophyseal arginine-vasopressin and arginine-vasotocin in man and sheep. Pediat. Res., 11: 627—628

Skowsky, W. R., Kikuchi, T. A.: (1978): The role of vasopressin in the impaired water excretion of myxedema. Am. J. Med. 64: 613—621

Sladek, C. D., Armstrong, W. E.: (1987): Effect of neurotransmitters and neuropeptides on vasopressin release. In: Vasopressin (edit: Gash, D. M., Boer, G. J.) Plenum Publ. Corp., 275—333

Smith, H. W.: (1959): From Fish to Philosopher.: The Story of our Internal Environment. Summit, N. J. CIBA, 1959

Smith, H. W.: (1951): The kidney: Structure and function in health and disease. London, Oxford Univ. Press

Smitz, S., Legros, J. J., Franchimont, P., LeMaire, M.: (1985): High molecular weight vasopressin: detection of a large amount in the plasma of a patient. Clin. Endocrinol., 23: 379—384

Snady, M.: (1987): Acute portal vein thrombosis, sclerotherapy and vasopressin: relationships and implications. Am. J. Gastroenterol. 82: 1292—1293

Snyder, N. A., Feigal, D. W., Arieff, A. I.: (1987): Hypernatremia in elderly patients. A heterogenous, morbid and iatrogenic entity. Ann. Int. Med., 107: 309—319

Sofroniew, M. V.: (1983): Vasopressin and oxytocin in the mammalian brain and spinal cord. Trends Neurosci., 6: 467—472

Sokol, H. W., Valtin, H.: (1982): The Brattleboro rat. Ann. NY Acad. Sci., 394: 1—828

Sørensen, P. S.: (1986): Studies of vasopressin in the human cerebrospinal fluid. Acta Neurol. Scand., 74: 81—102

Spruce, B. A., Baylis, P. H., Burd, J., Watson, M. J.: (1985a): Variation in osmoregulation of arginine-vasopressin during the human menstrual cycle. Clin. Endocrinol., 22: 37—42

Spruce, B. A., McCulloch, A. J., Burd, J., Orskov, H., Heaton, A., Baylis, P. H., Alberti, K. G. M. M: (1985b): The effect of vasopressin infusion on glucose metabolism in man. Clin. Endocrinol., 22: 463—468

Šrámková, J., Horký, K., Dvořáková, J.: (1979): Radioimmunoassay of arginine vasopressin in the plasma and urine. Physiol. bohemoslov., 28: 399—409

St-Louis, J., Parent, A. L., Lariviere, R., Schifrin, E. L.: (1986): Vasopressin responses and receptors in the mesenteric vasculature of estrogen treated rats. Am. J. Physiol., 251: H885—889

Stanton, B. A.: (1984): Regulation of ion transport in epithelia: Role of membrane reactivities from cytoplasmic vesicles. Lab. Invest., 51: 255—257

Stark, R. I., Daniel, S. S., Husain, M. K., Zubrow, A. B., James, L. S.: (1984): Effects of hypoxia on vasopressin concentrations in cerebrospinal fluid and plasma of sheep. Neuroendocrinology, 38: 453—460

Starling, E. H., Verney, E. B.: (1924): The secretion of urine as studied on the isolated kidney. Proc. Roy. Soc. London, Ser. B, 97, 1924: 321—363

Stephenson, J. L.: (1987): Models of the urinary concentrating mechanism. Kidney Int., 31: 648—664

Stephenson, J. L.: (1972): Concentration of urine in a central core model of the renal counterflow system. Kidney Int., 2: 85—94

Sterns, R. H.: (1987): Severe symptomatic hyponatremia: Treatment and outcome. Ann. Int. Med., 107: 656—664

Sterns, R. H., Riggs, J. E., Schochet, S. S.: (1986): Osmotic demyelination syndrome following correction of hyponatremia. New Engl. J. Med., 314: 1535—1542

Stoff, J. S., Kosa, R. M., Epstein, F. H.: (1979): The concentrating defect of acute potassium depletion in man is independent of renal prostaglandin (abstract). Kidney Int., 16: 874

Strupp, B., Weingartner, M., Goodwin, F. K., Gold, P. W.: (1984): Neurohypophyseal hormones and cognition. Pharmacol. Ther., 23: 267—279

Sulyok, E.: (1971): Relationship between electrolyte and acid base balance in premature infant during early postnatal life. Biol. Neonate, 17: 227—237

Sulyok, E.: (1988): Renal response to vasopressin in premature infants: what is new? Biol. Neonate, 53: 212—219

Sulyok, E., Kovács, L., Lichardus, B., Michajlovskij, N., Lehotská, V., Némethová, V.,

Varga, L.: (1985): Late hyponatremia in premature infants: Role of aldosterone and arginine vasopressin. J. Pediat., 106: 990—994

Sulyok, E., Németh, M., Tényi, I., Csaba, I. F., Varga, L., Varga, F.: (1981): Relationship between the development of the renin-angiotensin-aldosterone system and the electrolyte status in NaCl supplemented premature infants. Acta Paed. Hung., 22: 109—115

Sulyok, E., Németh, M., Tényi, I., Csaba, I. F., Varga, F., Györi, E., Thurzo, V.: (1979): Relationship between maturity, electrolyte balance and the function of the renin-angiotensin-aldosterone system in newborn infants. Biol. Neonate, 35: 60—65

Sulyok, E., Varga, F., Györy, K., Jobst., K., Csaba, F.: (1980): On the mechanism of renal sodium handling in newborn infants. Biol. Neonate, 37: 75—79

Sutor, A. H.: (1978): Intranasal application of dDAVP in severe hemophilia. Lancet, i: 446—448

Sutor, A. H.: (1980a): Intranasale Anwendung von dDAVP bei schwerer Hämophilie A und Körperhämophilie A. In: Minirin, Schattauer Verlag, Stuttgart: 109—114

Sutor, A. H.: (1980b): Anwendung von dDAVP bei Patienten mit mittelschwerer und schwerer Hämophilie B und Hemmkörperhämophilie. In: Minirin, Schattauer Verlag, Stuttgart, 1980, 137—144

Svenningsen, N. W., Aronson, A. S.: (1976): Postnatal development of renal concentration capacity as estimated by dDAVP-test in normal and asphyxiated neonates. Biol. Neonate, 25: 230—241

Swaab, D. F., Fliers, E., Hoogendijk, J. E.: (1987): Vasopressin in relationship to human aging and dementia. In: Vasopressin: principles and properties (Edit. Gash, D. M. and Boer, G. J.) Plenum Press, New York: 611—625

Swaab, D. F., Fliers, E., Partinan, T. S.: (1985): The suprachiasmatic nucleus in the human brain in relation to sex, age and senile dementia. Brain Res., 342: 37—44

Swanson, L. W., Kuypers, H. G. J. M.: (1980): The paraventricular nucleus of the hypothalamus. J. Comp. Neurol., 194: 555—570

Swanson, L. W., Sawchenko, P. E.: (1983): Hypothalamic integration: organization of paraventricular and supraopic nuclei. Annu. Rev. Neurosci., 6: 269—324

Szatalowicz, V. L., Goldberg, J. P., Anderson, R. J.: (1982): Plasma antidiuretic hormone in acute respiratory failure. Am. J. Med., 72: 583—587

Szatalowicz, V. L., Arnolda, P. E., Chaimowitz, C., Bichet, D., Berl, T., Schrier, R. W.: (1981): Radioimmunoassay of arginine-vasopressin in hyponatremic patients with congestive heart failure. New Engl. J. Med 305: 263—266

Tausch, A., Stegner, M., Leake, R. D., Artman, H. G., Fisher, D. A.: (1983): Radioimmunoassay of arginine vasopressin in urine: Development and application. J. Clin. Endocrinol. Metab., 57: 777—781

Thomas, T. H., Lee, M. R.: (1976): The specificity of antisera for the radioimmunoassay of arginine vasopressin in human plasma and urine during water loading and dehydration. Clin. Sci. Mol. med., 51: 526—536

Thomas, T. H., Morgan, D. B.: (1979): Post-surgical hyponatremia: the role of intravenous fluids and arginine-vasopressin. Br. J. Surg., 66: 540—542

Thompson, C. J., Baylis, P. H.: (1987): Reproducibility of osmotically stimulated thirst and vasopressin release (abstract). J. Endocrinol., 112, Suppl.: 69

Thompson, C. J., Burd, J. M., Baylis, P. H.: (1987): Acute suppression of plasma vasopressin and thirst after drinking in hypernatremic humans. Am. J. Physiol., 252: R1138—R1142

Thompson, D. A., Campbell, R. G., Lilavivat, U., Welle, S. L.: (1981): Increased thirst and plasma arginine vasopressin levels during 2-deoxy-d-glucose-induced glucoprivation in humans. J. Clin. Invest., 67: 1083—1093

Thrasher, T. N., Keil, L. C.: (1987): Regulation of drinking and vasopressin secretion: the role of organum vasculosum laminae terminalis. Am. J. Physiol., 253: R108—120

Thurston, J. H., Hauhart, R. E., Neslon, J. S.: (1987): Adaptive decreases in amino acids (taurine in particular), creatine and electolytes prevent cerebral edema in chronically hyponatremic mice. Metabol. Brain Dis., 2: 223—241

Tilders, F. J. H., Berkenbosch, F., Vermes, I., Linton, E. A., Smelik, P. G.: (1985): Role of epinephrine and vasopressin in the control of the pituitary-adrenal response to stress. Fed. Proc., 44: 155—160

Torda, T., Lichardus, B., Kvetňanský, R., Ponec, J.: (1978): Posterior pituitary dopamine and noradrenaline content: effect of thirst, ethanol and saline load. Endokrinologie, 72: 334—338

Trinh-Trang-tan, M. M., Bouby, N., Kriz, W., Bankir, L.: (1987): Functional adaptation of thick ascending limb and internephron heterogenity to urine concentration. Kidney Int., 31: 549—555

Tulassay, T., Rascher, W., Lang, R. E., Seyberth, H. W., Scharer, K.: (1987): Atrial natriuretic peptide and other vasoactive hormones in nephrotic syndrome. Kidney Int., 31: 1391—1395

Tulassay, T., Rasher, W., Seyberth, H. W., Lang, R. E., Toth, M., Sulyok, E.: (1986): Role of atrial natriuretic peptide in sodium homeostasis in premature infants. J. Pediatr., 109: 1023—1027

Turek, F. W.: (1985): Circadian neural rhythms in mammals. Ann. Rev. Physiol., 47: 49—64

Túri, S., Merth, I., Sztriha, L.: (1981): Indomethacin tratment of children suffering from nephrogenic diabetes insipidus or secondary tubulopathy associated severe polyuria. Int. J. Ped. Nephrol., 2: 262—268

Tyryskina, E. M., Ivanova, L. N., Finkinstein, Y. D.: (1981): Participation of liver receptors in the regulation of ion composition, osmolality and extracellular fluid volume. Pflügers Arch., 390: 270—277

Unger, T., Rohmeiss, P., Demmert, G., Luft, F. L., Ganten, D., Lang, R. E.: (1986): Differential actions of neuronal and hormonal vasopressin on blood pressure and baroreceptor reflex sensitivity in rats. J. Cardiovasc. Pharmacol., 8: (suppl. 7): 981—986

Usberti, M., Federico, S., Meccariello, S., Cianciaruso, B., Ballett a, M., Pecoraro, C.: (1984): Role of plasma vasopressin in the impairment of water excretion in nephrotic syndrome. Kidney Int., 25: 422—429

Usberti, M., Pecoraro, C., Federico, S., Cianciaruso, B., Guida, B., Romano, A., Grunetto, L.: (1985): Mechanism of action of indomethacin in tubular defects. Pediatrics, 75: 501—507

Uttley, W. S., Paxton, J., Thistlewaite, D.: (1972): Concentrating ability and grown failure in urinary tract disorders. Arch. Dis. Child., 47: 436—442

Vale, W., Spiess, J., Rivier, C., Rivier, J.: (1981): Characterization of a 4 1-residue ovine hypothalamic peptide that stimulates secretion of corticotropin and beta-endotoxin. Science, 213: 1394—1397

Vallotton, M. B., Favre, L., Dolci, W.: (1986a): Osmolar stimulation of vasopressin secretion in man: comparison of various protocols. Acta Endocrinol., 113: 161—167

Vallotton, M. B., Wuthrich, R. P., Lew, P. D., Capponi, A. M: (1986b): Effects of vasopressin and its analogs on rat aortic smooth muscle and renal medullary tubular cells: characterization of receptor subtypes. J. Cardiovasc. Pharmacol., 8 (suppl 7): S5—S11

Valtin, H.: (1967): Hereditary hypothalamic diabetes insipidus in rats (Brattleboro strain). Am. J. Med., 42: 814—827

Valtin, H.: (1984): Renal actions by which vassopressin may aid the concentration of urine. In: Nephrology (Edit. by R. R. Robinson), Proc. IX. Int. Cong. Nephrol., I, New York, Springer Verlag: 397—406

Valtin, H., Edwards, B. R.: (1987): GFR and the concentration of urine in the absence of vasopressin. Berliner-Davidson reexplored. Kidney Int., 31: 634—64.

Valtin, H., North, W. G., Edwards, B. R., Gellai, M.: (1985): Animal models of diabetes insipidus. In: Diabetes insipidus in man. (edit. Czernichow, P., Robinson, A. G.), Karger, Basel: 105—126

VanLeeuwen, F. W.: (1987): Vasopressin receptors in the brain and pituitary. In: Vasopressin, Principles and properties. Plenum Press, New York and London: 477—496

VanWimersma-Greidanus, Burbach, J. P. H., Veldhuis, H. D.: (1986): Vasopressin and oxytocin. Their presence in the central nervous system and their functional significance in brain processes. Acta Endocrinologica, 112: (suppl. 276): 85—94

Vávra, I., Machová, A., Holeček, V., Cort, J. H., Zaoral, M., Šorm, F.: (1968): Effect of a synthetic analogue of vasopressin in animals and in patients with diabetes insipidus. Lancet, i: 948—952

Veale, W. L., Cooper, K. E., Ruwe, W. D.: (1984): Vasopressin: Its role in antipyresis and febrile convulsion. Brain Res. Bull., 12: 161—165

Verbalis, J. G., Richardson, D. W., Stricker, E. M.: (1987): Vasopressin release in response to vasopressin producing agents and cholecystokinin in monkeys. Am. J. Physiol., 252: R749—R753

Verbalis, J. G., Robinson, A. G.: (1983): Characterization of neurophysin-vasopressin prohormones in human posterior pituitary tissue. J. Clin. Endorinol. Metab., 57: 115—123

Verbalis, J. G., Robinson, A. G.: (1985): (A) Neurophysin and vasopressin: Newer concepts of secretion and regulation. In: The Pituitary Gland (edit.: H. Imura), Raven Press, New York, 1985, 307—339

Verbalis, J. G., Robinson, A. G., Moses, A. M.: (1985): (B) Postoperative and post-traumatic diabetes insipidus. In: Diabetes insipidus in man (edit. T. P. Czernichow and A. G. Robinson) Karger, Basel, 1985: 247—265

Verney, E. B.: (1946): Absorption and excretion of water: The antidiuretic hormone. Lancet, ii: 781—783

Verney, E. B.: (1947): The antidiuretic hormone and the factors which determine its release. Proc. R. Soc. London. Ser. B, 135: 25—106

Vest, M., Talbot, N. B., Crawford, J. D.: (1963): Hypocaloric dwarfism and hydronephrosis in diabetes insipidus. Am. J. Child., 105: 175—181

Vieweg, W. V. R., David, J. J., Mowent, Wampler, G. J., Burns, W. J., Spradrin, V. W.: (1985): Death from self-induced water intoxication among patients with schizophrenic disorders. J. Nerv. Ment. Dis., 173: 161—165

Vieweg, W. V. R., Yank, G. R., Rowe, W. T., Hovermale, L. S.: (1987): Diurnal variations of sodium and water metabolism among patients with psychosis, intermittent hyponatremia and polydipsia (PIP syndrome). Biol. Psychiatry, 22: 224—227

Viinamaki, O., Erkkola, R., Kanto, J.: (1986): Plasma vasopressin concentrations and serum vasopressinase activity in pregnant and nonpregnant women. Biol. Res. in Pregnancy, 1: 17—19

Vilhardt, H.: (1988): The effect of vasopressin analogues on coagulation and fibrinolysis. Satellite symposium to the 8th Int. Congress of Endocrinology Kyoto, Japan

Villadsen, A. B., Pedersen, E. B.: (1987): Recumbant cranial diabetes insipidus. Acta Paed. Scand., 76: 179—183

Vincent, J. D., Legedre, P., Poulain, D., Arnauld, E., Teodosis, D.: (1985): Electrophysiology of vasopressin-secreting cells. In: Diabetes insipidus in man. (edit, P. Czernichow, A. G. Robinson), Karger, Basel: 52—68

Vokes, T., Aycinena, P. R., Robertson, G. L.: (1987): Effect of insulin on osmoregulation of vasopressin. Am. J. Physiol., 252: E538—548

Vokes, T. J., Robertson, G. L.: (1988): Disorders of antidiuretic hormone. Endocrinol. Metabol. Clin. North Am., 17: 281—299

Volhard, F.: (1910): Über der functionelle Untersuchung der Schrumpfnieren. Verh. dtsch. Ges. inn. Med., 27: 735

Van den Velden, R.: (1913): Die Nierenwirkung von Hypophysenextrakten beim Menschen. Biol. klin. Wochenschr., 50: 2083—2086

Vorherr, H., Massry, S. G., Fallet, R., Kaplan, L., Kleeman, C. R.: (1970): Antidiuretic principle in tuberculous lung tissue of a patient with pulmonary tuberculosis and hyponatremia. Ann. Int. Med., 72: 383—387

Wade, J. B.: (1985): Membrane structural studies of the action of vasopressin. Fed. Proc., 44: 2687—2692

Waggoner, R. W., Slonim, A. E., Armstrong, S. H.: (1978): Improved psychological status of children under dDAVP for central diabetes insipidus. Am. J. Psychiat., 135: 361—362

Walker, S. H.: (1981): Hypernatremia from oral rehydration solutions in infantile diarrhea. New Engl. J. Med., 304: 1238—1240

Watson, S. J. Akil, H., Fischli, W., Goldstein, A., Zimmermann, E., Nilaver, G., van Wimersma-Greidanus: (1982): Dynorphin and vasopressin: common localization in magnocellular neurons. Science, 216: 85—87

Weaber, B., Nussberger, J., Hofbauer, K. G., Nicod, P., Brunner, H. R.: (1986): Clinical studies with a vascular vasopressin antagonist. J. Cardiovasc. Pharmacol., 8 (suppl. 7): S111—S116

Weindl, A., Sofroniew, M.: (1985): Neuroanatomical pathways related to vasopressin. In: Neurobiology of vasopressin (edit: Ganten, D., Pfaff, D.), Springer Verlag, Berlin—Heidelberg, 137—196

Weiss, N. M., Robertson, G. L.: (1985): Effect of hypercalcemia and lithium therapy on the osmoregulation of thirst and vasopressin secretion. In: Vasopressin. (edit. Schrier, R. W.), Raven Press, New York: 281—289

Weitzman, R. E., Fisher, D. A.: (1977): Log linear relationship between plasma arginine-vasopressin and plasma osmolality. Am. J. Physiol., 233: E37—E40

Weitzman, R. E., Fisher D. A., DiStefano, J. J., Bennett, G. M.: (1977): Episodic secretion of arginine vasopressin. Am. J. Physiol., 233: E32—E36

Weitzman, R. E., Fisher, D. A., Robillard, J. E., Erenberg, A., Kennedy, R., Smith, F. G.: (1978a): Arginine vasopressin response to an osmotic stimulus in the fetal sheep. Pediat. Res., 12: 35—38

Weitzman, R. R., Glatz, T. H., Fisher, D. A.: (1978b): The effect of hemorrhage and hypertonic saline upon plasma oxytocin and arginine vasopressin in conscious dogs. Endocrinology, 103: 2154—2160

Whitnall, M. H., Gainer, H.: (1988): Major pro-vasopressin-expressing and pro-vaso-pressin deficient subpopulations of CRF-neurons in normal rats. Neuroendocrinology, 47: 176—180

Wijdicks, E. F. M., Vermeulen, M., van Brummelen, P., den Boer, N. C., van Gijn, J.: (1987): Digoxin-like immunoreactive substance in patients with aneurysmal subara-chnoid hemorrhage. Br. Med. J., 294: 729—732

Williams, T. D. M., Dacosta, D., Mathias, C. J., Bannister, R., Lichtman, S. L.: (1986): Pressor effects of arginine vasopressin in progresive autonomic failure. Clin. Sci., 71: 173—178

Wille, S.: (1986): Comparison of desmopressin and enuresis alarm for nocturnal enuresis. Arch. Dis. Child., 61: 30—33

Wintour, E. M., Congin, M., Hardy, K. J., Henessy, D. P.: (1982): Regulation of urine osmolality in fetal sheep. Quart. J. Exp. Physiol., 67: 427—435

Wiriyathian, S., Rosenfeld, C. R., Arant, B. S., Porter, J. C., Faucher, D. J., Engle, W. D.: (1986): Urinary arginine vasopressin: pattern of excretion in the neonatal period. Pediat. Res., 20: 103—108

Wirz, H., Hargittay, B., Kuhn, W.: (1951): Lokalisation des Konzentrierungsprocesses in der Niere durch direkte Kryoskopie. Helv. Physiol. Acta, 9: 196—207

Wolfson, B., Manning, R. W., Davis, L., Arentzen, R., Baldino, F.: (1985): Co-localization of corticotropin releasing factor and vasopressin mRNA in neurons after adrenalectomy. Nature, 315: 59—61

Woods, L. L., Cheung, C. Y., Power, G. G., Brace, R. A.: (1986): Role of arginine vasopressin in fetal renal response to hypertonicity. Am. J. Physiol., 251: F156—F163

Yamaji, T., Ishibashi, M., Katayama, S.: (1981): Nature of the immunoreactive neurophysins in ectopic vasopressin producing oat cell carcinomas of the lung. J. Clin. Invest., 68: 388—398

Yancey, P. H., Clark, M. E., Hand, S. C., Bowlus, R. D., Somero, G. N.: (1982): Living with water stress: Evolution of osmolyte systems. Science, 217: 1214—1222

Yang-Te Tsai, Chii-Shyan Lay, Kwok-Hung Lai, Wai-Wah Ng, Yeong-Shyan Yeh., Jiin-YuWang: (1986): Controlled trial of vasopressin plus nitroglycerin vs. vasopressin alone in the treatment of bleeding esophageal varices. Hepatology, 6: 406—409

Zaoral, M., Kolc, J., Šorm., F.: (1967): Amino acids and peptides LXXXI. Synthesis of 1-deamino-8-D-gamma aminobutyrine-vasopressin, 1-deamino-8-D-lysine and 1-deamino-8-D-arginine vasopressin. Coll. Czechoslov. chem. Commun., 32: 1250—1256

Zerbe, R. L.: (1985): Genetic factors in normal and anormal regulation of vasopressin secretion. In: Vasopressin (edit: Schrier, R. W.) Raven Press, New York, 213—220

Zerbe, R. L., Henry, D. P., Robertson, G. L.: (1983): Vasopressin response to orthostatic hypotension: Etiological and clinical implications. Am. J. Med., 3: 265—271

Zerbe, R. L., Robertson, G. L.: (1981): A comparison of plasma vasopressin measurements with a standard indirect test in the differential diagnosis of polyuria. New Engl. J. Med., 305: 1539—1546

Zerbe, R. L., Robertson, G. L.: (1983): Osmoregulation of thirst and vasopressin secretion in human subjects: effect of various solutes. Am. J. Physiol., 244: E607—E614

Zerbe, R., Stropes, L., Robertson, G.: (1980): Vasopressin function in the syndrome of inappropriate antidiuresis. Ann. Rev. Med., 31: 315—327

Ziegler, E. E., Fomon, S. J.: (1971): Fluid intake, renal solute load and water balance in infancy. J. Pediat., 78: 561—568

Zikmund, V., Lichardus, B.: (1962): Effects of psychic stimuli on water economy in man. Activ. nerv. super., 4: 383—387

Zimmerhackl, B. L., Robertson, C. R., Jamison, R. L.: (1986): The medullary microcirculation. Kidney Int., 31: 641—647

Zimmermann, D., Green, D. C.: (1975): Nephrogenic diabetes insipidus type II: Defect distal to adenyl-cyclase step. Pediat. Res., 9: 381—384

Zimmermann, E. A., Carmel, P. W., Husain, M. K., Ferin, M., Tannenbaum, M., Frantz, A. G., Robinson, A. G.: (1973): Vasopressin and neurophysin: high concentrations in monkey hypophyseal portal blood. Science, 198: 925—927

Zimmermann, E. A., Li-Yun, M. A., Milaver, G.: (1987): Anatomical basis of thirst and vasopressin secretion. Kidney Int., 32 (suppl. 21): S14—S19

SUBJECT INDEX

Developments in Nephrology

1. Cheigh, J. S., Stenzel, K. H. and Rubin, A. L. (eds.): Manual of Clinical Nephrology of the Rogosin Kidney Center. 1981   ISBN 90-247-2397-3
2. Nolph, K. D. (ed.): Peritoneal Dialysis. 1981 ed.: out of print
   3rd revised and enlarged ed. 1988 (not in this series)   ISBN 0-89838-406-0
3. Gruskin, A. B. and Norman, M. E. (eds.): Pediatric Nephrology. 1981
   ISBN 90-247-2514-3
4. Schück, O.: Examination of the Kidney Function. 1981
   ISBN 0-89838-565-2
5. Strauss, J. (ed.): Hypertension, Fluid-electrolytes and Tubulopathies in Pediatric Nephrology. 1982   ISBN 90-247-2633-6
6. Strauss, J. (ed.): Neonatal Kidney and Fluid-electrolytes. 1983
   ISBN 0-89838-575-X
7. Strauss, J. (ed.): Acute Renal Disorders and Renal Emergencies. 1984
   ISBN 0-89838-663-2
8. Didio, L. J. A. and Motta, P. M. (eds.): Basic, Clinical, and Surgical Nephrology. 1985   ISBN 0-89838-698-5
9. Friedman, E. A. and Peterson, C. M. (eds.): Diabetic Nephropathy: Strategy for Therapy. 1985   ISBN 0-89838-735-3
10. Dzúrik, R., Lichardus, B. and Guder, W. (eds.): Kidney Metabolism and Function. 1985   ISBN 0-89838-749-3
11. Strauss, J. (ed.): Homeostasis, Nephrotoxicity, and Renal Anomalies in the Newborn. 1986   ISBN 0-89838-766-3
12. Oreopoulos, D. G. (ed.): Geriatric Nephrology. 1986
    ISBN 0-89838-781-7
13. Paganini, E. P. (ed.): Acute Continuous Renal Replacement Therapy. 1986   ISBN 0-89838-793-0
14. Cheigh, J. S., Stenzel, K. H. and Rubin, A. L. (eds.): Hypertension in Kidney Disease. 1986   ISBN 0-89838-797-3
15. Deane, N., Wineman, R. J. and Benis, G. A. (eds.):Guide to Reprocessing of Hemodialyzers. 1986   ISBN 0-89838-798-1
16. Ponticelli, C., Minetti, L. and D'Amico, G. (eds.): Antiglobulins, Cryo-globulins and Glomerulonephritis. 1986   ISBN 0-89838-810-4
17. Strauss, J. (ed.), with the assistance of L. Strauss: Persistent Renal-genitourinary Disorders. 1987   ISBN 0-89838-845-7

18. Andreucci, V. E. and Dal Canton, A. (eds.): Diuretics: Basic, Pharmaco-logical, and Clinical Aspects. 1987   ISBN 0-89838-885-6
19. Bach, P. H. and Lock, E. H. (eds.): Nephrotoxicity in the Experimental and Clinical Situation, Part 1. 1987   ISBN 0-89838-977-1
20. Bach, P. H. and Lock, E. H. (eds.): Nephrotoxicity in the Experimental and Clinical Situation, Part 2. 1987   ISBN 0-89838-980-2
21. Gore, S. M. and Bradley, B. A. (eds.): Renal Transplantation: Sense and Sensitization. 1988   ISBN 0-89838-370-6
22. Minetti, L., D'Amico, G. and Ponticelli, C. (eds.): The Kidney in Plasma Cell Dyscrasias. 1988   ISBN 0-89838-385-4
23. Lindblad, A. S., Novak, J. W. and Nolph, K. D. (eds.): Continuous Am-bulatory Peritoneal Dialysis in the USA. 1989   ISBN 0-7923-0179-X
24. Andreucci, V. E. and Dal Canton, A. (eds.): Current Therapy in Nephrology. 1989   ISBN 0-7923-0206-0
25. Kovács, L. and Lichardus, B.: Vasopressin — Disturbed secretion and its effects. 1989   ISBN 0-7923-0249-4
26. De Broe, M. E. and Coburn, J. W. (eds.): Aluminium and Renal Failure. 1989   ISBN 0-7923-0347-4
27. Gardner, Jr., K. D. and Bernstein, J. (eds):
The Cystic Kidney. 1989   ISBN 0-7923-0392-X

Kluwer Academic Publishers

DORDRECHT / BOSTON / LONDON